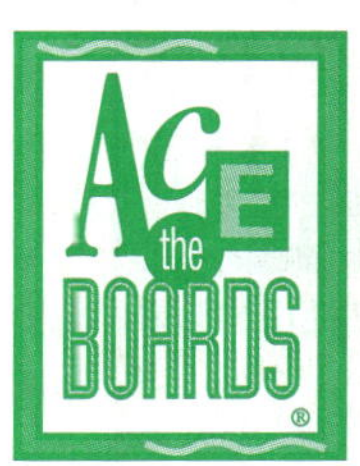

Microbiology & Immunology

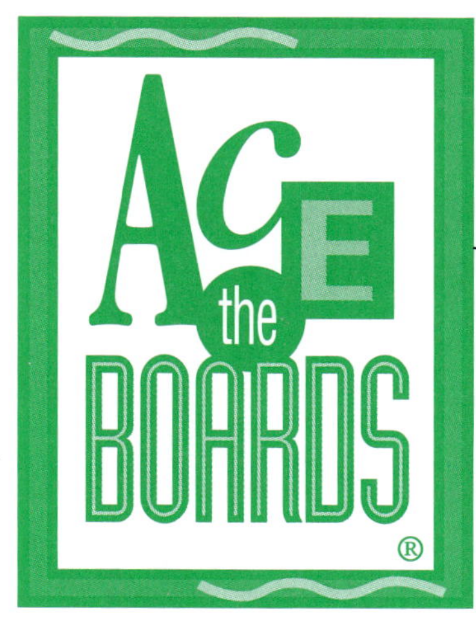

MOSBY'S USMLE step 1 REVIEWS

Microbiology & Immunology

Ken S. Rosenthal, Ph.D.
Professor,
Department of Microbiology and Immunology,
Northeastern Ohio Universities College of Medicine,
Rootstown, Ohio

James S. Tan, M.D., F.A.C.P.
Professor of Internal Medicine,
Head/Infectious Disease Section,
Northeastern Ohio Universities College of Medicine;
Chairman/Program Director,
Department of Medicine,
Summa Health System,
Akron, Ohio

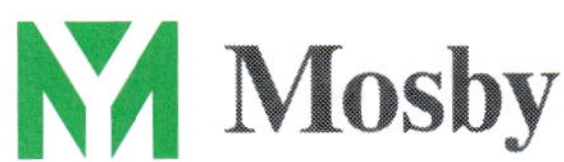

St. Louis Baltimore Boston Carlsbad Chicago Naples New York Philadelphia Portland
London Madrid Mexico City Singapore Sydney Tokyo Toronto Wiesbaden

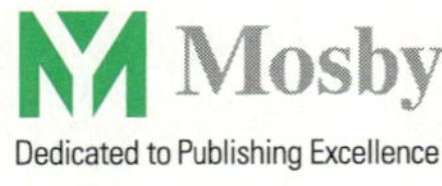

A Times Mirror Company

Vice-President and Publisher *Anne S. Patterson*
Editor *Emma D. Underdown*
Developmental Editor *Christy Wells*
Project Manager *Dana Peick*
Production Editor *Jeffrey Patterson*
Manufacturing Supervisor *Tony McAllister*
Book Designer *Amy Buxton*
Cover Designer *Stacy Lanier/AKA Design*

Printed in the United States of America
Composition by Graphic World, Inc.
Printing/binding by R.R. Donnelly

Mosby-Year Book, Inc.
11830 Westline Industrial Drive
St. Louis, Missouri 63146

Library of Congress Cataloging-in-Publication Data

Rosenthal, Ken S.
Mosby's USMLE step 1 reviews—microbiology and immunology/Ken S. Rosenthal, James S. Tan.
p. cm.—(Ace the boards)
Includes index.
Other title: Microbiology and immunology.
1. Medical microbiology—Examinations, questions, etc. 2. Immunology—Examinations, questions, etc. I. Tan, James S. II. Title. III. Series.
[DNLM: 1. Viruses—examination questions. 2. Bacteria—examination questions. 3. Communicable Diseases—immunology—examination questions. QW 18.2 R815m 1996]
QR46.R755 1996
DNLM/DLC
for Library of Congress 95-52095
CIP

ISBN 0-8151-7349-0 (IBM)
ISBN 0-8151-8670-3 (MAC)

96 97 98 99 00 / 9 8 7 6 5 4 3 2 1

Contributors

Jere Boyer, Ph.D.
Adjunct Professor of Microbiology and Immunology,
Northeastern Ohio Universities College of Medicine;
Director of Clinical Research,
Aultman Hospital, Canton, Ohio

Richard E. Depew, Ph.D.
Professor Microbiology/ Immunology,
Northeastern Ohio Universities College of Medicine

Josephine Dick, Ph.D.
Northeastern Ohio Universities College of Medicine

Sandra Klespies, Ph.D.
Clinical Associate Professor of Microbiology and Immunology,
Northeastern Ohio Universities College of Medicine;
Department of Pathology and Laboratory Medicine,
Children's Hospital Medical Center of Akron, Akron, Ohio

Edgardo Rozenbom, B.S.
Northeastern Ohio Universities College of Medicine;
Kent State University

Preface

"READ ME," said the first page of the book to Alice (and all the other medical students).

ACE THE BOARDS: Microbiology and Immunology is an aid for remembering and a guide for relearning the basic concepts and clinical data tested on the USMLE exams. Our goal is to make recall and review as easy as possible. As teachers, we looked at the curriculum and boiled it down to "What do I need to know?"

ACE THE BOARDS: Microbiology and Immunology provides summary tables, lists, charts, and two color illustrations to help you grab the important material. The informatiion is presented in an easily accessible, • bulleted, *colorized* format. Icons help to find information quickly. Space is provided for notes.

ACE THE BOARDS: Microbiology and Immunology includes USMLE style questions to reinforce the information and to prepare and practice for the Board exam. The questions are in best answer, matching, and extended matching formats, similar to the Board exam.

Extensive explanations are provided for all possible answers. You learn not only why the right answer is correct but why other choices are *incorrect*.

The computer diskette of questions will allow you to customize your own review exams to provide immediate feedback on areas requiring further study and practice in taking the Boards.

- Board-style questions will reinforce the clinical utility of the information and are a direct way to help you prepare for the Boards.
- The perforated answer sheets can be torn out and placed next to the questions to help you review the material.
- The computer-question bank allows you to customize exams, which test specific subjects or the entire discipline.

Every student asks what they need to know for the exam. Believe it or not, the USMLE exam is not a total trivia exam. No one knows what will be on the exam except the people at USMLE who make up the exam. Logically, the major portion of the questions on the exam will cover the most important material, the most common diseases, the "in the news" topics, and the most basic concepts.

A useful approach to studying for the exam is to remember that the exam tests your preparation for becoming a physician. Basic recall of facts and problem solving are both required. We developed this book to help you THINK LIKE A PHYSICIAN when preparing for the exam. Each of the infectious agents is presented in a format to answer the following questions relevant to a physician.

What is the organism?
  What is it structure?
  What are the key distinguishing features?
How does it cause disease?
  What are the mechanism(s) of pathogenesis:
    interaction with the host?
    host response?
    immune response?
Which diseases?
  What are the key distinguishing symptoms?
Risk:
  Who?
  How spread?
  Where?
  When?
Is it treatable?
  Antibiotic?
Is it preventable?
  Vaccine?
  Sanitation?

Finally, be sensible in your approach to review and study. Give yourself enough time to review the material. Practice taking tests. Ask friends or faculty for clarification when necessary.

Studying and taking a test of this magnitude is like training for a big race. You must be prepared and mentally fit. Maintain your physical fitness throughout the term. Get a good night's sleep and eat sensibly before the exam. Enter the exam with a "Go get 'em" attitude. *Answer all the questions.* Don't worry if some of the questions are unfamiliar.

ACE THE BOARDS: Microbiology and Immunology was developed by two teachers, a basic scientist of medical microbiology and immunology, and an infectious disease specialist. We both have worked hard to promote the success of our students in microbiology and on the Boards.

The development of several sections of the book was facilitated by student input. Medical and graduate students were consulted throughout the development of this book to ensure that it would present the material in the most useful, "to the point" manner.

Acknowledgments

We would like to acknowledge the following reviewers for their suggestions:

Michael Edwards
SUNY Health Science Center at Syracuse

David L. McCorvey
University of Wisconsin Medical School

Wilson Tang
Harvard Medical School

This book could not have been written without the expert organization and editing of Christy Wells and Emma Underdown. Finally, we must acknowledge the tolerance of our families, Judy, Joshua and Rachel Rosenthal and June Tan, who gave up their husbands and fathers for many weekends and evenings.

Test-Taking Strategies

Suzanne F. Kiewit, M.Ed.

To perform well on the USMLEs, it is imperative that you begin with a **plan.** Preparation time is at a premium, so you will want to be as efficient and effective as possible by planning well.

MONTHS AHEAD OF THE EXAM

- Sit down with a blank calendar and block in your commitments: classes, final exams, scheduled events.
- Include time for activities of daily life: eating, sleeping, exercising, socializing, banking, maintaining your home, and so forth.
- The remaining time is available for study/review.
- Determine an orderly approach to the material you need to cover that fits your particular set of needs (e.g., subject-by-subject approach, systems approach, pathologic state approach).
- Assign the remaining time to content areas. This is done in various ways: material covered freshman year first, easiest first, least comfortable material first, detailed subjects last, whatever. Your plan should reflect your goal: to maximize your score.
- Establish a warm-up, which may consist of breaking the tension in major muscle groups (neck rolls, shoulder rolls, etc.), a quick visualization of you performing successfully, or a brief meditation. Practicing this warm-up routine before each of your study sessions will make it a familiar activity that helps you learn effectively, as well as take exams effectively.
- Designate time at the end of your study period for panoramic review. Depending on your needs, that might be a week or just several days before the exam.
- Plan for feedback on your efforts. Schedule time for answering questions on the material you are reviewing and for taking at least one mock comprehensive exam.
- Do the comprehensive exam midway through your study period so that you can refine your efforts to reflect the degree of your performance.

DAYS AHEAD OF THE EXAM

- Divide each day into thirds: morning block, afternoon block, and evening block.
- Consider the time of day that is most productive for you and do the most difficult or least favorite material at that time.
- Assign more blocks of study to those areas requiring the most review to reach a comfortable knowledge level.
- A popular way to use blocks is to pair subjects or materials. For instance, pair strong content with weaker content so that you are not always in the position of not knowing material (which would invite negative feelings or ineffectiveness). Or pair a conceptual subject with a detail subject, such as physiology with anatomy, so that you are not always doing the same kind of thinking (this invites positive effort).
- Use your most productive blocks of time for actual study/review. Use the nonpeak times for reinforcement of material covered or feedback by answering questions on material that you have covered.

Planning the Blocks

- Once you determine time allocations for each content area and an orderly approach that fits your needs and goals, you want to specify what you plan to do during each block.
- Be specific as to content area, material to study, and task; for example, MICRO: review chart on viruses; PHYS: answer questions on renal; and so forth.
- Each study block will last approximately 3 to 4 hours. To be most efficient and effective, plan to take a 5- or 10-minute break every hour. If you are having difficulty getting into the study mode, plan to study for 25 minutes, then take a 5-minute break. Reserve longer breaks for switches between subjects. Get up and move around on breaks.

BEFORE THE EXAM

Knowing about the USMLEs helps demystify them. In general, the USMLE exams are a 2-day, four-book examination. Approximately 3 hours are allotted per exam book. Each day you will complete one book of about 200 items in the morning and another book in the afternoon.

In each exam book, questions are organized by question type, not content. Specific directions precede each set of questions. Only two question formats are used: one-best-answer multiple choice items (which typically come first on the exam) and matching items (toward the end of the exam). Students have reported that one-best-answer items make up the bulk of the exam (70% to 75%) and negatively stemmed items make up only 10% to 15% of the questions (Bushan, Le, and Amin, 1995). Matching sets, which make up about 15% to 20% of the items, may include short leading lists or long leading lists of up to 26 items from which to choose.

From year to year there may be variations in the organization and presentation of both content and item formats. It would be wise to read the National Board of Medical Examiners' *General Instructions* booklet, which you will receive when you register. This booklet contains descriptions of content, item format, and even a set of practice items. Be certain you read this booklet and familiarize yourself with the questions.

You can further maximize exam performance by taking control. Adults tend to perform better when they feel that they have a measure of control. For the USMLE it is easy to feel out of control. You are told what time to arrive, where to go, what writing instrument to use, when to break the seal, and so on. You want to assume control of as many aspects as possible to maximize your performance:

STUDY Follow the sage advice of planning your work and working your plan to maintain satisfactory preparation with regard to study.

SLEEP Get a good night's rest. Sleep needs vary, but 6 hours is usually minimum. Try to get the appropriate amount of sleep that you require.

NUTRITION Maintain proper nutrition during both study time and exam time. Eat breakfast. Choose foods that help keep you on an even energy level. Eat light lunches on exam days. If you have a favorite food and can take it with you, treat yourself.

MEDICATION It may be cold, flu, or allergy season. Take no medications that may make you drowsy.

CLOTHING Heating and cooling systems are rarely balanced enough to suit everyone. Wear articles of clothing that can be added or removed as necessary. Strive for personal comfort.

READINESS Develop physical, mental, emotional, and psychologic readiness for the exam. Keep your thoughts about the exam and your preparation efforts running positively. You must believe that *you can do this!*

ARRIVAL Plan to arrive as close to the designated time as possible and still allow yourself sufficient time to check in. Keep to yourself so that other people's anxieties will not affect you. Take care of personal needs. Find your seat.

ACCLIMATION Settle in and get comfortable. Take several deep breaths . . . RELAX. A relaxed mind thinks better than a tense one—it's that old "fight-or-flight" syndrome. Do your warm-up routine to help you relax.

ATTENTION Pay attention to the proctor. Complete all identification material as required. Read all instructions carefully. Ask for clarification as needed. Do not open your booklet until told to do so. After you are told to break the seal, quickly glance through the whole test to see how it is set up and how questions are organized. Again, you want to take control of the situation. A quick purview eliminates surprises and allows you to develop a plan.

DURING THE EXAM

Plan Your Approach

There are numerous approaches to answering questions. Answer questions in the order that appeals to you. Doing the easier ones first may give a psychologic boost; however, the ones you skip may stay on your mind and cloud your thinking.

Another approach is to answer each question in sequence. Start with the first one in the section with which you begin and fill in an answer for each question. Do not leave any blanks! The theory behind this is that if you spend any time at all on an item, you should mark your best response at that time and go on. If you are not certain of your choice, mark "R" in the test booklet for review and return to it later as you have time.

Some students plan to do the matching items first. Matching items are the last set of questions in the booklets. If you prefer matching items, this is a reasonable plan because it helps you get started with items about which you feel confident. It is also reasonable because matching items are not good items on which to guess if you run short of time. **You** must decide the order in which you want to do the questions.

Complete the Bubble Sheet or Answer Card Carefully

There are two schools of thought on this matter. One is to fill in the bubble sheet **item by item** as you go. This method minimizes transcription errors. The other method is **block transfer.** Complete a logical chunk of questions in the test booklet (one or two pages) and then transfer responses to the bubble sheet. Be sure that the last question number on the page is the last numeral you blacken. This method saves time and offers a mini-mental break at the end of each block. Such minibreaks help decrease fatigue during a long exam. Choose the method that will work for you and *practice* it as you take prep questions.

Budget Your Time

If only the allotted time and the number of questions were considered, you would have approximately 54 seconds per question. Obviously, some questions may go more quickly and balance out the ones that take longer. To keep track, you need a pacing strategy. A good strategy is to establish checkpoints at 30-minute intervals. When you overview the booklet, circle the numerals corresponding to where you should be at 30 minutes, 60, 90, 120, and so on. For example, if you have 200 questions on a 3-hour exam, you should be at question number 33 at 30 minutes. As you complete the exam, check your time at the circled items. This technique keeps you from watching the clock too much, yet permits multiple opportunities to adjust your pacing.

If you find yourself spending too much time on any one question, select your best choice at that time, mark an answer, and "R" it for later review. The point is to keep going. Laboring too long on one question limits you from responding to other items you may know well. Remember, controlling your time helps you maximize your points.

ANSWERING THE QUESTIONS

- **Read and *understand* the stems and alternatives.**
  The most frequent error made on exams is misreading or misinterpreting the various aspects of a question. The **stem** is the introductory question or statement. The **alternatives** are the options from which you select the one best response. To encourage reading and understanding, use a process.
- **Follow a process to answer questions.**
  1. Quickly read the stem.
  2. Quickly read the options. (Combined, the first two steps create a preview of the item.)
  3. Carefully read, underline, and mark the stem in a timely fashion.
     - Selectively underline key words and phrases.
     - Pay attention to nouns, verbs, and modifiers.
     - Circle age and gender.
     - Note data in telescopic form (e.g., ↑ BP).
     - Graphically represent material if it helps you to understand (e.g., diagram the renal tubule to answer a question about reabsorption).
  4. Carefully read each alternative. Mark as appropriate.
- **Consider each alternative as one in a series of true, false, or not sure (?) statements.**
  Read each alternative. Rather than slashing out the ones you eliminate, work with each one and designate it as **true, false,** or varying degrees of **true/false/?.** This marking strategy requires you to make judicious decisions about alternatives relative to the stem. It also provides a record of your original thinking, which will save you rethinking time if you need to reconsider a question. Practice this strategy on preparation questions so it becomes second nature.
- **Avoid premature closure.**
  Sometimes you may read a question and anticipate a response. Such a reaction helps focus your attention. However, be sure to read *all* the options so that you are selecting the *best* response. In one-best-answer multiple choice questions, there is one *best* and several *likely* responses. Avoid being misled; consider all the alternatives.
- **Be leery of negative stems.**
  Negative stems require shifting to a negative thinking mode to determine which alternatives are not correct. You can avoid this shift by using this strategy:
  - Circle such words as *except, least, false, incorrect, not true* to raise your awareness of them.
  - Cross out the negative and read the stem as though it were a positive.
  - Mark each option as T/F/?. The F option will then be the appropriate choice.
- **Keep your original answers.**
  To change or not to change answers is a difficult decision. The answer depends on a person's previous history. If you are the kind of student who, if you change answers, changes them from wrong to right, then selectively changing answers may be worthwhile. If, on the other hand, your past experience has been to change right answers to wrong answers, selectively changing answers is probably not a good idea. Good performers change answers, but only if they have reason, such as acquired insight or discovery of misreading or misinterpretation.

- **Maintain an even emotional keel.**
If a question upsets you, calm yourself. Take several deep breaths. Tell yourself, "I can do this!" Give yourself a mental or physical break. Pay special attention to the next two or three questions after a bout of emotional uneasiness. It is possible to miss items when attention is diffused.

THINKING THROUGH QUESTIONS

- **Use logical reasoning and sound thinking.**
  - Read the item carefully. After careful reading, ask "What is this question really asking?" Restate it so that you know what is being asked.
  - Engage in a mental dialogue with the question. Talk to yourself about what you do know. Always start with what **you** know. Verbalize your thinking.
  - If a diagram or graphic representation is included, orient yourself to it **first** so that the options do not lead your thinking.
- **Use information found within the questions themselves to help you answer others.**
There will not be "gimmes" on a nationally standardized exam. However, there may be items or graphics that trigger remembrances.
- **Create a diagram, chart, map, or graphic representation of given information.**
Material that is visually presented usually helps clarify thinking. Use selective, quick sketching as warranted.
- **Reason through information like a detective.**
  - Sift through the details (preview).
  - Determine the relevant information (selectively mark).
  - Put the clues together as in solving a puzzle (reason).
- **Read carefully and note key descriptors.**
  - Note words such as *chronic, acute, greater than, less than, adult, child.*
  - Attend to prefixes such as *hyper-, hypo-, non-, un-, pre-, post-.*
- **Analyze base words and affixes.**
Studying a question at the word level may help you remember salient information. Look for base words or related words. Determine Latin or Greek word parts and use their meanings to assist you.
- **Consider similar options equally.**
If you mark one alternative as "false" for a particular reason and another option is qualified for the same reason, it's probably "false" as well.
- **Trust the questions.**
The questions are designed to determine if you have a working knowledge of the material. They are not written to trick you. You need to believe that your medical school curriculum and your study efforts prepared you for most of the questions.
- **Meet the challenge of clinical vignettes.**
Longer, vignette items challenge you to discern the relevant from the irrelevant material. In doing so, you are given multiple clues to consider. To effectively handle the vignette item, follow this strategy:
  - Scan the stem and read the first several lines.
  - Skip to the end of the stem and read the last several lines.
  - Check the alternatives to narrow your focus.
  - Now that you know what the question is about, go back to the stem; read and mark what's important to your informed decision making.
  - Make good T/F/? decisions.
- **Reread your underlines and markings when you are down to two choices, at 50/50.**
By the time you work through a stem and numerous alternatives, it is easy to lose the gist of the question. Checking your focus by rereading only the underlines ensures that you are answering the question being posed.

ANSWERING MATCHING ITEM SETS

Matching items are used to measure your ability to distinguish among closely related items. They require knowledge of specific sets of information. As you study, be alert to potential material that could be tested in this way.

Matching items can be formatted in two ways. **Short leading list matching** items include a set of five lettered options followed by a lead-in statement and then several numbered stems. **Long leading list matching** items include a set of up to 26 lettered options, followed by a lead-in statement and then several numbered stems.

To efficiently deal with a short leading list item, consider it as an upside-down multiple choice item with the same repeated options. To handle it effectively, do the following:

- Scan the list; determine the topic.
- Read the lead-in statement; determine the focus.
- Quickly read the stem; then read and mark key words.
- In the left margin, create a grid with A, B, C, D, E at the top.

- Make good T/F/? decisions about each stem, marking them in the grid. In this way you can see the pattern of your responses. Similarly, a grid with the item numbers can be drawn beside the leading list and responses marked there.

Handling long leading list matching items effectively requires some modifications in the process. It is not efficient to make T/F/? decisions about each option, so follow this strategy:

- Scan the list; determine the topic.
- Read the lead-in; determine the focus.
- Read a stem and generate your own response.
- Narrow the focus. Put a check mark by those related options in the long list.
- Read and mark specifics in the stem to differentiate among those alternatives you marked.
- Make good T/F/? decisions.

For each stem, mark the narrowed-list options with a different symbol (star, dash, etc.). Items are listed in logical order, alphabetically or numerically. When looking for an option such as "xanthinuria," do not start at the beginning of the list. Looking in the appropriate place saves valuable seconds.

TEST WISENESS

How a question is worded can often influence your response to it. Most clues about "test psychology" are a function of the way in which a question is worded—test constructors cannot rename body parts, drugs, diseases, and so forth. Being aware of the psychology behind the wording can often help you answer the test question.

Using techniques of test psychology to arrive at a correct answer has limited value on standardized exams because those who construct the exams are well aware of the use of these techniques. Nonetheless, being wise to these techniques of test psychology may add another point or two to your score, and they can also enhance your sense of control. Knowing these techniques provides additional strategies to employ should the question temporarily stump you.

The best way to take any exam is to be totally prepared with a strong knowledge base and personal test confidence. The following techniques should be used only if you have exhausted your knowledge base, eliminated all distractors, and cannot come up with the answer even with logical thinking and sound reasoning. Such techniques are **not** a substitute for knowledge, nor are they foolproof.

- **Identify common ideas or themes within the options and between the stem and options.**
  - Circle repeated words in the options.
  - Select the option with the most repeated words or phrases.
  - Circle words repeated in both stem and options.
  - Select the option that contains key words or related words from the stem. This is a stem/option repetition.
- **Beware of words that narrow the focus or are too extreme because they tend to be incorrect.**
  Circle such words as **all, always, every, exclusively, never, no, not, none.**
- **Options that are look-alikes are good candidates for exclusion.**
- **Note qualifiers that broaden the focus because they may be correct.**
  Circle words such as *generally, probably, most, often, some, usually.*
- **Identify antonyms or two opposing statements as potentially correct options.**
  Test constructors may use pairs of opposites, so this tip may lose its effectiveness.
- **Select the most familiar-looking option.**
  Always go from what you know. Alternatives with unknown terms may be likely distractors.
- **Select the longest, most inclusive answer.**
  This would include "All of the above" as a strong potential response.
- **In numerical items, knock out the high and low alternatives and select one in the middle that seems most plausible.**
- **In negatively stemmed questions, categorize responses; the one that falls out of the category is a likely candidate.**
- **Mark the same alternative consistently throughout the test if you have no best guess and cannot eliminate distractors.**
  Before the test, decide which letter (A, B, C, D, E) will be your choice. In this way, if you have given a question your best effort and cannot decide, mark your favorite response and move to questions that cover more comfortable material.

AFTER THE EXAM

- **Between booklets and overnight:**
  - Take a well-deserved break. Eat nutritionally.
  - If you feel the urge to study, study material that is comfortable, from a source with which you are familiar (e.g., personally developed study cards or your annotated review book).
  - If you discovered a recurring "theme," you might desire to consult that set of information.

   - Do something pleasurable. Relax. Get a good night's rest.
- **After the final booklet:**
   - Recognize that this exam is a measure of what you know on a given day for a given set of information at a given point in time. Keep a reasonable perspective.
   - **Celebrate!**

References

Bushan V, Le T, Amin C: First aid for the USMLE Step 1, ed 5, Norwalk, Conn., 1995, Appleton & Lange.

Contents

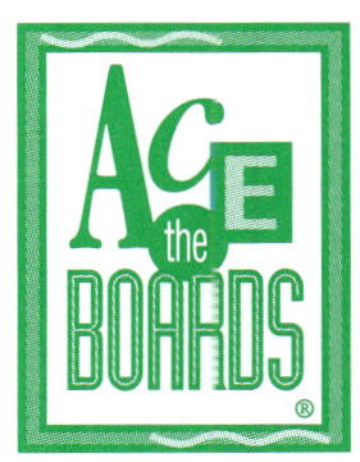

Microbiology
& Immunology

Chapter 1

Immunology and Basic Concepts in Pathogenesis

Section 1.1 Elements of the Immune Response

Immune responses are mediated by specific cells with defined functions. The characteristics of the main cells of the immune system are presented in Figure 1.1 and Table 1.1.

- **Hematopoietic Cell Differentiation** Understanding the relationship of the different cell types is facilitated by an awareness of their development. Lymphocytes undergo antigen-independent and antigen-dependent differentiation.

  Differentiation generally requires specific lymphokines and specific cell-surface interactions. These interactions occur in defined body locations (Fig. 1.2).

Section 1.2 Antigen Nonspecific Immune Responses

- **Natural Immunity**
  - **Barriers and blockers** Skin, secretions (e.g., mucus, basic proteins in saliva), ciliated mucoepithelium, body temperature, and fever act as physical and chemical barriers.

  - **Complement system** This system inactivates and promotes clearance of bacteria and other infectious agents and promotes inflammatory responses. It consists of two pathways: the alternative pathway (properdin system; see section 1.5) and the classical pathway. *C3 is the central component of both complement cascades.*
  - **Inflammation** The increased permeability of blood vessels allows neutrophils, proteins, and other elements to leak into the infected site. Chronic inflammation causes accumulation of lymphocytes, polymorphonuclear neutrophils (PMNs), and macrophages and proliferation of fibroblasts (scarring).
- **Phagocytic Clearance of Infectious Agents** Phago means "to eat." Initially, PMNs, such as neutrophils and eosinophils and later, monocytes or macrophages, engulf, internalize, and inactivate the bacteria. *The presence of neutrophils implies bacterial infection.*
  - **Steps in phagocytosis**
    - *1. Attachment* This is promoted by **opsonins** that bind to the bacteria (or other particles) and then to specific receptors on the phagocyte. Dead cells can also be taken up by phagocytes.

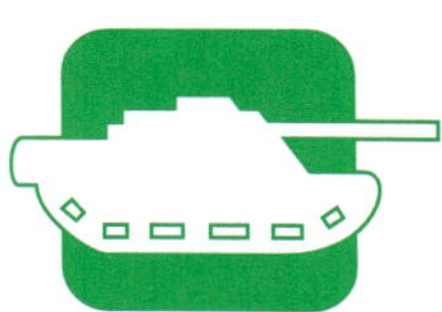

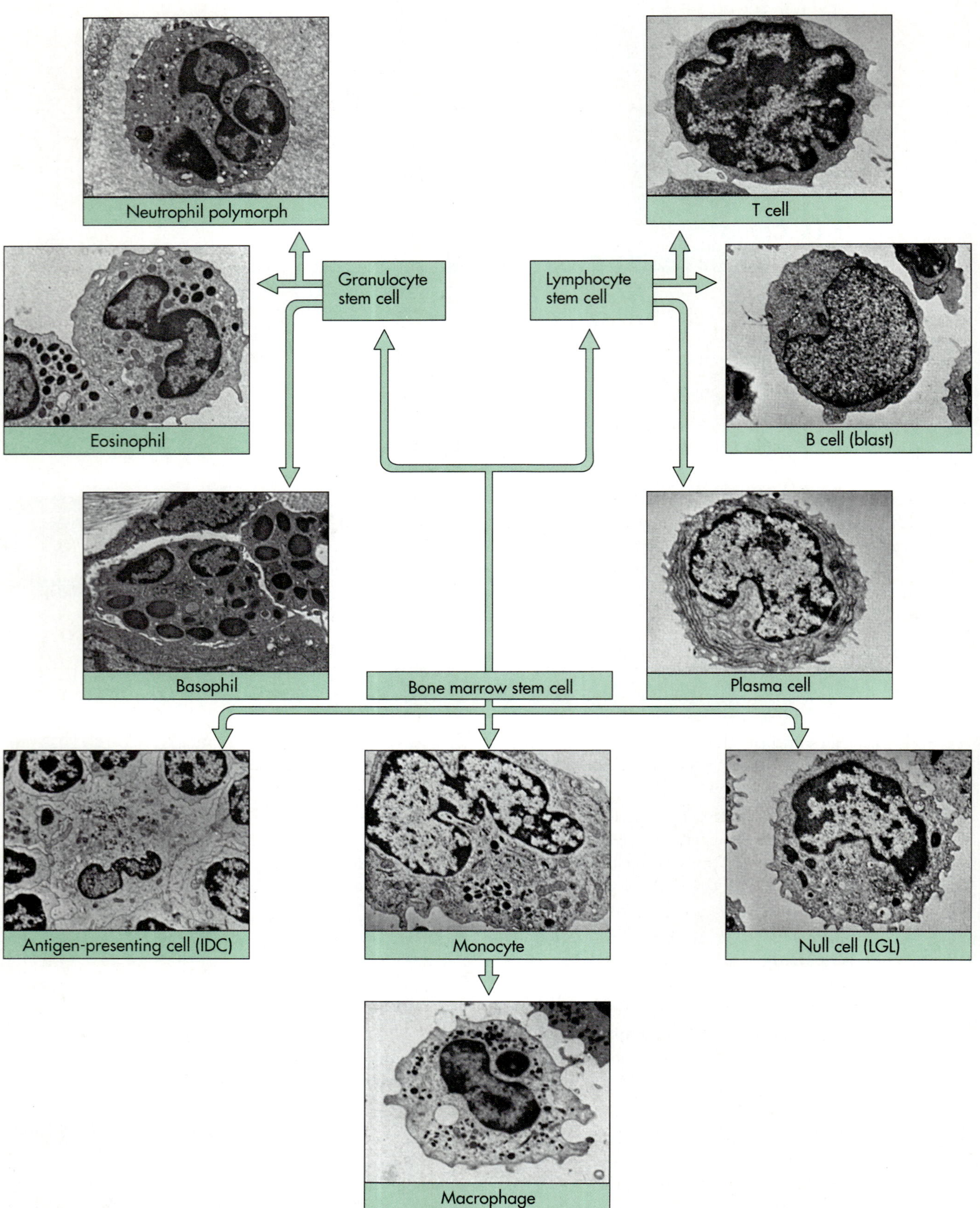

Fig. 1.1 Morphology of cells involved in the immune response. Mononuclear cells include lymphocytes, monocytes, and macrophages. Polymorphonuclear leukocytes include neutrophils, eosinophils, basophils, and mast cells.

Table 1.1 *Cells of the Immune Response*

Cells	Characteristics	Markers	Functions
Natural Cytolytic Cells			
Killer (K) cells	Large granular lymphocytes	Fc receptors for antibody	Kill antibody decorated cells, e.g., virus-infected cells
Natural Killer (NK) cells	Large granular lymphocytes		Kill malignant or virus-infected cells (**no MHC restriction**)
Phagocytic Cells			
Neutrophils	Granulocytes or polymorphonuclear leukocytes (PMN), short life span Segmented Bands (more immature)	Multilobed nucleus and granules	*Phagocytise* and kill *bacteria*
Eosinophils	Bilobed nucleus, heavily granulated cytoplasm	Stains with eosin Y	Defend against parasites
Macrophages	(See below)		
Antigen Presenting Cells		MHC class II–expressing cells	Present antigen to CD4$^+$ T helper cells
Monocytes	5% of circulating blood cells, precursors of macrophages	Horse-shoe–shaped nucleus, lysosomes, granules	Found in lymph nodes, lungs, blood
Macrophages	May be resident in tissues, also capable of activation; activated by interferon γ	Large, granular	Found in lymph nodes, lungs, blood, spleen, and other organs Produces lymphokines such as IL-1, TNF, IL-6, GM-CSF, and interferon α, and complement; activated macrophages are cytolytic for tumor and virus-infected cells
Langerhans cells			Found in skin and transport antigen to lymph nodes
Dendritic cells			Found in lymph nodes, tissues
Microglial cells			Found in brain
Kupffer cells			Found in liver
B lymphocytes	(See below)		
Antigen Responsive Cells			
Lymphokine producing cells (CD4$^+$ T lymphocytes)	Mature in thymus; activated by APC/antigen through **MHC class II antigen presentation**	CD2, CD3, T-cell receptor, CD4	Helper T cells Release IL-2 and other lymphokines, activate other T cells and promote growth and class switching of B lymphocytes Delayed-type hypersensitivity T cells Promotes inflammatory responses; essential for elimination of fungal and intracellular bacterial infections
Cytolytic cells (CD8$^+$ T lymphocytes)	Mature in thymus; recognition of antigen presented by **MHC class I antigens**	CD2, CD3, T-cell receptor, CD8	Cytolysis of virus-infected, tumor, and transplant cells

Continued.

Table 1.1 *Cells of the Immune Response—cont'd*

Cells	Characteristics	Markers	Functions
Suppressor cells ($CD8^+$ T lymphocytes)	Recognition of antigen presented by **MHC class I antigens**	CD2, CD3, T-cell receptor, CD8	Suppression of T and B cell responses
Antibody producing cells			
B cells	Mature in Peyer's patches, bone marrow, bursal equivalent Large nucleus, small cytoplasm; activated by antigens with repeating units (e.g., flagellin, LPS, capsular polysaccharide) and T cell factors	Surface Ig, **MHC class II antigens**	Antibody production and antigen presentation
Plasma cells	Small nucleus, large cytoplasm		Terminally differentiated, antibody factories
Other Cells			
Eosinophils	Bilobed nucleus		Anti-parasitic cells
Mast cells		Fc receptors for IgE	Release histamine

MHC, Major histocompatibility complex; *APC,* atrial premature complex; *TNF,* tumor necrosis factor; *GM-CSF,* granulocyte-macrophage–stimulating factor; *LPS,* lipopolysaccharide.

Types of opsonins

- C3b produced via the alternative or the classical complement pathway binds to C3 receptors on the phagocyte.
- IgG bound to bacteria, viruses, or other particles binds to Fc receptors on the phagocyte. IgG can also activate the classical complement cascade to produce C3b.

2. Ingestion The particle is surrounded and internalized into a phagosome (Fig. 1.3).

3. Digestion (Box 1.1)

a) Degranulation: cytoplasmic granules that contain enzymes fuse with the phagosome.
b) Oxygen burst and glucose utilization
c) Production of H_2O, superoxide, activated halides

Defects in digestion

1. Bacterial production of catalase
    - breaks down hydrogen peroxide
    - examples are staphylococci, *Neisseria* spp., Enterobacteriaciae, and *Candida albicans*
2. Bacterial or viral inhibition of phagosome–granule fusion
    - prevents antimicrobial activity
    - allows intracellular growth or replication
3. Genetic deficiencies

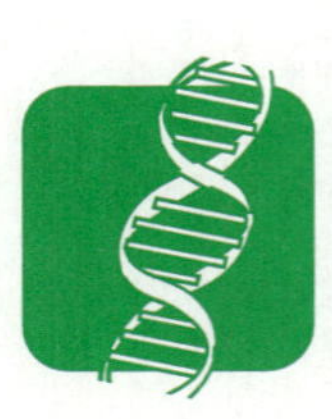

Chronic granulomatous disease (CGD):
- defective hydrogen peroxide and superoxide production
- inability to kill bacteria that produce catalase

Chediak-Higashi disease:
- defective phagocytes incapable of degranulation
- increased susceptability to bacterial infections

Myeloperoxidase deficiency:
- delayed killing of staphylococci and *C. albicans*

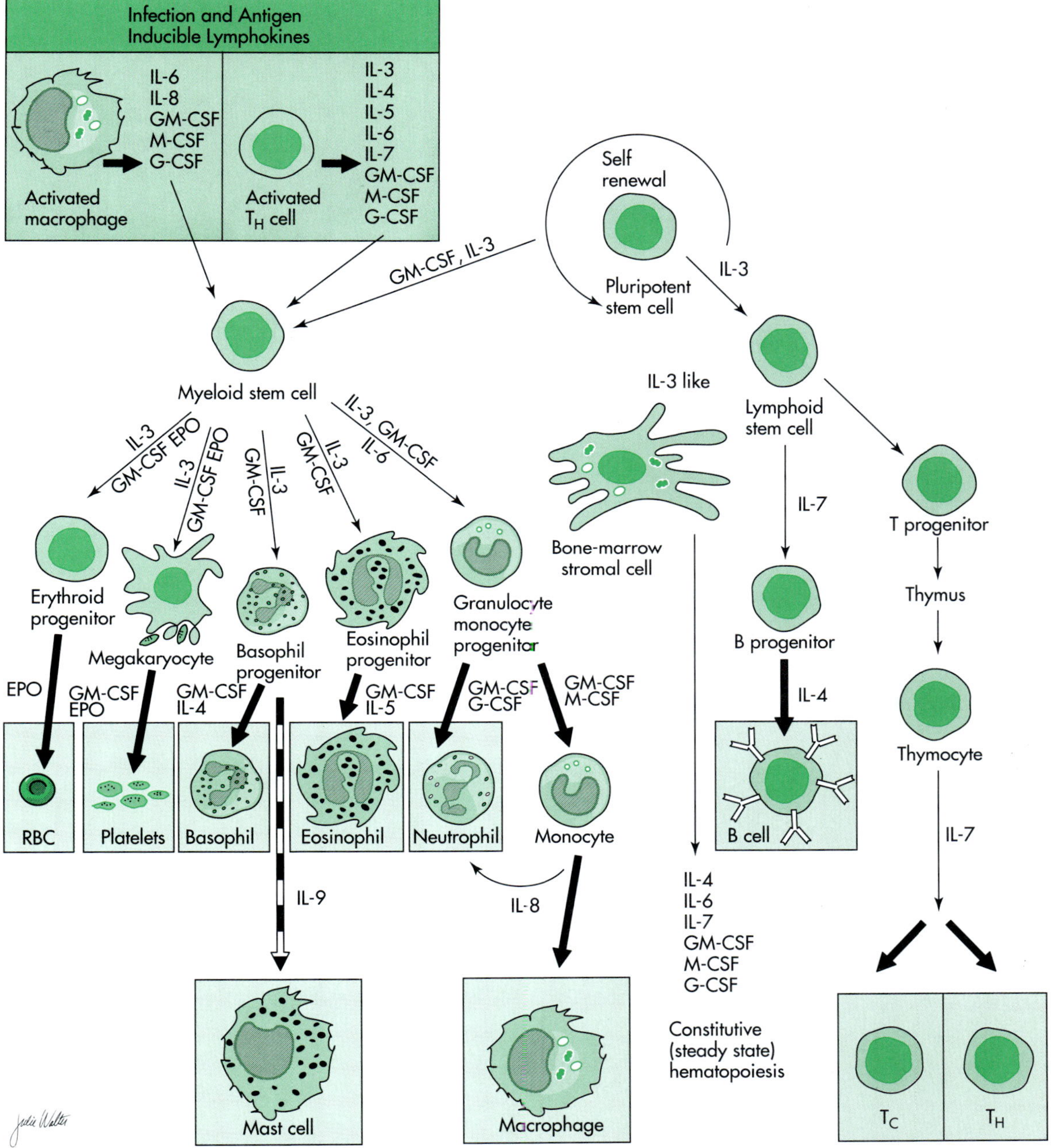

Fig. 1.2 Hematopoietic cell development. Differentiation is promoted by environmental factors and lymphokines, as indicated. The pluripotent stem cell is the source of all hematopoietic cells, which develop along two main pathways, the lymphoid and the myeloid paths of development. Differentiation may be continuous or induced by lymphokines in response to infection. *GM-CSF,* Granulocyte-macrophage–colony stimulating factor; *M-CSF,* macrophage–colony stimulating factor; *G-CSF,* granulocyte–colony stimulating factor; *EPO,* erythropoietin; *RBC,* red blood cell.

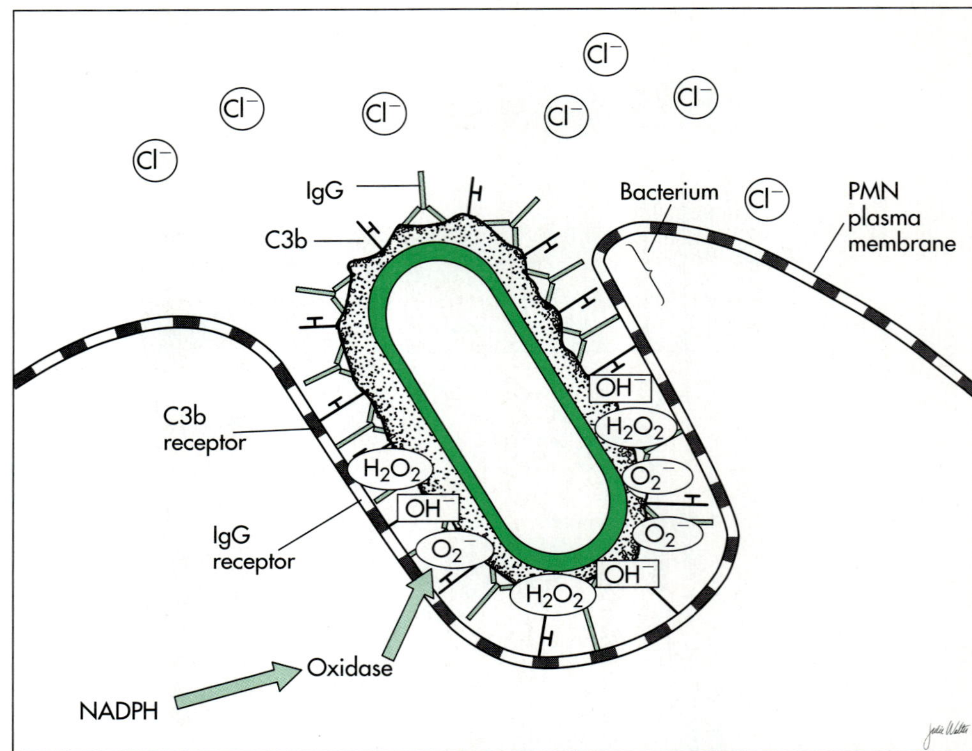

Fig. 1.3 Killing of bacteria by a phagocyte. Bacteria are opsonized by IgG and C3b, promoting their adherance and uptake by phagocytes. Bactericides and hydrogen peroxide are produced and released in response to bacterial adherance to kill the bacteria. *PMN,* Polymorphonuclear neutrophil leukocytes; *NADPH,* reduced nicotinamide-adenine dinucleotide phosphate.

Box 1.1

ANTIBACTERIAL COMPOUNDS OF THE PHAGOLYSOSOME

Oxygen Dependent Compounds

Hydrogen peroxide: NADPH oxidase
NADH oxidase
Superoxide
Hydroxyl radicals (OH)
Activated halides (Cl^-, I^-, Br^-): myeloperoxidase

Oxygen Independent Compounds

Acids
Lysozyme (degrades bacterial peptidoglycan)
Lactoferrin (chelates iron)
Defensins and other cationic proteins (damage membranes)
Proteases: elastase, cathepsin, G

NADH, Nicotinamide-adenine dinucleotide phosphate; *NADPH,* reduced NADH.

Table 1.2 *Functional Components of the Antibody Molecule*

Structural Region	Function
Variable/Idiotype region	Interacts with antigens
Fc region	Interacts with immune components to promote activation of other immune functions, killing of infectious agents, and clearance of antigen from the body
Membrane-spanning region	Found only on surface immunoglobulin; antibody acts as an antigen receptor to promote antigen-specific activation of B cells

Table 1.3 *Fc Interactions with Immune Components*

Immune Component	Interaction	Function
Membrane Fc receptor	B cells	Activation of B cells
	Macrophages	Opsonization
	PMNs	Opsonization
	T cells	Activation
	Cells responsible for antibody dependent cellular cytotoxicity (ADCC)	Killing
	Mast cells for IgE	Allergic reactions, antiparasitic response
Complement	Complement system	Opsonization, killing (especially bacteria)

PMN, Polymorphonuclear neutrophil leukocytes.

Section 1.3 Immunoglobulins

Antibodies bind specifically to antigens and block or neutralize their function (e.g., viruses) or promote their destruction or clearance from the body.

Antibody molecules have two major structural regions (Tables 1.2 and 1.3):

- **Variable region** or antigen combining site: *Binds antigen*
- **Fc portion:** *Interacts with host systems for antigen clearance (e.g., complement, Fc receptors)*

All antibody molecules have heavy and light chains that are encoded by separate genes.

- **Light chains** have one variable and one constant domain. There are two types of light chains, κ and λ.
- **Heavy chains** have one variable and three constant domains. There are five major types of heavy chains, one for each type of antibody (μ, γ, δ, α, ϵ). Each of the heavy chains also comes in a membrane and a soluble form.

The immunoglobulin chains are held together by disulfide bonds.

Immunoglobulin Types, Functions, and Structures

Vocabulary

Isotypes: Antibody molecules that are distinguished by the Fc portion of the molecule (e.g., IgM, IgD, IgG, IgA, IgE). *(The isotype is the same for all individuals.)*

Allotypes: Isotype antibody molecules have regions that differ among individuals (in addition to the antigen binding region). *("Allo" them have different IgG.)*

Idiotypes: Different antibodies of the same isotype and allotype that differ in the antigen binding region (the variable region). *(There are lots of different types of idiots.)*

Hinge region: The flexible part of the molecule defined by disulfide bonds and found only in IgG and IgA.

- **Isotypes (IgM, IgD, IgG, IgA, and IgE)** Structural distinctions between the isotypes result in different functions and roles in immunity (Fig. 1.4 and Table 1.4).

  — *IgM*
  - largest antibody; pentameric, held together with J chain
  - first antibody produced during an immune response
  - T cell independent
  - too large to spread into tissue from serum
  - effective antibacterial, complement-binding antibody

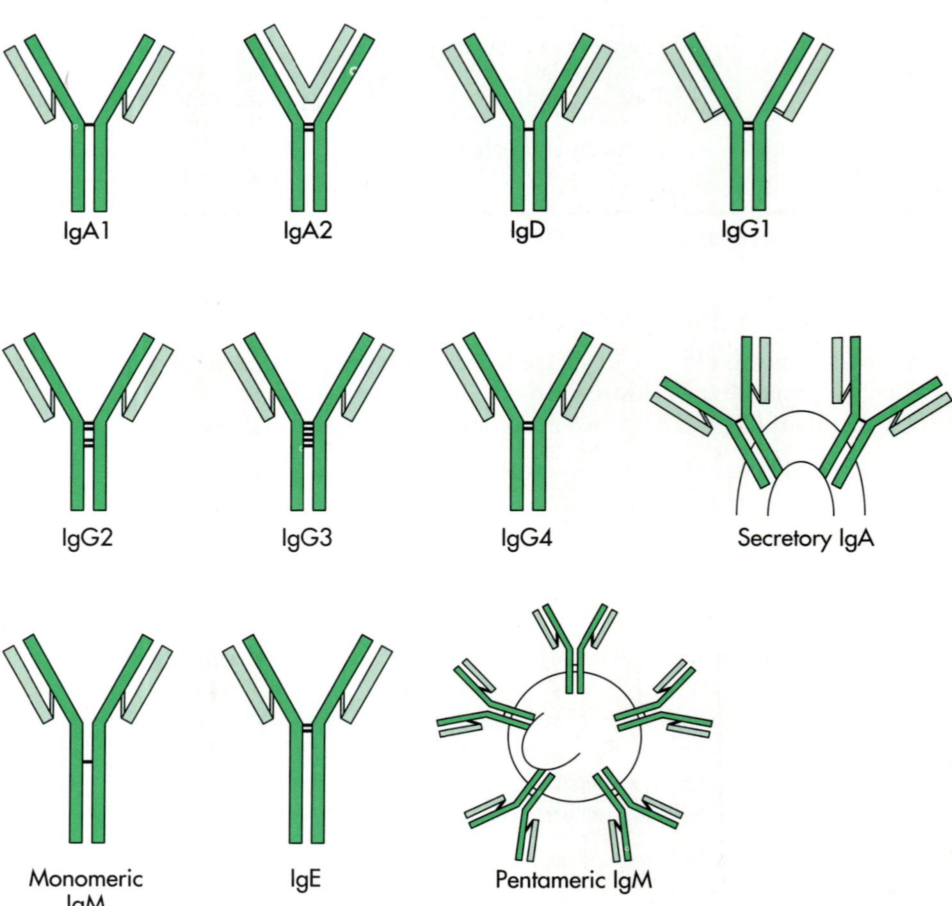

Fig. 1.4 Comparative structures of the immunoglobulin classes and subclasses in humans. IgA and IgM are held together in multimers by the J chain. IgA can acquire the secretory component for traversal of epithelial cells.

Table 1.4 *The Immunoglobulins*

Ig	IgG	IgM	IgA	IgD	IgE
Serum concentration (mg/dl)	800-1700	50-190	140-420	0.3-0.40	<0.001
Total Ig (%)	85	5-10	5-15	<1	<1
Complement fixation	+	++++	–	–	–
Principal biological effect	Resistance—opsonin; secondary response	Resistance—precipitin; primary response	Resistance—prevents movement across mucous membranes	?	Anaphylaxis
Principal site of action	Serum	Serum	Secretions	?; Receptor for B cells	Mast cells
Molecular weight (kd)	154	900	160 (+ dimer)	185	190
Serum half-life (days)	23	5	6	2-3	2-3
Antibacterial lysis	+	+++	+	?	?
Antiviral lysis	+	+	+++	?	?
H-chain class	γ	μ	α	δ	ϵ
Subclass	$\gamma_1\gamma_2\gamma_3\gamma_4$	$\mu_1\mu_2$	$\alpha_1\alpha_2$		

- monomeric IgM present on surface of early B cell
- major component of rheumatoid factor (an autoantibody)

— *IgD*
- membrane immunoglobulin present with IgM

— *IgG*
- major antibody form (constitutes 85% of all antibodies)
- longest half-life
- crosses placenta
- fixes complement, stimulates chemotaxis, acts as opsonin
- present on cell surface of B cell

— *IgA*
- secretory or serum antibody
- divalent, held together with J chain
- secretory component promotes release through epithelial cells

— *IgE*
- constitutes less than 1% of total antibody
- involved in allergic response
- antiparasitic
- binds to Fc receptors on mast cells
- antigen binding to cell-bound IgE promotes histamine, prostaglandin, platelet activating factor, and cytokine release

- **Subtypes of IgG (see Fig. 1.4)** Structural distinctions between the subtypes of IgG result in different functions and roles for these subtypes in immunity.
- **Proteolytic digestion of IgG**

Proteases cut immunoglobulins into defined functional fragments (Fig. 1.5).

- pepsin cleavage: $F(ab')_2$—bivalent antigen binding

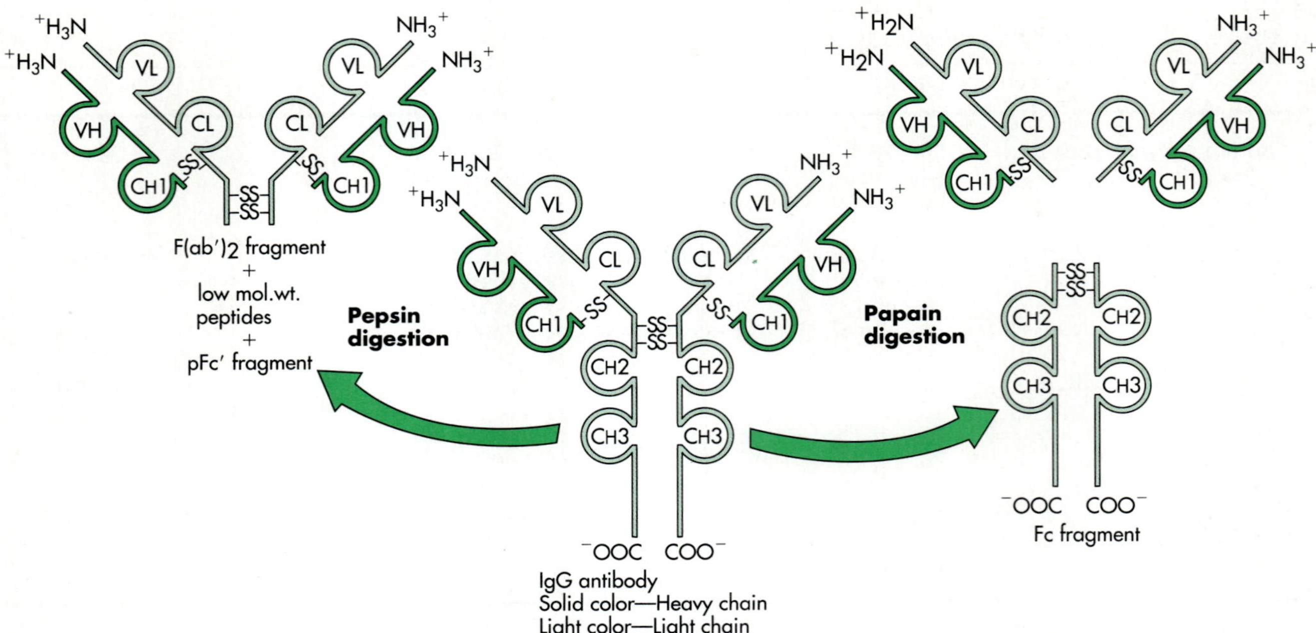

Fig. 1.5 Proteolytic digestion of IgG. Pepsin treatment produces a *dimeric* F(ab′)$_2$ fragment. Papain treatment produces *monovalent* Fab fragments and the Fc fragment. The F(ab′)$_2$ and the Fab fragments bind antigen but lack a functional Fc region.

- papain cleavage: Fab—monovalent antigen binding
- papain or pepsin cleavage: Fc—binds to cellular Fc receptors

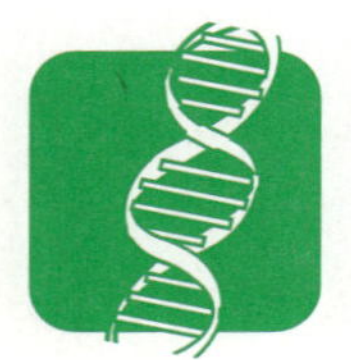

- **Immunogenetics (Figs. 1.6 to 1.9)**
  - The immunoglobulin genes are generated by combining different sets of genetic building blocks. Mutation adds diversity. Final processing occurs at the mRNA level.
  - The light chain is encoded by the V, J, and C genes.
  - The heavy chain is encoded by the V, D, J, and C genes.
  - There are more than 100 V genes, 12 D (heavy chain) genes, 5 (light chain) or 6 (heavy chain) J genes, but only 8 C genes (one for each of the isotypes: μ, γ1-γ4, δ, α, ε). *Random combination of the V, D, and J genes, together with somatic mutation generates great diversity.*

The C genes are arranged in the following order: μ, δ, γ4, γ2, γ3, γ1, ε, α. These genes associate with the V, D, and J region genes in the same order.

Immunoglobulin gene rearrangements occur during differentiation of the pre-B cell to an immunocompetent B cell.

The μ and δ genes are present together in the pre-B cell and in the early B cell. The final mRNA for membrane IgM or IgD or for secreted IgM is produced by splicing the μ, δ, or membrane-spanning segment from the mRNA.

Class switching (IgM to IgG, IgE, or IgA) occurs by deletion of the C region genes that precede the final C gene.

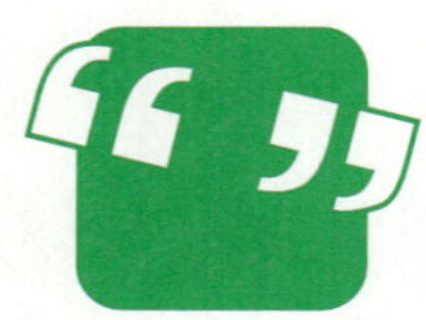

- **Functional regions of antibody** Antibody molecules have defined functional regions that accomplish three major tasks (see Table 1.2).

— ***Vocabulary***

Neutralization: Attachment of antibody to any material, for ex-

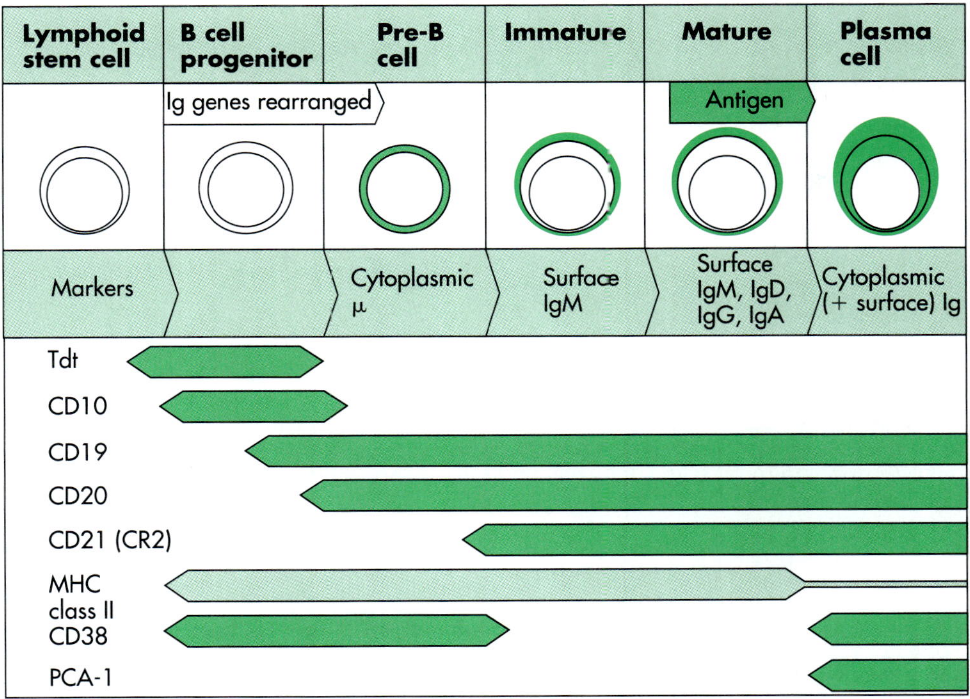

Fig. 1.6 Differentiation of the B lymphocyte. The development of the B cell is initiated by rearrangement of the immunoglobulin genes that constitute the initial antibody repertoire. Different forms of immunoglobulin and other markers distinguish the phases of development, culminating in the terminally differentiated plasma cell. The plasma cell is an antibody factory with a large cytoplasm and a small nucleus. *TdT,* Terminal deoxynucleotide transferase; *MHC,* major histocompatibility complex.

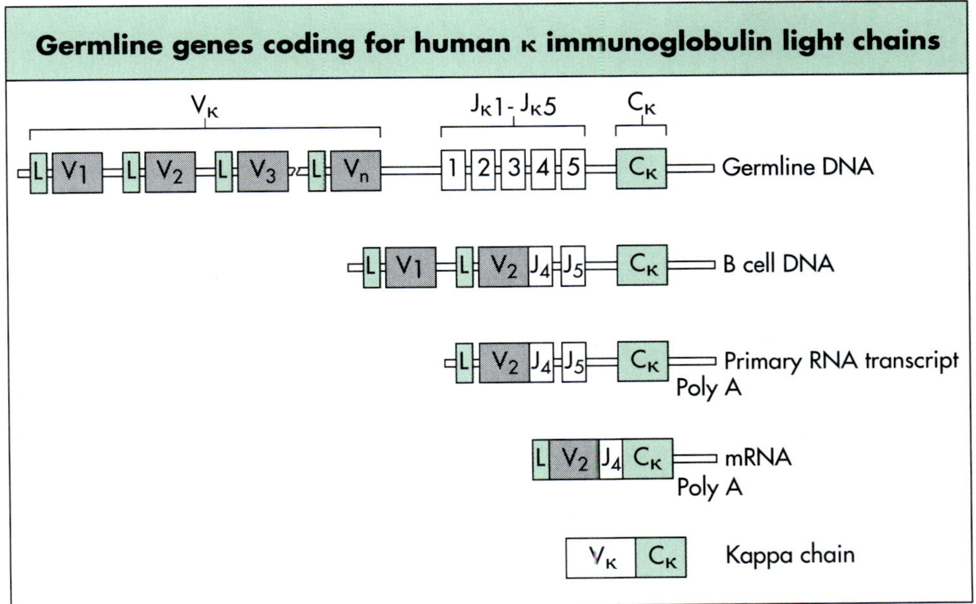

Fig. 1.7 Rearrangement of the germline genes to produce the four human immunoglobulin light chains. Genetic recombination juxtaposes one of 100 V region genes with a J region gene and a C_{κ} gene during differentiation into a pre-B cell. The remaining intervening sequences are removed by splicing the mRNA. (*L,* leader sequence).

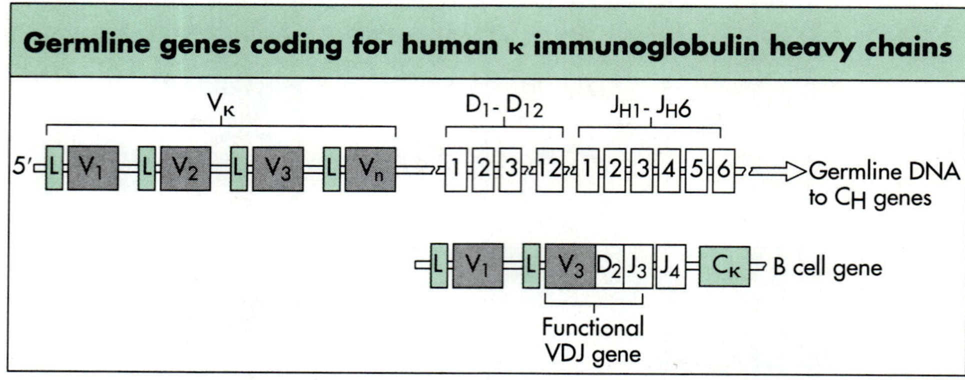

Fig. 1.8 Rearrangement of the germline genes to produce the human immunoglobulin heavy chains. A V region gene (out of 100 possible) combines with a D region gene (out of 12 possible) and a J region gene (out of 6 possible). Constant region genes μ, δ, γ, ϵ, or α (corresponding to IgM, IgD, IgG, IgE, and IgA) are attached to the VDJ region.

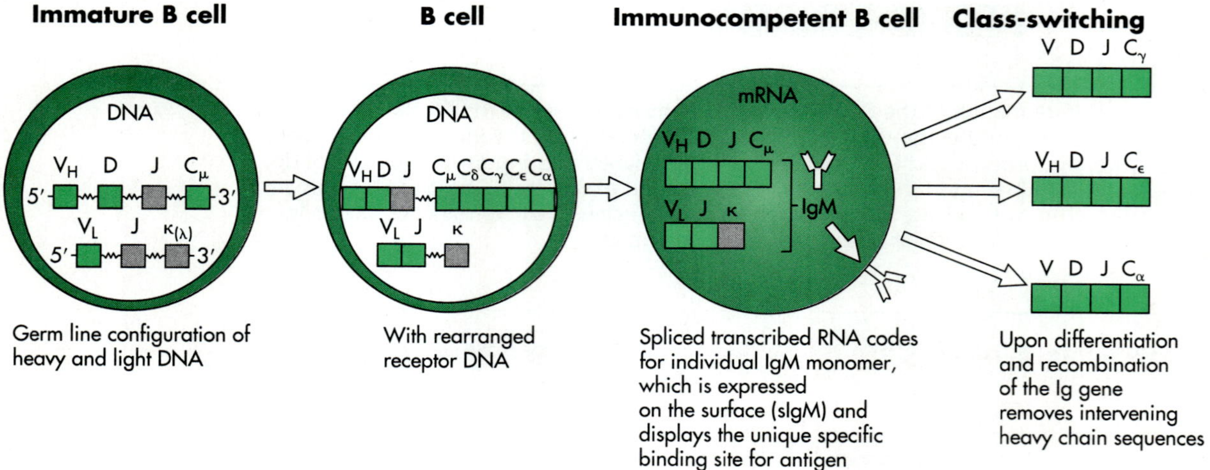

Fig. 1.9 Differentiation of the B cell promotes genetic recombination and class switching. Switch regions in front of the constant region genes (including IgG subclasses 1 to 4) allow recombination of the VDJ region with different heavy chain constant region genes, genetically removing the μ and other intervening genes. This produces the different heavy chain genes. Splicing of the mRNA produces the final IgmRNA.

ample, a toxin or a virus, that results in inactivation by preventing it from binding to its receptor or by promoting its destruction.

Opsonization: Promoting uptake by phagocytes bearing Fc receptors.

- **Antigen-antibody interactions** During an immune response, antibodies are made against different epitopes of the foreign object, protein, or infectious agent. Each antibody may recognize a different structure **(epitope)** on the larger unit. Each B cell produces only one type of antibody molecule **(monoclonal)**. However, many different B lymphocytes will be producing antibodies that bind with different strengths **(affinities)** for the same antigen.

Specific antiserum is therefore a mixture of many different antibody molecules that differ in the epitope that they recognize and in the strength of the interaction (unless it is a monoclonal antibody).

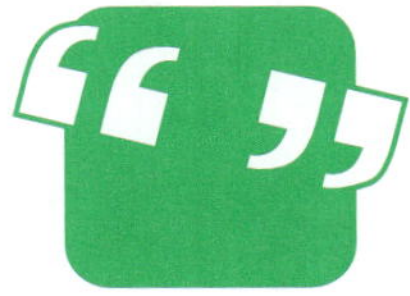

— ***Vocabulary***

Affinity: Binding strength of the variable or idiotype region of antibody for its epitope on the larger antigen structure.

Avidity: Binding strength of the multivalent antibody molecules for the entire antigen (all epitopes); the sum of all the interactions with the antigen.

Polyclonal antibody: Normal antibody produced by many different B cells; a mixture of many different antibody molecules.

Monoclonal antibody: Antibody produced by a single clone of B cells, which unlike polyclonal antibodies, recognizes only one epitope. As a result, monoclonal antibodies *do not* usually promote agglutination reactions (see below).

Agglutination reactions: At appropriate concentrations of antibody and antigen **(equivalence)** each antibody molecule will bind more than one antigen molecule and crosslink it into a large complex that may precipitate from the solution.

— ***Antigen-antibody reactions***

Immune complex disease: Antigen-antibody complexes formed in blood under certain pathogenic conditions can initiate hypersensitivity reactions (Type III) and tissue destruction. Examples are chronic hepatitis B infection, poststreptococcal glomerulonephritis, and lupus erythematosus.

— ***Diagnostic test***

The *Ouchterlony test* is a precipitin reaction in agar in which antibody and antigen are placed in opposing wells and allowed to diffuse towards each other. *At the equivalence concentration, they will precipitate and form a line.* The Ouchterlony test is used to determine identity, partial identity, or nonidentity between antigens (Fig. 1.10).

Section 1.4 T Cells

T cells are defined by their cell surface molecules.

- T cells respond to antigens but the antigens must first be digested and then presented to the T cell in association with a major histocompatability complex (MHC) molecule (i.e., it must be presented "in the context of a MHC molecule") (Fig. 1.11).
- Helper T cells ($CD4^+$ cells) interact with and help other lymphoid cells and therefore respond to peptide antigens in association with *MHC class II molecules on antigen presenting cells (APC).*
- Cytolytic and suppressor T cells ($CD8^+$ cells) patrol the body for cells expressing viral antigens or tumor related abnormal proteins, presented by the *MHC class I molecules.* MHC class I molecules are found *on all nucleated cells.*
- T cells bind different peptides through an antibody-like cell surface *T cell receptor (TCR).* Binding to the T cell receptor initiates cell activation and T cell functions.
- T helper cells release lymphokines (protein molecules that act as soluble messengers), which activate other cells.
- Cytolytic T cells act directly on the target cells expressing the foreign peptide antigen.

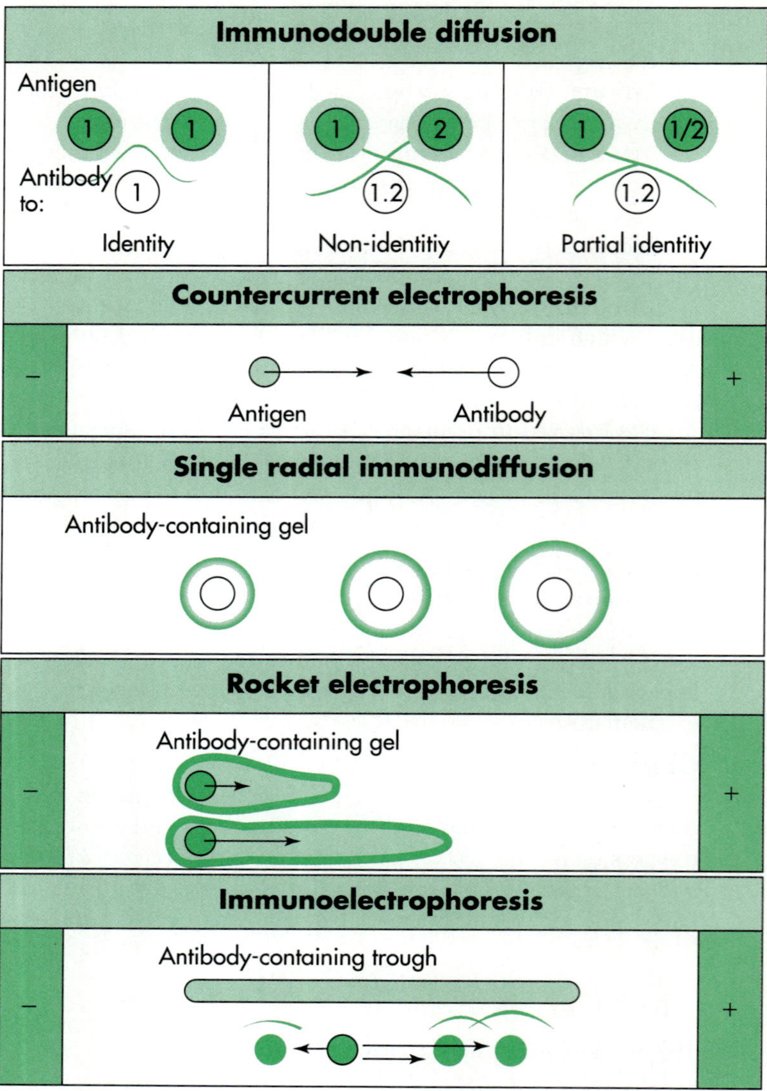

Fig. 1.10 Analysis of antigens and antibodies by immunoprecipitation. Precipitation of protein occurs at the equivalence point when multivalent antibody forms large complexes with antigen. **Immunodouble diffusion (Ouchterlony):** Antigen and antibody diffuse from wells, meet, and form a precipitin line. If *identical antigens* are used, then the concentration of antigen between the wells is doubled and precipitation does not occur in this region. If different antigens are used, two different precipitin lines are produced. **Countercurrent electrophoresis:** Similar to the Ouchterlony method, but facilitated by electrophoresis. **Single radial immunodiffusion:** Diffusion of antigen into an antibody containing gel. Precipitin rings are indicative of an immune reaction and area of the ring is proportional to the concentration of antigen. **Rocket electrophoresis:** Radial immunodiffusion with electrophoresis. **Immunoelectrophoresis:** Antigens are first separated by electrophoresis, antibody is added to a trough and then diffusion of antibody and separated antigen produce area of precipitation.

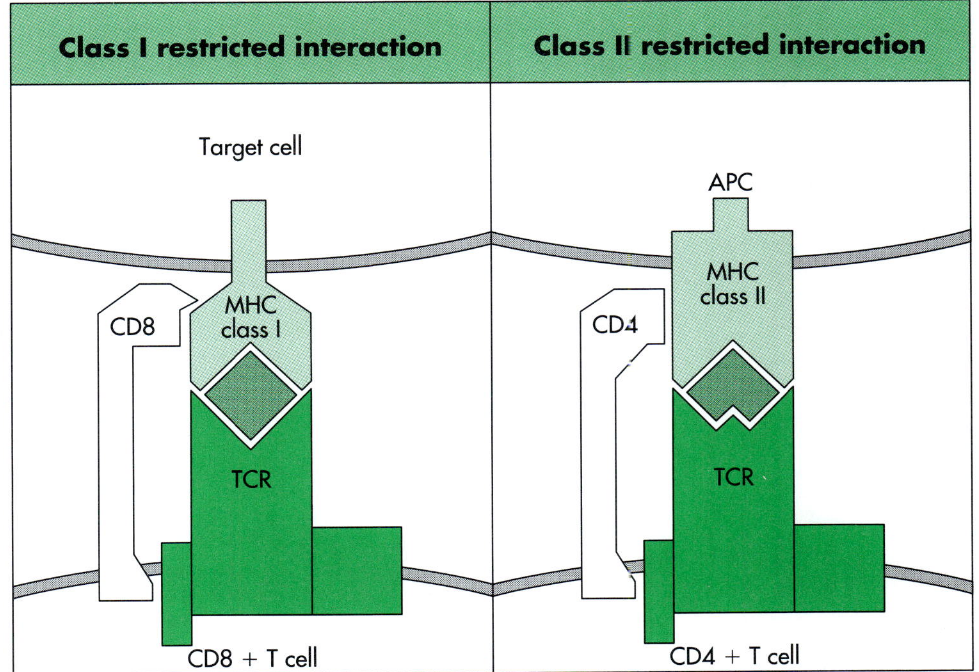

Fig. 1.11 Major histocompatibility complex (MHC) restriction and antigen presentation to T cells. *Left,* Antigenic peptides bound to MHC class I molecules are presented to the T cell antigen receptor (TCR) on $CD8^+$ T killer/suppressor cells. *Right,* Antigenic peptides bound to MHC class II molecules on the antigen presenting cell (atrial premature complex [APC]; B cell or macrophage) are presented to $CD4^+$ helper and DTH T cells.

T Cell Development Differentiation of T cells occurs mainly in the thymus (Fig. 1.12).

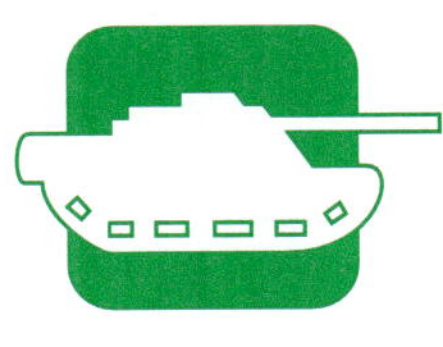

The markers found on both $CD4^+$ and $CD8^+$ T cells are present early in cell differentiation. These include CD2, CD3, the T cell receptor, CD5, and CD7.

- T cell surface molecules
  - ***Antigen recognition molecules***

T cell receptor. Antigen recognition occurs through the T cell receptor, which is similar to the antibody molecule in structure, with diversity for different antigens, and with genetic mechanisms for developing that diversity. Binding to the T cell receptor promotes but is not sufficient for proper activation of the T cell.

The T cell receptor is a multivalent complex and consists of different subunits (Fig. 1.13).

ANTIGEN RECOGNITION UNITS

- $\alpha\beta$ subunits: present in most T cell receptors, only one clonal molecule per cell, recognizing only one antigen
- $\gamma\delta$ subunits: rare occurrence, present mainly on T cells found in mucosal epithelium

ACTIVATION UNIT

- CD3 complex: consists of the γ, δ, ϵ, and ζ chains that associate with the $\alpha\beta$ subunits; binding to antigen promotes phosphorylation of CD3 and activation of T cell

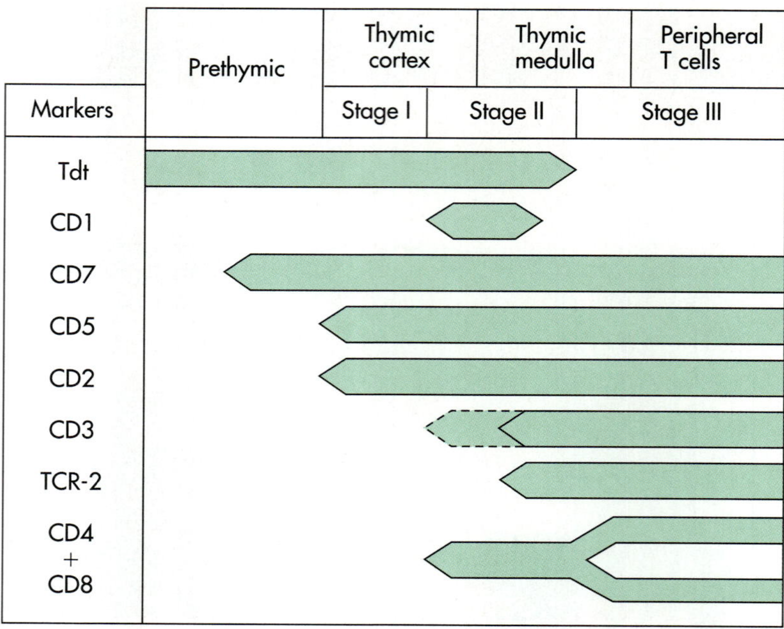

Fig. 1.12 Human T cell development. T cell markers are useful for identification of the differentiation stages of the T cell and for characterizing T cell leukemias and lymphomas. *TdT,* Terminal deoxynucleotide transferase.

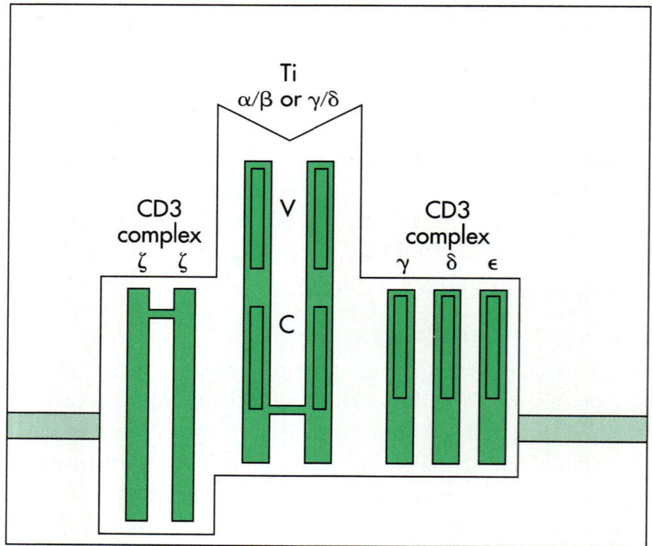

Fig. 1.13 The T cell receptor. The T cell receptor consists of different subunits. Antigen recognition occurs through the αβ or γδ subunits. The CD3 complex of γ, δ, ϵ, and ζ subunits promote T cell activation.

— *Accessory molecules*

- CD5: present on all T cells, promotes activation
- CD28: promotes activation
- CD45: CD45RA present on naive T cells; CD45RO present on memory T cells

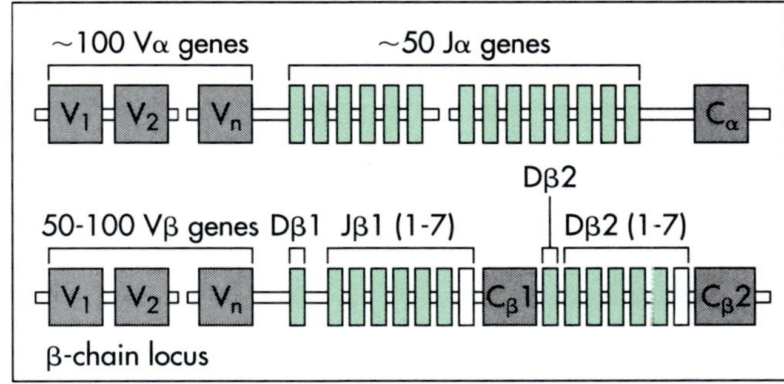

Fig. 1.14 T cell receptor α and β gene loci. Note the similarity to immunoglobulin genes.

— *Adhesion molecules*
  - CD2: found on all T cells; sheep erythrocyte receptor; promotes adhesion to LFA-3 molecule on target cell
  - LFA-1: binds to ICAM-1 and -2 on target cells
  - VLA-4: binds to fibronectin on target cells
  - VLA-5: binds to fibronectin

— *Functional determinants*
  - CD4: binds to MHC class II molecules on the surface of antigen presenting cells; defines T cell as a helper or a delayed type hypersensitivity T cell (DTH)
  - CD8: binds to MHC class I molecules on the surface of all nucleated cells; defines T cell as a killer or a suppressor T cell

— *Genetics of the T cell receptor (Fig. 1.14)*

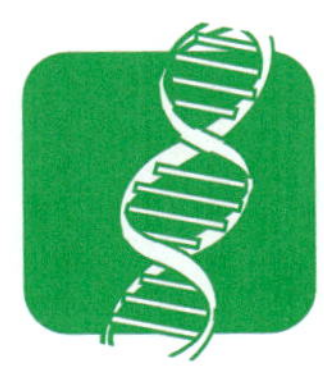

  - The diversity of the T cell receptor is generated in a manner similar to that for antibody.
  - The T cell receptor gene consists of multiple V, D, and J segments, similar to the antibody gene.
  - Different V, D, and J segments recombine to form different T cell receptor genes.
  - More than one D segment can be present in the T cell receptor gene unlike the antibody genes, and this increases the diversity.
  - Somatic mutation does not occur for the T cell receptor genes, in contrast to the antibody genes.

■ **Structure and Genetics of the MHC Antigens (Figs. 1.15, 1.16)** The MHC antigens are termed HLAs (human leukocyte antigens) in humans and H-2 antigens in mice. Differences in HLA molecules between individuals **(allogeneic differences)** prevent transplantation.

● MHC class I antigens

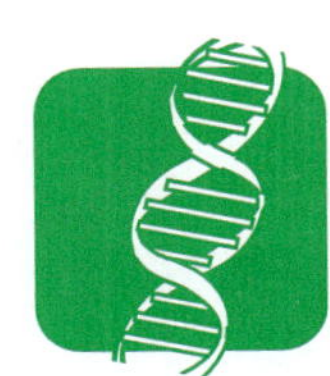

  - found on all nucleated cells and are the major determinants of "self"
  - are dimers consisting of a variable heavy chain and a light chain which is called β_2-microglobulin
  - encoded by three separate HLA genes—HLA-A, HLA-B, and HLA-C
  - pairs of different HLA-A, HLA-B, and HLA-C genes (inherited from each parent) expressed in each individual
  - present antigenic peptides to CD8-expressing T cells

● MHC class II antigens
  - found mainly on antigen presenting cells (e.g., macrophages, B cells) (also on activated T cells)

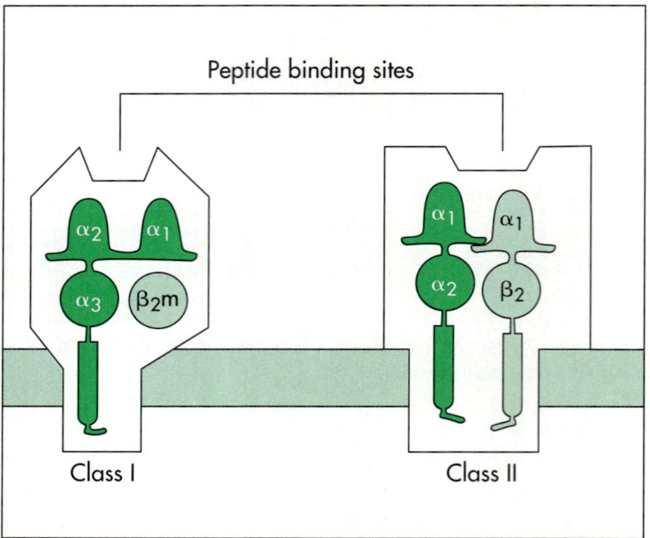

Fig. 1.15 Structure of MHC class I and II molecules. The MHC class I molecules consist of two subunits: the heavy chain and β_2-microgobulin. MHC class II molecules consist of two subunits: α and β.

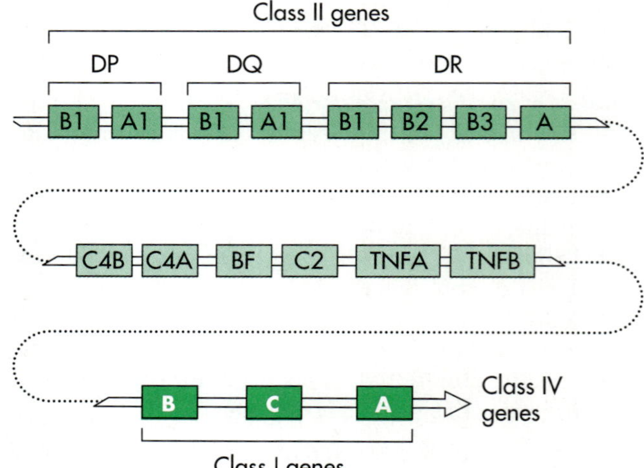

Fig. 1.16 Genetic map of the human major histocompatability complex (MHC). Genes for tumor necrosis factor (TNF) are also within the MHC gene complex.

- encoded by the HLA-DP, HLA-DQ, and HLA-DR loci (originally termed HLA-D)
- dimeric in structure, consisting of α and β subunits
- present antigenic peptides to CD4-expressing T cells
- bind the antigenic peptide in a cleft formed by the α and β subunits

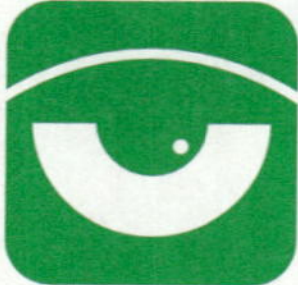

- **Mechanism of peptide presentation by MHC class I and MHC class II molecules (Fig. 1.17)**

All cells degrade their protein "trash" and then display it on the cell surface on MHC class I molecules as if to say, "This is who I am" to the neigh-

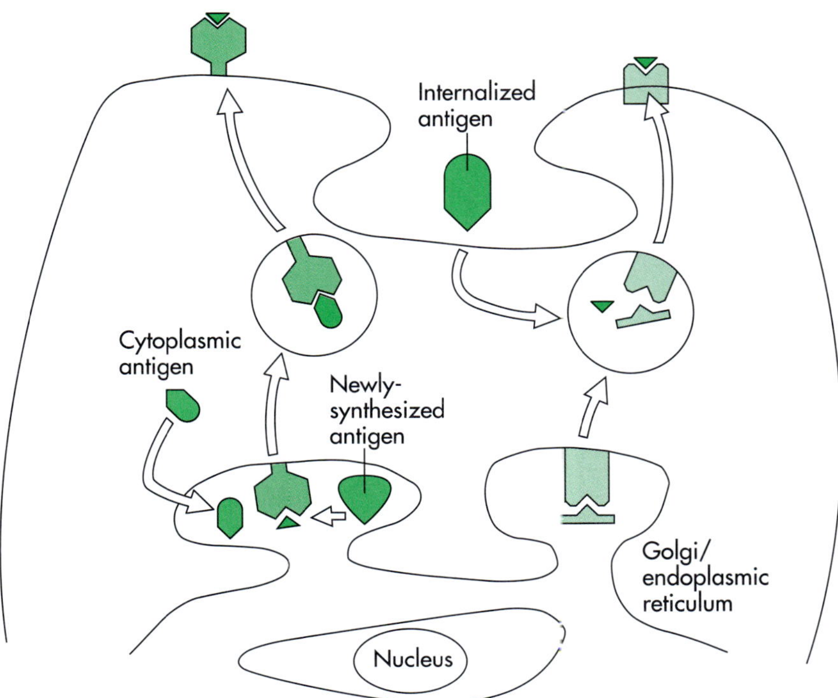

Fig. 1.17 Antigen presentation by MHC molecules. *Endogenous* antigen (produced by the cell and analogous to cell trash), is proteolyzed in the endoplasmic reticulum, binds to a groove in the MHC class I molecule, allowing the complex to move to the cell surface for presentation to $CD8^+$ T cells. *Exogenous* antigen (phagocytized) is degraded in lysosomes, transferred to endosomes containing the MHC class II molecules, binds to the MHC class II molecule, and is presented at the cell surface to $CD4^+$ T cells.

borhood-policing $CD8^+$ cytolytic T lymphocytes. If a viral intruder were to enter the cell, its trash would also be presented and would alert the policing $CD8^+$ T cells. Foreign cells (transplants) would also alert the $CD8^+$ cells.

Antigen presenting cells phagocytose protein trash, degrade it, and display it on MHC class II molecules and alert the helping "civil servants," the $CD4^+$ T cells, to activate the system and respond to the trash present in the neighborhood.

— ***Endogenous antigen presentation***

- MHC class I molecules present peptides from proteins synthesized within a cell.
- MHC I molecules present peptides resulting from degradation of cellular proteins, which are shuttled into the endoplasmic reticulum for disposal as trash. These peptides are often derived from nuclear proteins, glycoproteins, and other proteins.
- Peptide binding to the MHC class I molecule is required for the MHC class I molecule to move from the endoplasmic reticulum to the cell membrane.

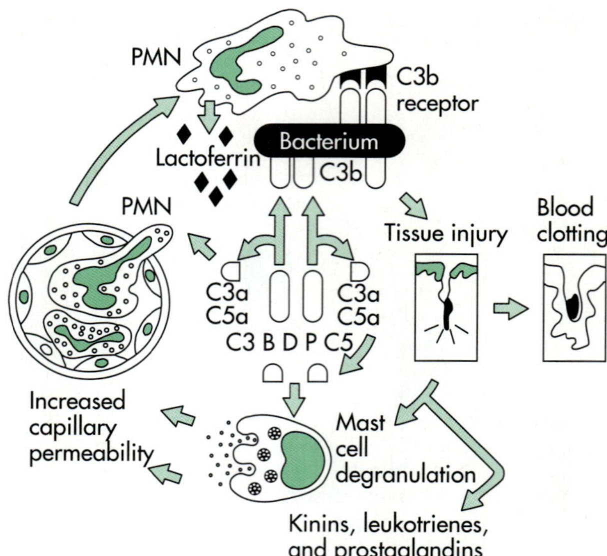

Fig. 1.18 Alternative pathway for activation of complement. Activation of the alternative complement pathway by bacterial cell surfaces produces C3b, which opsonizes the bacteria and C5a, which is chemotactic for polymorphonuclear neutrophil leukocytes (PMNs) and macrophages and triggers mast cell degranulation. Other agents increase capillary blood flow and permeability.

- The peptide-binding cleft of the MHC class I molecule holds a nine-amino acid peptide.

— ***Exogenous antigen presentation***

- MHC class II molecules present peptides from proteins that are phagocytosed and degraded in lysosomes by antigen presenting cells.
- The MHC class II peptide–binding cleft holds a 12-amino acid or longer peptide.

Section 1.5 Immune Responses

Overview Immune responses to antigen generally proceeds with the following cascade of events:

1. Activation of antigen nonspecific responses
   - alternative complement pathway (Fig. 1.18)
   - interferon (generally for viral infections [see Section 3.3, p.158])
   - phagocytes: neutrophils, macrophages
   - release of IL-1 and tumor necrosis factor (TNF) by macrophages
   - mobilization of antigen-presenting cells to lymph nodes
2. Initial activation of antigen-specific responses
   - T-helper ($CD4^+$) cell activation—release of IL-2, IL-4, interferon-γ, and other lymphokines
   - activation and proliferation of IgM-producing B cells; production of antigen-specific IgM
3. Maturation of the response

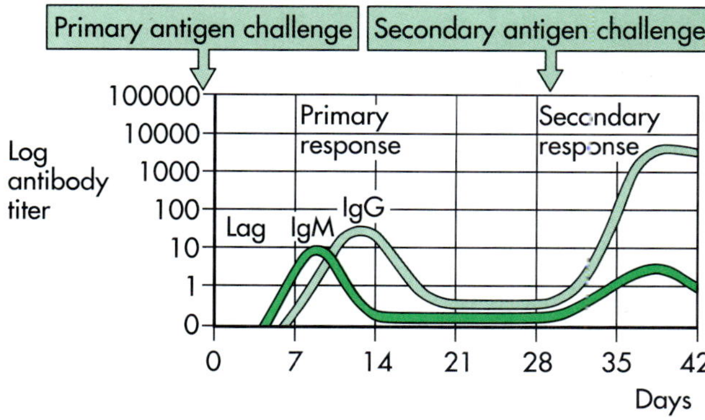

Fig. 1.19 Time course of immune responses. The primary response occurs after a lag period. The IgM response is the earliest response. The secondary immune response (anamnestic response) reaches a higher titer, lasts longer, and consists predominantly of IgG.

- B cell growth and differentiation induced by lymphokines from helper T cells results in IgG, IgA, or IgE class switch in antibody production
- expansion of $CD4^+$ T cells and helper function or DTH responses
- release of IL-2, interferon γ, and other lymphokines
- activation of macrophages by interferon gamma
- enhancement of phagocytic, antiviral and antitumor activities after macrophage activation
- cytolytic and suppressor T cell ($CD8^+$ T cell) growth and activation
- swelling of lymph nodes because of lymphoid proliferation
- increased mobilization of T cells and macrophage to location of antigen (e.g., site of infection)

4. Development of memory B and T cells
   - rechallenge with antigen produces a secondary response that is faster and stronger (anamnestic response) because of immunologic memory (Fig. 1.19)

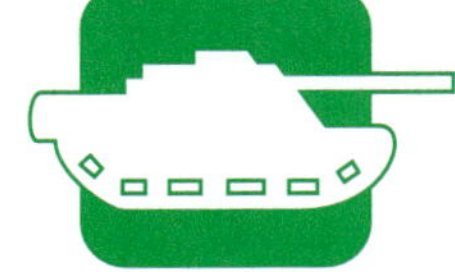

T Cell Activation Several interactions between the T cell and its target are *required* for activation (Figs. 1.20 and 1.21).

Proper activation of the T cell requires **two signals.**

Signal 1: Antigen-specific binding and cell surface crosslinking

- Binding of antigen-specific T cell receptor to the peptide in association with the MHC molecule
- CD4 (on T cell) binding to MHC class II molecules on antigen presenting cell OR CD8 (on T cell) binding to MHC class I molecules on target cell
- Binding of adhesion proteins to their receptors on antigen-presenting cells or target cells holds the two cells together; for example, CD2 and LFA-1 on T cells respectively bind LFA-3 and ICAM-1 on antigen presenting cells and target cells
- Binding of the T cell receptor to the MHC-peptide complex activates hydrolysis of phosphatidyl inositol and induces a calcium flux

Signal 2: Lymphokine binding

- Interleukin-1 (IL-1) (produced by macrophages) binding to its receptor on T cells
- Interleukin-2 (IL-2) (produced by helper T cells) binding to its receptor on T cells

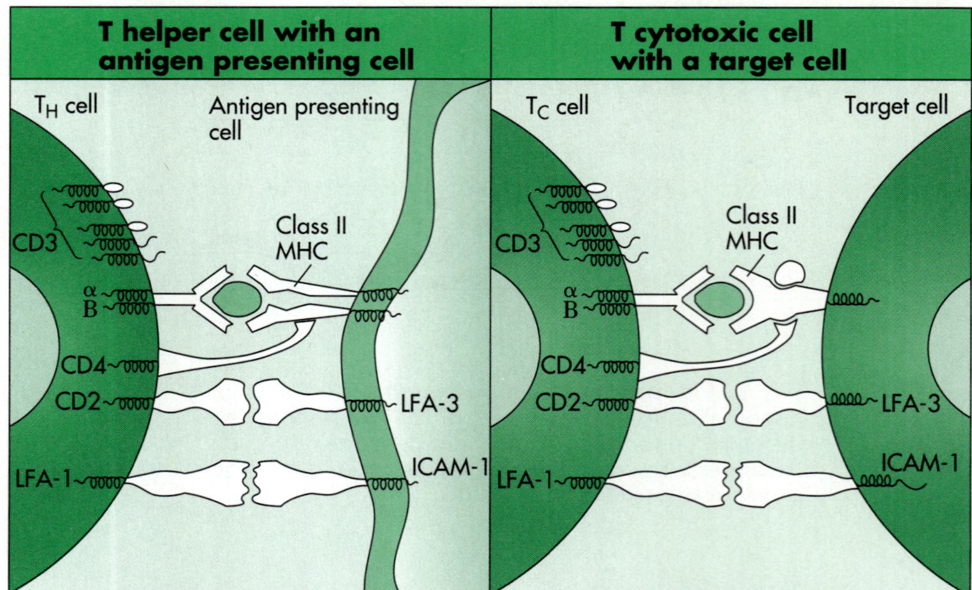

Fig. 1.20 Interaction of T cell with antigen presenting cell or target cell. The T cell receptor (TCR) interacts with antigenic peptides presented by major histocompatibility complex (MHC) molecules. The CD3 complex activates the T cell, and the other molecules tighten the cellular interaction.

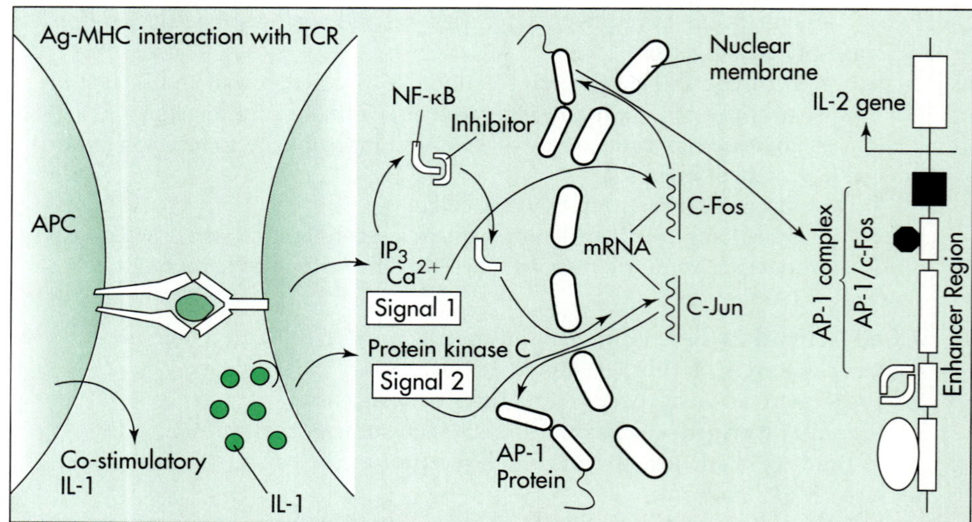

Fig. 1.21 T cell activation requires two signals. The costimulation of the T cell by antigen binding to the TCR and IL-1 binding to its receptor activates the T cell via calcium release, inositol phosphate production, and protein kinase C activation. Phosphorylation of messenger molecules activates transcription of IL-2.

- Binding of interleukins stimulates the protein kinase C pathway and calcium release. These actions promote IL-2 gene transcription and other events (see Fig. 2.21)

Proper activation of the T-helper cell promotes the production of interleukin-2, which activates other T cells and also increases its own expression of IL-2 receptors, thereby enhancing its ability to bind and maintain activation by IL-2.

- **Activation of T helper cells** The T cell receptor binds to antigenic peptide associated with a MHC class II molecule on an antigen presenting cell (macrophage, B cell).

  Note: The B cell is an antigen presenting cell. The B cell specifically binds antigen (via surface Ig), takes it up, and presents a peptide portion of the antigen to the T helper cell responsive to the same antigen.

- **Lymphokine release**
  - Lymphokines are hormonelike regulators of immune cell growth, differentiation, activation, and suppression.
  - Lymphokines produced by activated $CD4^+$ T helper cells activate and control the function and development of other T cells, B cells, macrophage, and inflammatory cells (Table 1.5 and Fig. 1.22).
  - Two classes of T helper cells are distinguished by the types of lymphokines that they secrete: *T_H1 (DTH:inflammatory T cells) and T_H2 (helper T cells)* (Fig. 1.23).
  - IL-2 activates T cell growth and differentiation as well as B cell growth.
  - Lymphokines stimulate B cell activation and development. IL-2, IL-4 and IL-5 stimulate B cell growth, whereas IL-4, IL-5, and IL-6 effect differentiation.

- **Activation of cytotoxic T cells (CTLs)**
  - The T cell receptor binds to antigenic peptide linked to MHC class I molecules on target cells (virus-infected cells, tumor cells, or transplanted tissue).
  - IL-2 produced by T helper cells binds to IL-2 receptors.
  - Signals from *both* IL-2 and antigen are required for differentiation of the pre-CTL to the cytotoxic T cell.

— ***Killing by cytotoxic T cells***

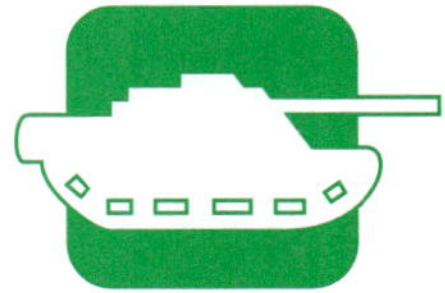

- The T cell receptor on an activated CTL binds to an antigenic peptide linked to MHC class I molecules.
- The CD8 molecule binds to the outside of the MHC class I molecule, thereby strengthening the interaction.
- Fas ligand on T cells binds to Fas receptor on the target cell and stimulates apoptosis (cell suicide characterized by breakdown of DNA) in the target cell.
- Adhesion proteins on T and target cells bind to each other creating a space.
- Granules in the T cell release toxic substances into the space between the two cells created by the adhesions. These toxic substances include the following:
  - **perforin** (pokes holes in the membrane similarly to complement component C9)
  - serine esterases

Tolerization

Partial activation (i.e., receptor interaction with MHC-peptide without interleukin stimulation) leads to the death of the T cell. This is a mechanism for eliminating self-reactive T cells in the developing thymus (thereby inducing **tolerance** to self antigens).

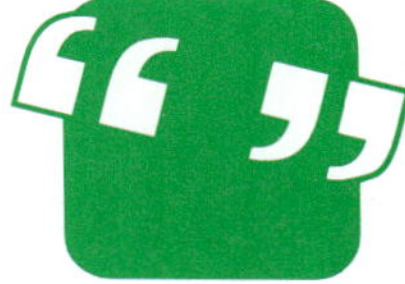

- **Antibody production**
  - B cells are responsible for antibody production.

Table 1.5 *Lymphokines*

Factor	Function	Source
Lymphokines	T cell, B cell, and hematopoietic growth factors; multiple effector functions	Lymphocytes
α-Interferon	Inhibits cell proliferation and tumor growth, enhances natural killer cell activity and phagocytosis	Leukocytes
Interleukin-1	Induces lymphokine production, enhances B cell proliferation and antibody production, increases phagocytosis, acts as chemoattractant, increases T cell activation and IL-2 receptor expression	Macrophages, dendritic cells, B lymphocytes, PMNs, endothelial and smooth muscle cells, and others
Tumor necrosis factor α	Many functions shared with IL-1	Activated macrophages, others
Colony-stimulating factors	Specific factors stimulate the growth of specific cell lines such as neutrophils, monocytes, eosinophils, erythrocytes, megakaryocytes and basophils	Monocytes, fibroblasts, T cells, B cells, endothelial and epithelial cells, kidney cells
γ-Interferon	Activates macrophages, increases MHC class II expression on cell surfaces, inhibits cell proliferation, enhances accessory cell function of macrophages, inhibits virus replication	Stimulated T lymphocytes, natural killer cells
Lymphotoxin (tumor necrosis factor β)	Target cell destruction	Lymphocytes
Interleukin-2	Induces proliferation of activated T cells, B cells, and natural killer cells, stimulates lymphokine and immunoglobulin production	Activated $CD4^+$ T cells
Interleukin-3	Acts on pluripotent stem cells to stimulate growth of neutrophils, monocytes, erythrocytes, basophils, eosinophils, and megakaryocytes	Activated T lymphocytes
Interleukin-4	Stimulates B cells, promotes immunoglobulin subtype switching, stimulates mast cells and hemopoiesis, activates macrophages	T helper cells, mast cells
Interleukin-5	Helps stimulate B cell proliferation and growth, stimulates eosinophils, promotes immunoglobulin subtype switching, enhances expression of IL-2 receptor	T helper cells
Interleukin-6	Increases immunoglobulin secretion, stimulates production of acute phase proteins, stimulates T cells and thymocytes, enhances differentiation of myelomonocytic cell lines	T and B cells, monocytes, fibroblasts, epithelial and endothelial cells
Interleukin-7	Stimulates pre-B cells and thymocytes, stimulates mature T cells, stimulates megakaryotes and myeloid precursors	Bone marrow stromal cells
Interleukin-8	Stimulates migration of monocytes and neutrophils, stimulates release of superoxide anions and lysosomal enzymes, chemotactic for basophils and T lymphocytes, stimulates release of histamine from basophils	Monocytes, fibroblasts, epithelial and endothelial cells, synovial cells
Interleukin-9	Enhances mast cell growth and $CD4^+$ T cell	T cells, spleen cells
Interleukin-10	Regulates the class of immune response, modulates accessory cell (APC) function	T cells
Interleukin-11	Acts as a megakaryocyte potentiator, stimulates IgG production	Fibroblasts, stromal cells

From Murray PR, Kobayashi GS, Pfaller MA, Rosenthal KS: *Medical microbiology*, ed 2, St Louis, 1994, Mosby.
PMNs, Polymorphonuclear neutrophilic leukocytes; *APC,* antigen presenting cells.

- Maturation of the immunoglobulin gene accompanies the differentiation of the B cell (Fig. 1.24).
- IgM is the first type of antibody produced in an antibody response.
- Unstimulated B cells express IgM and IgD on the cell surface.

— ***Antigen driven antibody production*** Cell surface IgM and IgD are antigen-specific receptors. Binding of antigen to these re-

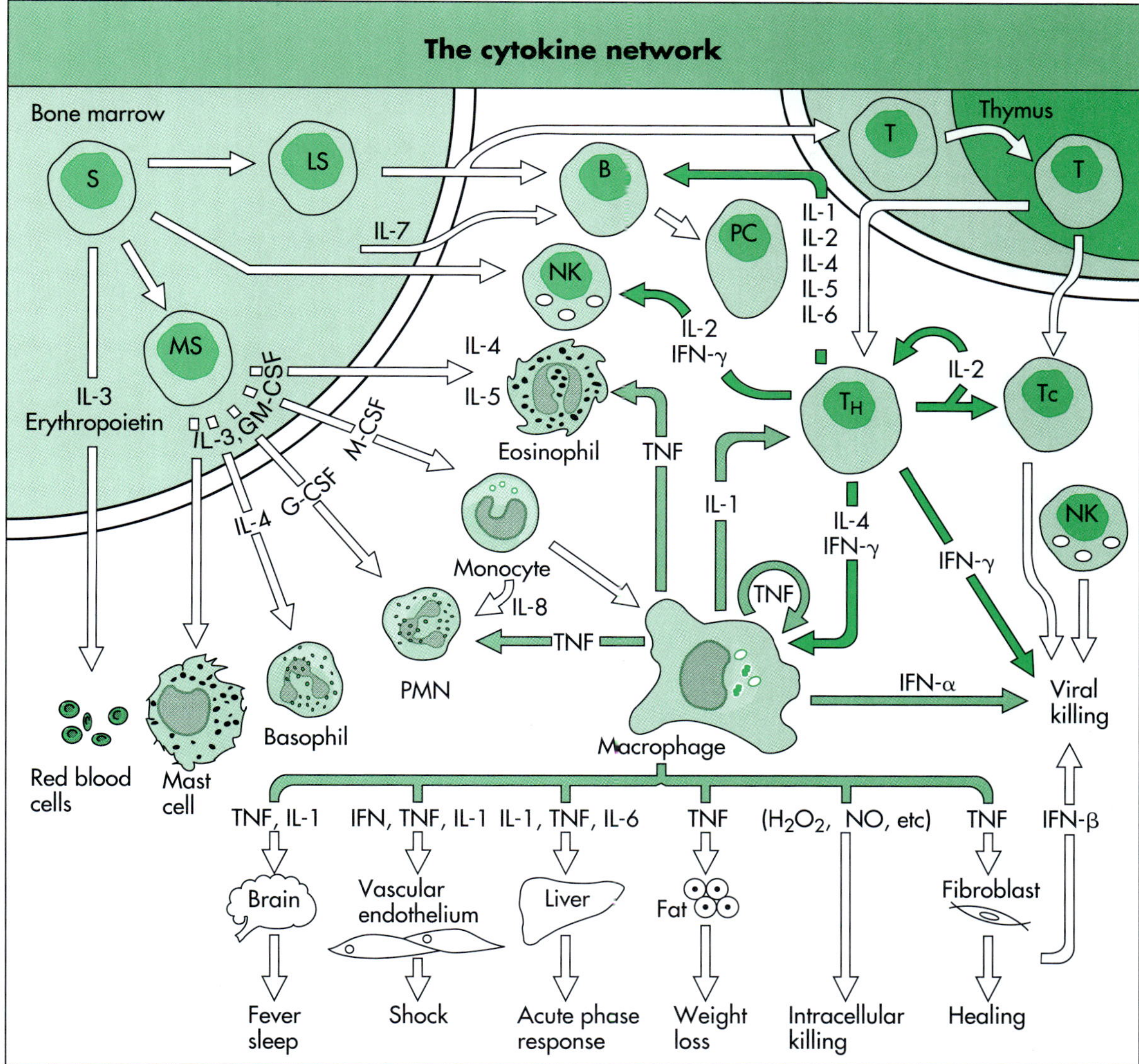

Fig. 1.22 Cytokines. Cytokines (lymphokines) are primarily produced by T cells (dark arrows) and macrophages (light arrows) and promote activation or differentiation of blood cells. Constituative and immune response-induced activities are indicated. *S,* Stem cell; *LS,* lymphoid stem cell; *MS,* myeloid stem cell; T_H, T helper cell; T_c, T cytotoxic cell; *NK,* natural killer cell; *PC,* plasma cell; *PMN,* polymorphonuclear leukocyte; *TNF,* tumor necrosis factor; *GM-CSF,* granulocyte-macrophage colony-stimulating factor.

ceptors stimulates growth *(blast transformation)* and antibody production.

— ***Repetitive antigens promote T cell independent stimulation of B cells*** by cross-linking the cell surface antibody. Examples are bacterial surfaces, flagellin, and dextran.

— ***Lymphokines*** produced by **T helper cells** are required for proliferation and the final differentiation from IgM to IgG, IgA, or IgE production.

• During blast transformation, B cells get larger and differentiate into effector cells. Terminal (end of the line) differentiation of B cells produces **plasma cells** (antibody factories) (Fig. 1.25).

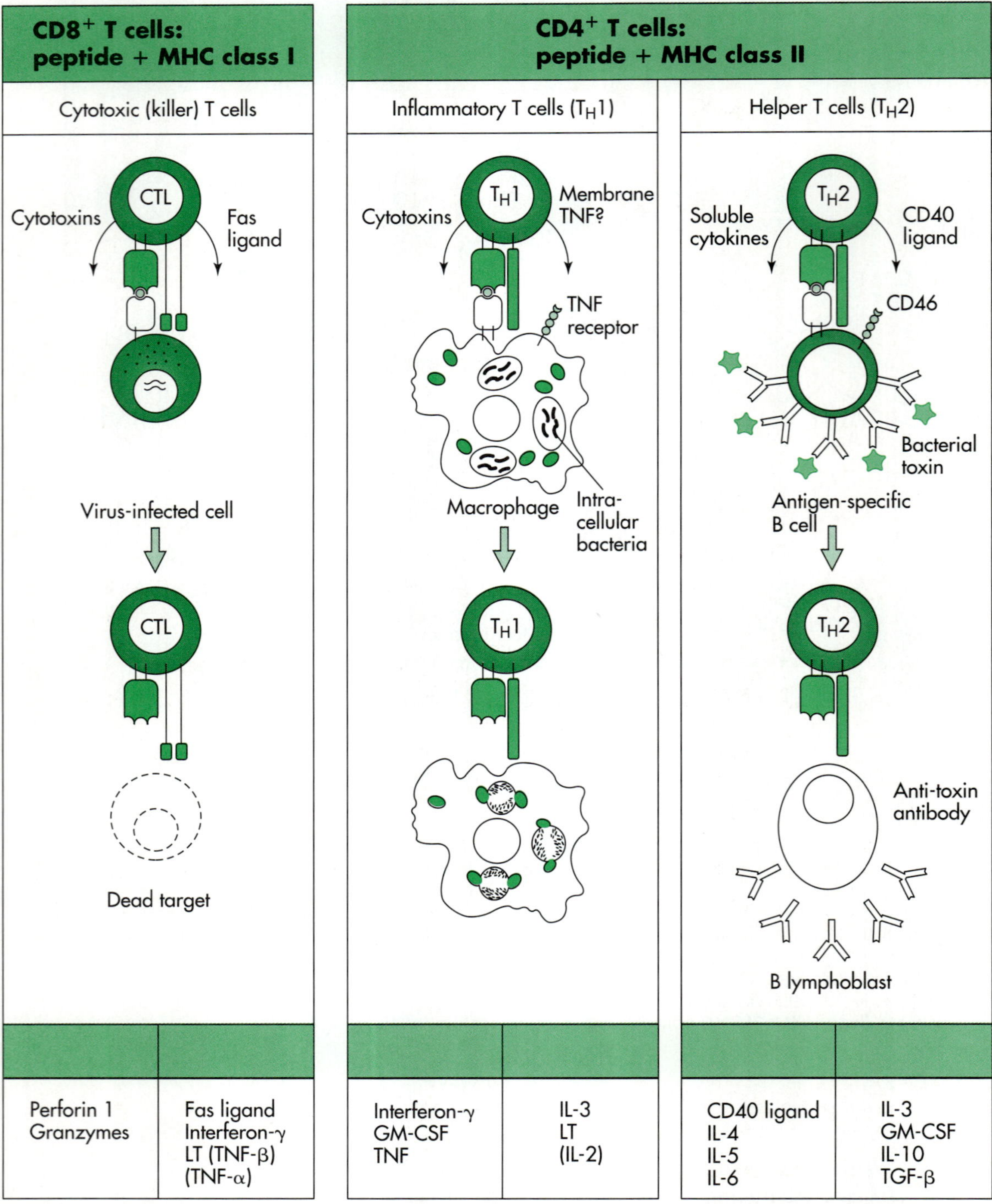

Perforin 1 Granzymes	Fas ligand Interferon-γ LT (TNF-β) (TNF-α)	Interferon-γ GM-CSF TNF	IL-3 LT (IL-2)	CD40 ligand IL-4 IL-5 IL-6	IL-3 GM-CSF IL-10 TGF-β

Fig. 1.23 T cell responses. CD4+ T cells are activated by antigen presenting cells. MHC class II antigen plus peptide on B cells plus second signal (CD40) activate classic helper cells (T_H2) which produce lymphokines (e.g., IL-2, IL-10) to promote B cell differentiation, and T cell activation. MHC class II antigen plus peptide on macrophages plus second signal (TNF or IL-1) activate classic DTH cells (T_H1) that produce interferon-γ and promote inflammation. CD8+ T cells are activated by MHC class I antigens plus peptide. They release perforin molecules to permeabilize the membrane and stimulate the FAS receptor to promote apoptosis in the target cell.

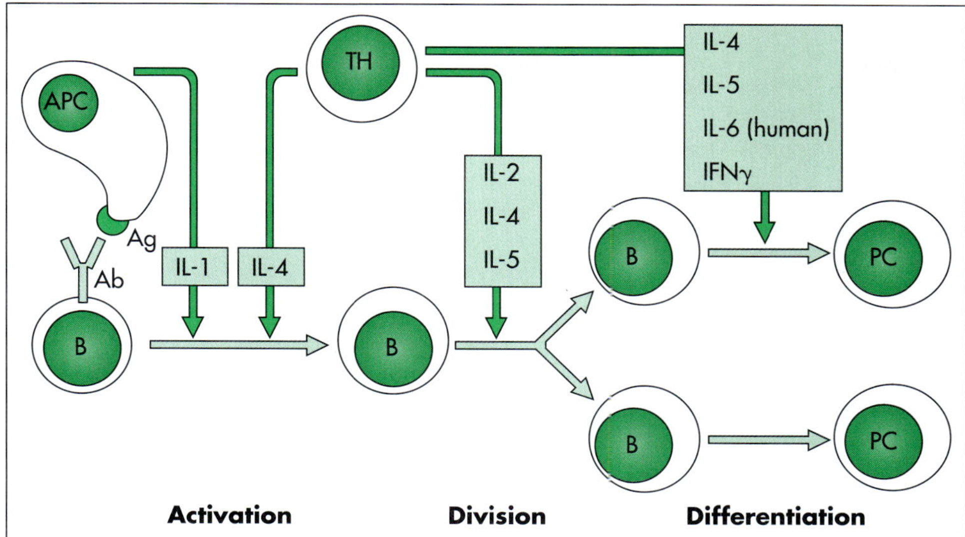

Fig. 1.24 B lymphocyte activation. Crosslinking of cell surface receptors activates lymphocytes. Multivalent molecules, such as lectins, that stimulate cell growth are termed mitogens. Lymphokines activate or stimulate growth on differentiation of B cells.

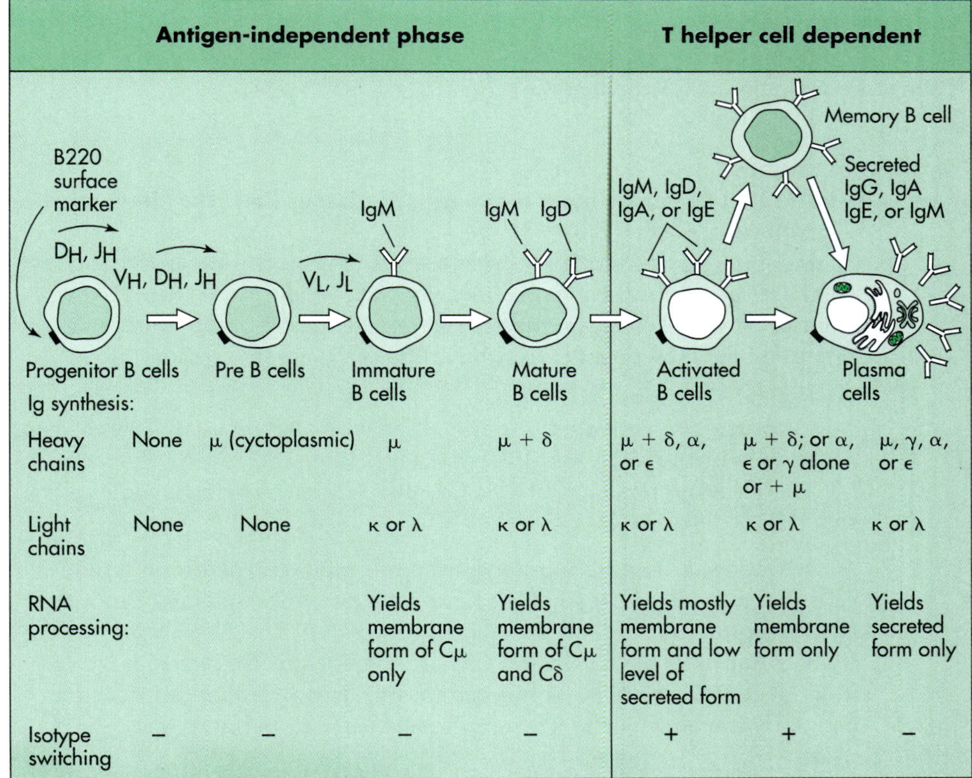

Fig. 1.25 Development of the B cell and antibody procuction. Different phases of B cell development are distinguished by the structure of the antibody genes and by the type of antibody produced by the cell. Genetic changes in the B cell require lymphokines, e.g., T cell help.

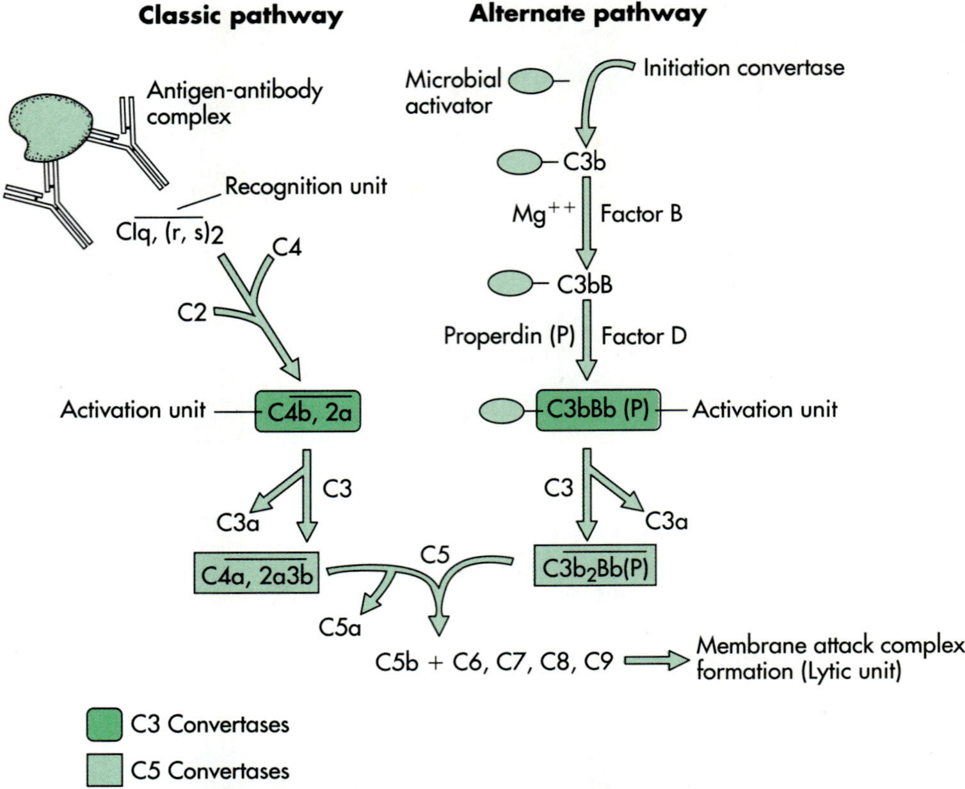

Fig. 1.26 The classical and alternative complement pathways. The center point of both pathways is activation of C3 and then C5.

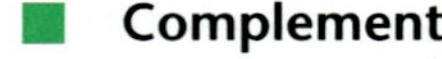

Complement

- There are two complement pathways: the **classical** and the **alternative (properdin)** (Fig. 1.26).
- The complement cascade produces a series of specific proteases that cleave and activate the subsequent element in the cascade.
- Both pathways produce proteases that cleave the C3 component, which is required for subsequent activation of the complement cascade.

Biological activities

Cytotoxic components C5 to C9, when deposited on a cell surface, form a hole in the cell membrane, killing the cell (Fig. 1.27).

The cleavage products of C3, C4, and C5 have the following activities (Fig. 1.28):

- **Opsonic:** binding to receptors on macrophages, neutrophils, and B cells. For example, **C3b** and **C4b** bind CR1 receptors, and **C3d** binds the CR2 receptor.
- **Anaphylotoxic: C3a** and **C5a** are chemotactic for neutrophils, promote degranulation of basophils and mast cells, and release of histamine and leukotriene, which mediates increased vascular permeability.

Genetic deficiencies in complement components increase the risk for bacterial infection.

- **Deficiency in components C1 to C4: pyogenic infections**
- **Deficiency in components C5 to C8: neisserial infections**

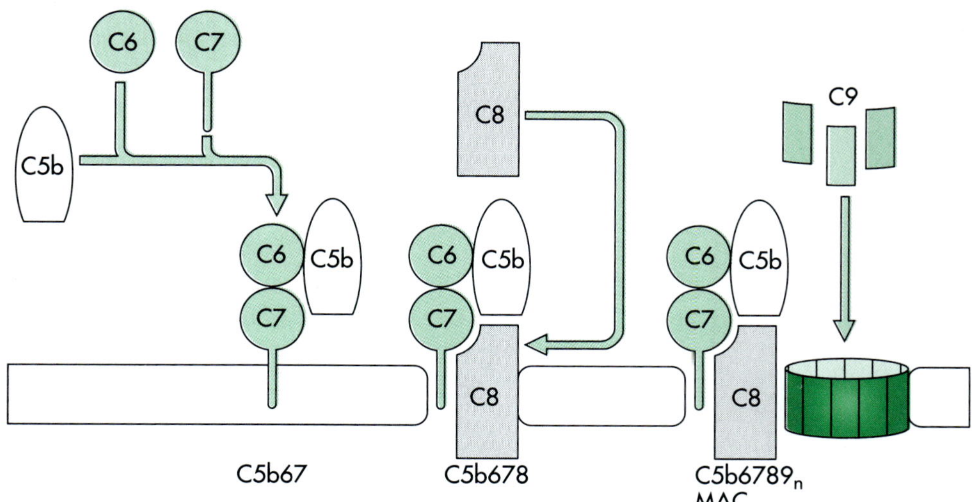

Fig. 1.27 Cell lysis by complement. Activation of C5 initiates the molecular construction of an oil-well–like membrane attack complex (MAC).

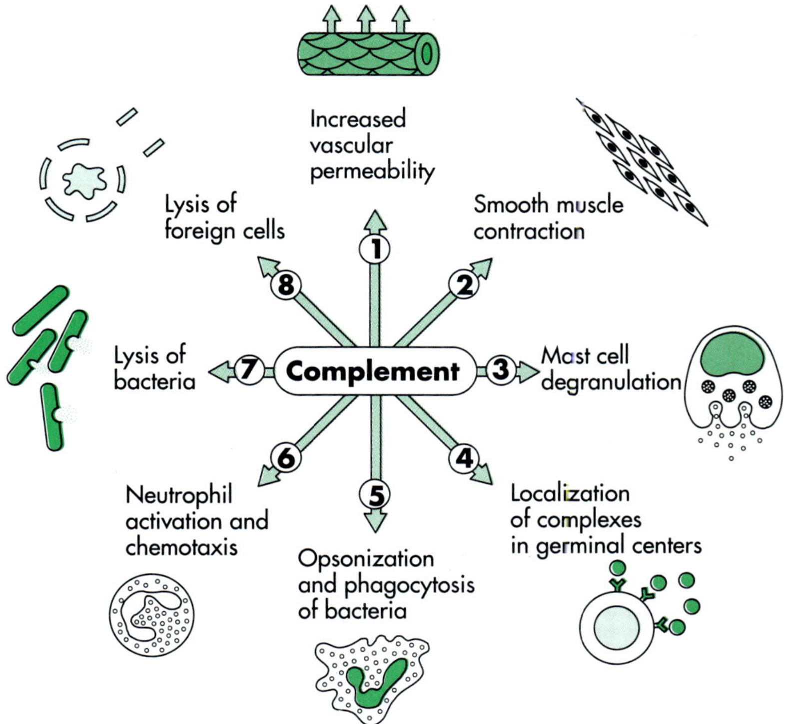

Fig. 1.28 Activities of complement components. The activities 1-8 are induced by the following components: 1-3 by C3a and C5a; 4 and 5 by C3; 6 by C5a; and 7 and 8 by C5 to C9 (MAC).

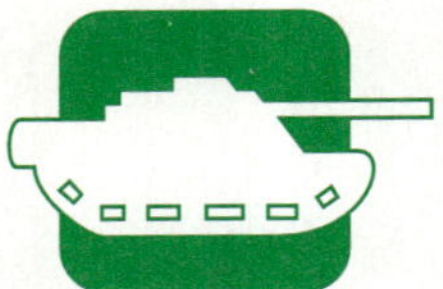

Other Cells Involved in the Immune Response

Macrophages (cells of the monocyte/macrophage lineage)

- Macrophages are phagocytic cells capable of presenting antigen, producing lymphokines (IL-1 and tumor necrosis factor) and interferon-α, and of being activated into killer cells by interferon-γ produced by T and NK cells.
- Macrophages are early initiators of the immune response because they present antigen and produce IL-1.
- Macrophages use Fc and complement C3b/C4b receptors to bind opsonized antigen (e.g., bacteria coated with antibody or with C3b produced by the alternative [antibody independent] or classical complement pathways).
- Activated macrophages (activated by interferon-γ), are larger, take up antigen more readily, have more receptors for opsonized antigen, secrete higher levels of antibacterial lytic substances, IL-1, tumor necrosis factor, prostaglandins, and complement components, and can kill phagocytized microbes.
- Macrophages kill by secretion (either into vacuoles or extracellularly) of superoxide and peroxide ions, tumor necrosis factor, and digestive enzymes.

Natural killer/killer cells (NK/K cells)

- NK/K cells are large granular lymphocytes, previously called null cells because they lack the major B and T cell markers.
- NK/K cells resemble T cells in that they produce interferon-γ kill cells by contact and by mechanisms similar to those of $CD8^+$ cells.
- NK/K cells are activated by interferons.
- NK cells kill virus-infected and tumor cells. The target antigen recognized is unknown but **killing is not MHC restricted.**
- K cells express antibody Fc receptors and kill target cells decorated by antibody.

Lymphokine-activated killer (LAK) cells

- LAK cells are generated by IL-2 treatment of lymphocytes in culture.
- These cells include NK and T cells.
- LAK cells have enhanced **antitumor activity.**

Hypersensitivity Responses

Once activated, the immune response is sometimes difficult to control and causes tissue damage. Hypersensitivity responses are responsible for many of the symptoms associated with microbial infections, especially viral infections.

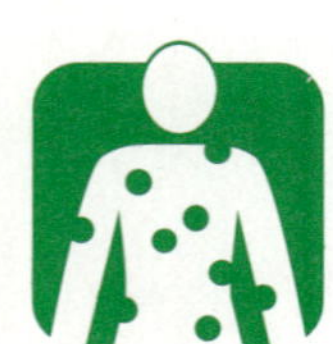

Type 1 hypersensitivity: IgE-mediated allergies (atopic or anaphylactic reactions) (Fig. 1.29)

- IgE helps defend against parasitic infections.
- IgE binds to Fc receptors on mast cells and thus becomes the cell surface receptor for allergens. Crosslinking of the IgE triggers degranulation of mast cells.
- IgE-mediated allergic reactions can occur within minutes.
- The immediate reaction is caused by **histamine,** SRS-A (leukotrienes), ECF-A, serotonin, and prostaglandins.
- The late-phase reaction is caused by SRS-A (slow reacting substance of anaphylaxis, consisting of leukotrienes C_4 and D_4).

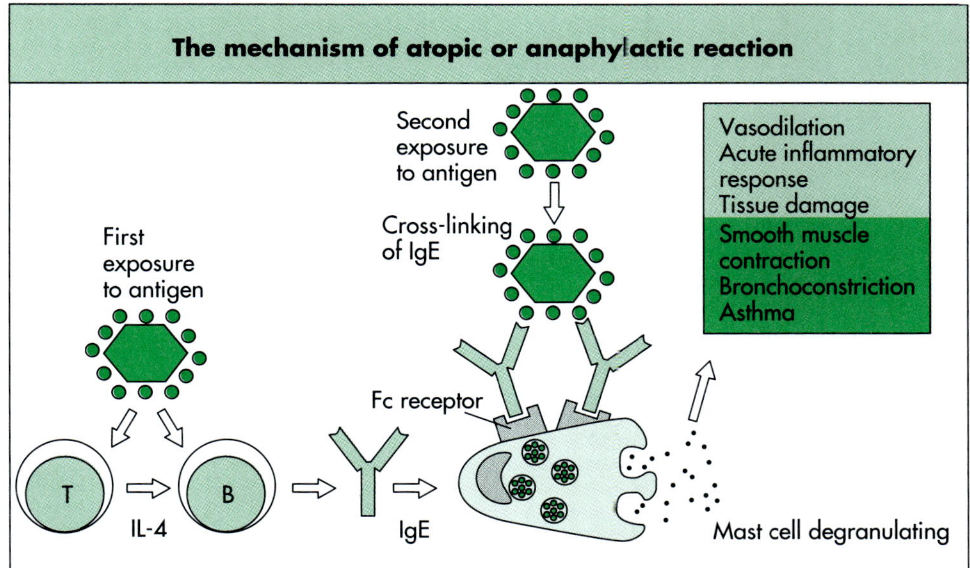

Fig. 1.29 Type 1 hypersensitivity: IgE-mediated atopic and anaphylactic reactions. IgE produced in response to initial challenge binds to Fc receptors on mast cells and basophils. Allergen binding to the cell-surface IgE promotes release of histamine and prostaglandins from granules to produce symptoms. Examples are hay fever, asthma, penicillin allergy, and reaction to bee stings.

- During desensitization therapy (allergy shots), IgG is produced. The IgG binds the allergen and prevents binding to IgE.

- **Type 2 hypersensitivity: antibody and complement (Fig. 1.30)** Antibody to cell-surface molecules promotes cell lysis either by activating complement or by binding Fc receptors on effector cells. Clinical examples of Type 2 hypersensitivity reactions are:

  - Myasthenia gravis—antibodies to acetylcholine receptors
  - Autoimmune hemolytic anemia—antibodies to red cell antigens
  - Goodpasture's syndrome—antibodies to lung and kidney basement membrane
  - Hemolytic disease of the newborn (blue babies)— maternal antibody to fetal erythrocytes; affects a second baby (Rh incompatability)

- **Type 3 hypersensitivity: immune complexes and complement (Fig. 1.31 and Table 1.6)** Excess soluble antigen in the bloodstream binds antibody, gets trapped in capillaries, especially in the kidney, and initiates the complement cascade.

  Activation of the complement cascade initiates inflammatory reactions. Responses occur within 3 to 6 hours.

  Initiators: insect bites; infection with hepatitis B virus elicits large amounts of HbsAg, which forms immune complexes.

  Examples of immune complex disease are the following:

  - **Arthus reaction**—skin reaction to intradermally injected antigen, consisting of redness and swelling
  - Serum sickness
  - Glomerulonephritis
  - Farmer's lung—reaction to inhalation of actinomycetes

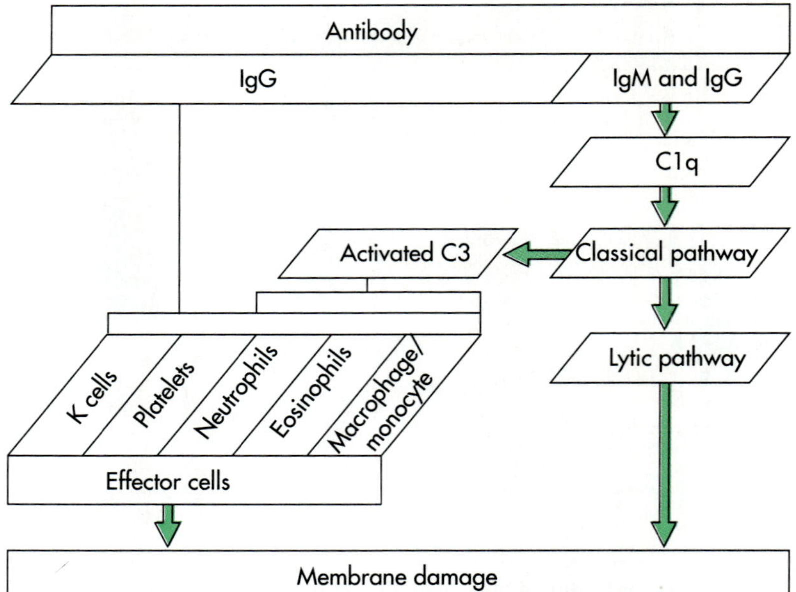

Fig. 1.30 Type II hypersensitivity: mediated by antibody and complement. Complement activation promotes direct cell damage through the complement cascade and by activating effector cells. Examples are Goodpasture's syndrome, response to Rh factor in newborns, and autoimmune endocrinopathies.

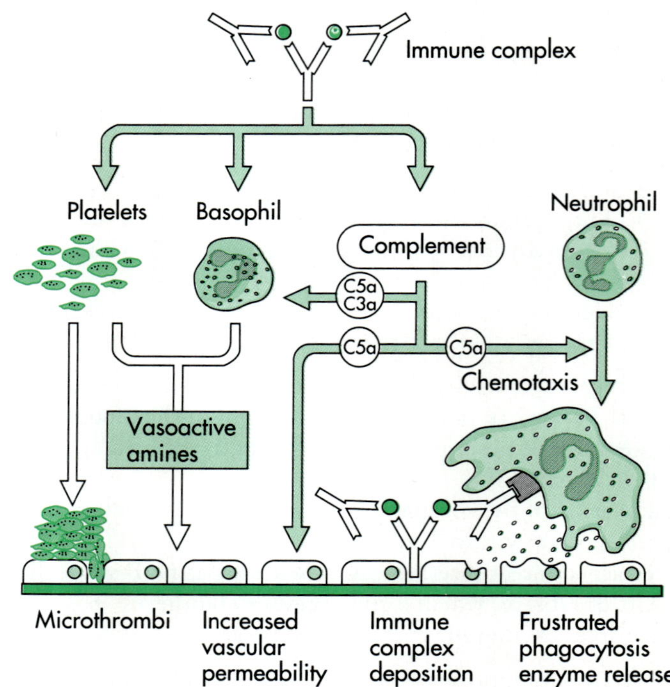

Fig. 1.31 Type III hypersensitivity: immune complex deposition. Immune complexes can be trapped in the kidney and elsewhere in the body, can activate complement, and cause other damaging responses. Examples are serum sickness, nephritis associated with chronic hepatitis B virus infection, and Arthus reaction.

Table 1.6 ***Immune Complex Diseases: Sites of Deposition***

	Circulating Complexes	Vasculitis	Nephritis	Arthritis	Skin Deposits
Rheumatoid arthritis	+	+		+	
Systemic lupus erythematosus (SLE)	+	+	+	+	+
Polyarteritis	+	+	+		
Polymyositis dermatomyositis		+			+
Cutaneous vasculitis	+	+			+
Leprosy	+		+	+	+
Malaria	+		+		
Trypanosomiasis	+	+	+		
Bacterial endocarditis	+	+	+		
Hepatitis	+	+	+		

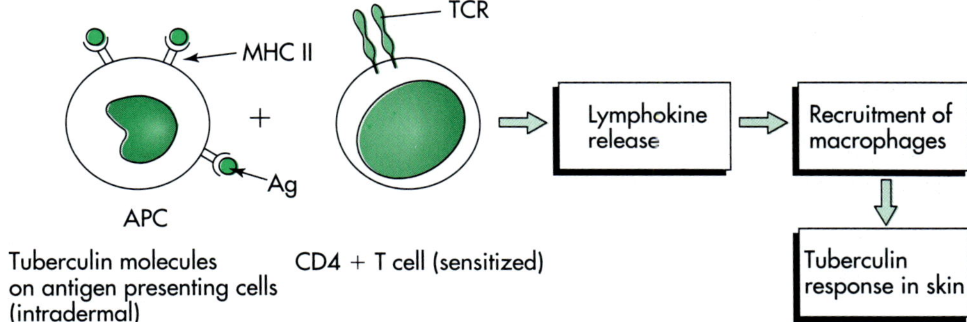

Fig. 1.32 Type IV hypersensitivity: delayed type hypersensitivity mediated by $CD4^+$ T cells (T_H1). Activation of the $CD4^+$ T cells releases lymphokines, including interferon γ, which promote inflammation. Examples are the tuberculin response (PPD test) and contact sensitivity to poison ivy and metals, such as nickel.

- **Type 4 hypersensitivity: $CD4^+$ T cell-induced delayed-type hypersensitivity (DTH) (Figs. 1.32 and 1.33)** The DTH response is **essential** for controlling **fungal infections** and **intracellular bacteria** (e.g., mycobacteria). It results from lymphokines and other effector molecules released by $CD4^+$ T cells. The four types of DTH reactions are described in Table 1.7.

Section 1.6 Summary of Specific Immune Responses

Transplant Rejection

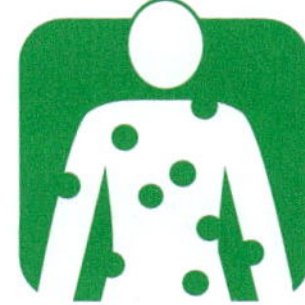

- **Allograft rejection:** This is primarily a T cell response mediated by T cell recognition of foreign MHC class I antigens.
- **Host-versus-graft response:** This is an immune response that results in rejection of foreign tissue.
- **Graft-versus-host response:** Lymphocytes present in transfused blood or in a transplanted tissue react against the new host.

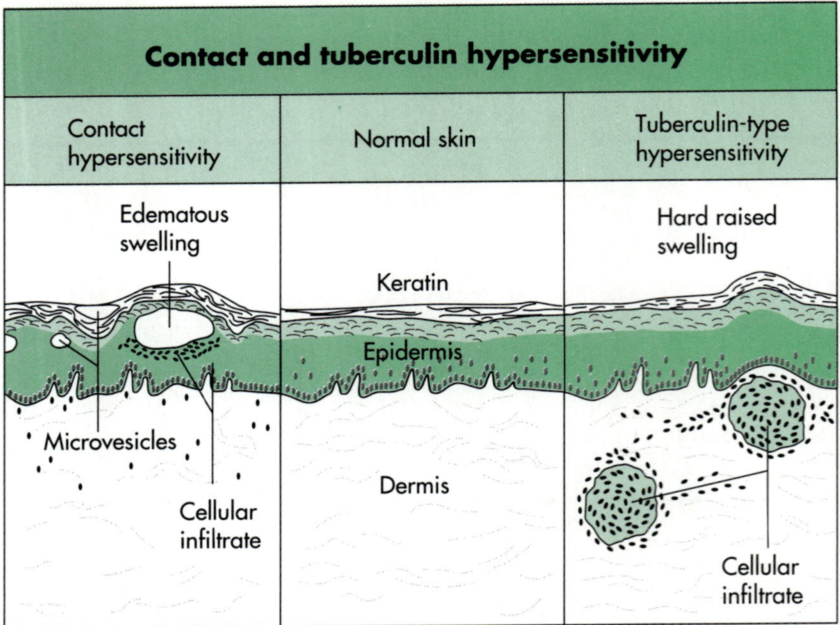

Fig. 1.33 Contact and tuberculin hypersensitivity responses. These Type IV responses are cell-mediated but differ in the site of cell infiltration and in the symptoms. Contact hypersensitivity occurs in the epidermis and leads to formation of blisters; tuberculin-type hypersensitivity occurs in the dermis and is characterized by swelling.

Table 1.7 ***Summary of the Important Characteristics of Four Types of Delayed Hypersensitivity Reaction***

Type	Reaction Time	Clinical Appearance	Histological Appearance	Antigen
Jones-Mote	24 hours	Skin swelling	Basophils, lymphocytes, mononuclear	Intradermal antigen, e.g., ovalbumin
Contact	48 hours	Eczema	Mononuclear cells, edema, raised epidermis	Epidermal: e.g., nickel rubber, poison ivy, etc.
Tuberculin	48 hours	Local induration and swelling ± fever	Mononuclear cells, lymphocytes and monocytes, reduced macrophages	Dermal: tuberculin, mycobacterial and leishmanial antigens
Granulomatous	4 weeks	Skin induration	Epithelioid cell granuloma, giant cells, macrophages, fibrosis, ± necrosis	Persistent Ag or Ag/Ab complexes in macrophages or "nonimmunological" (e.g., talcum powder)

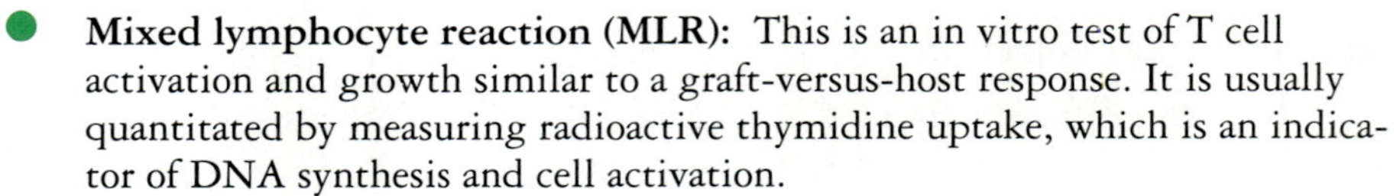

- **Mixed lymphocyte reaction (MLR):** This is an in vitro test of T cell activation and growth similar to a graft-versus-host response. It is usually quantitated by measuring radioactive thymidine uptake, which is an indicator of DNA synthesis and cell activation.

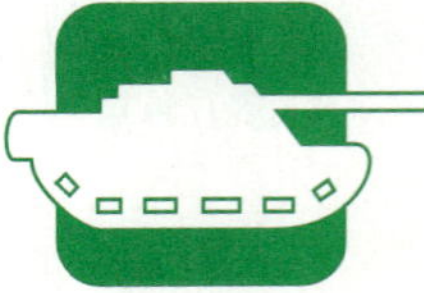

Antibacterial Responses

- This response is initiated by macrophages and other phagocytic cells.
- Complement bacterial surfaces may activate the alternative pathway of complement to cleave C3 and produce C5 to C9.

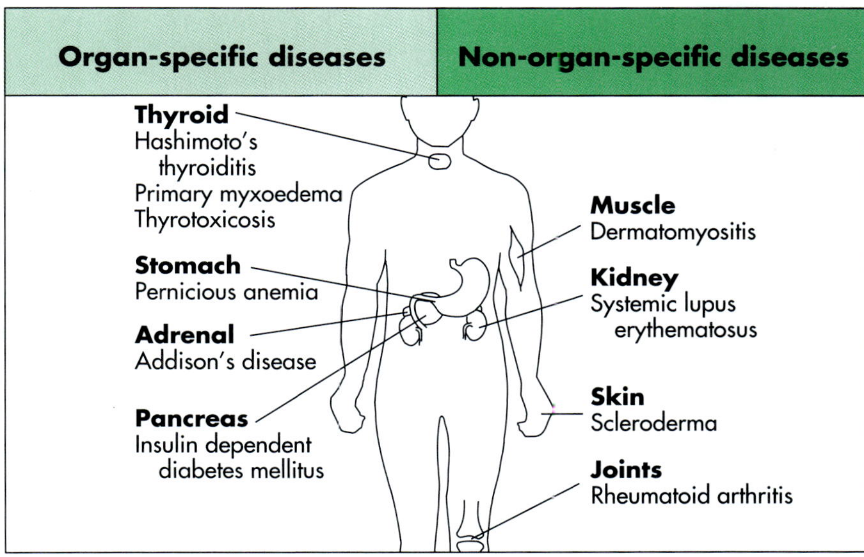

Fig. 1.34 Types of autoimmunity.

- C3a and C5a are chemoattractants for neutrophils.
- C3b is an opsonin and causes enhanced clearance.
- Antibody production is the primary specific immune response for bacteria.
- Antibody acts mainly as an opsonin to promote clearance by phagocytic cells.
- Neutrophils and other PMNs are important antibacterial agents.
- DTH responses for clearance of intracellular bacteria.

Antiviral Responses

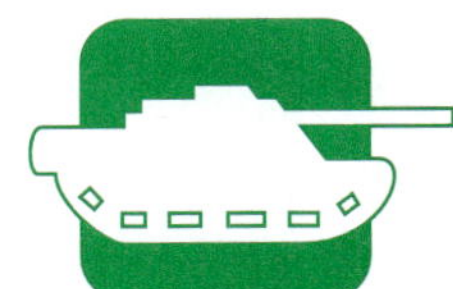

- Production of interferons α and β is the earliest response in the infected cell.
- Interferons trigger local responses (promote an antiviral state in surrounding cells), as well as systemic activation of immune responses.
- NK cells activated by interferon are active against virus-infected cells.
- Antibody is important for neutralizing (inactivating, preventing binding to target cells) and opsonizing extracellular virus and especially for limiting viremia.
- T cell and cytolytic responses are essential for nonlytic viruses and enveloped viruses (e.g., the herpes, paramyxo, and influenza viruses).
- Immunopathology is often the predominant symptom of viral infection.

Antitumor Responses

- A primarily T cell-mediated killing of tumor cells results from altered MHC expression or from tumor antigens
- LAK (lymphokine [IL-2] activated killer) cells and NK cells may respond to reductions in MHC class I molecules on tumor cell surfaces.
- Activated macrophages also have antitumor activity.

Autoimmune Responses (Fig. 1.34)

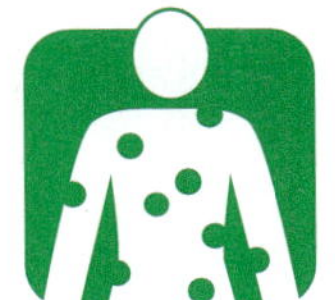

Disregulation of immune response or lack of self-tolerance can be caused by the following:

- cross reactivity with microbial antigens (e.g., Group A streptococci and rheumatic fever)

- polyclonal activation induced by tumors or infection (e.g., malaria, Epstein-Barr virus infection)
- genetic predisposition resulting from lack of tolerization

Agents of autoimmune pathology:

- Autoantibodies
- Activated T cells: CTL, DTH T cells (cytokine/lymphokine release)
- Hypersensitivity responses due to antibody or DTH

MHC association: Individuals with certain MHC antigens are at higher risk for autoimmune responses. For example, HLA B27 antigen is associated with juvenile rheumatoid arthritis and ankylosing spondylitis. This may be a result of **genetic linkage** (close proximity of the two genes on the chromosome) of the disease-related gene to HLA-B27. Alternatively, HLA-B27 may bind and present antigenic peptides, which elicit autoimmune reactions.

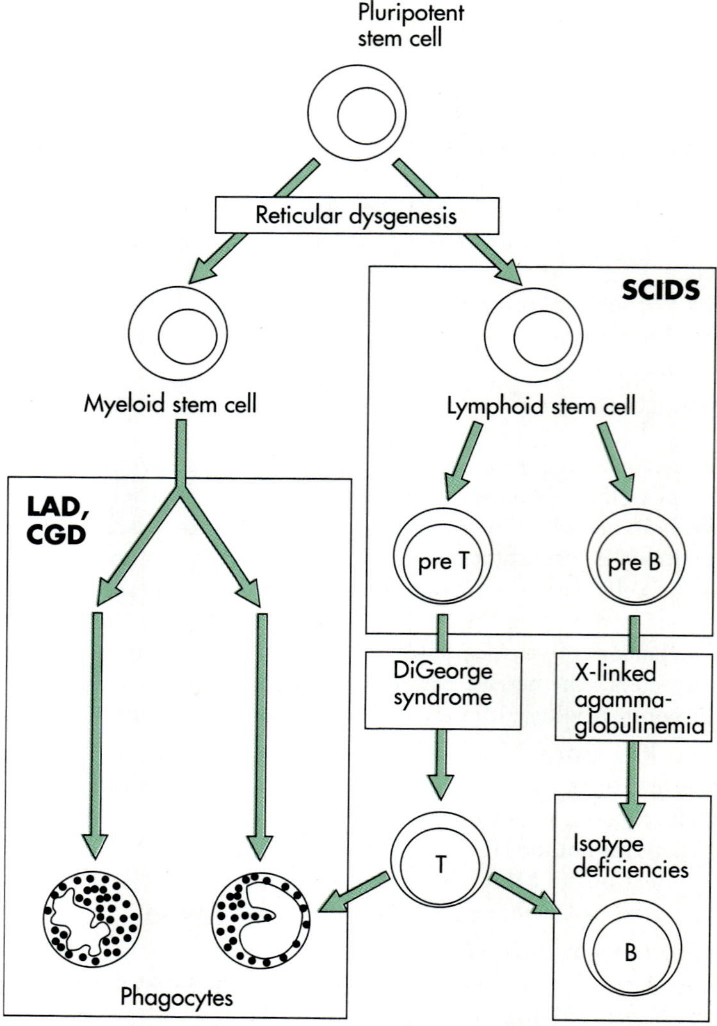

Fig. 1.35 Immunodeficiency resulting from defects in lymphocytes and phagocytes. *SCID,* Severe combined immunodeficiency; *LAD,* leukocyte adhesion disease; *CGD,* Chédiak-Higashi syndrome.

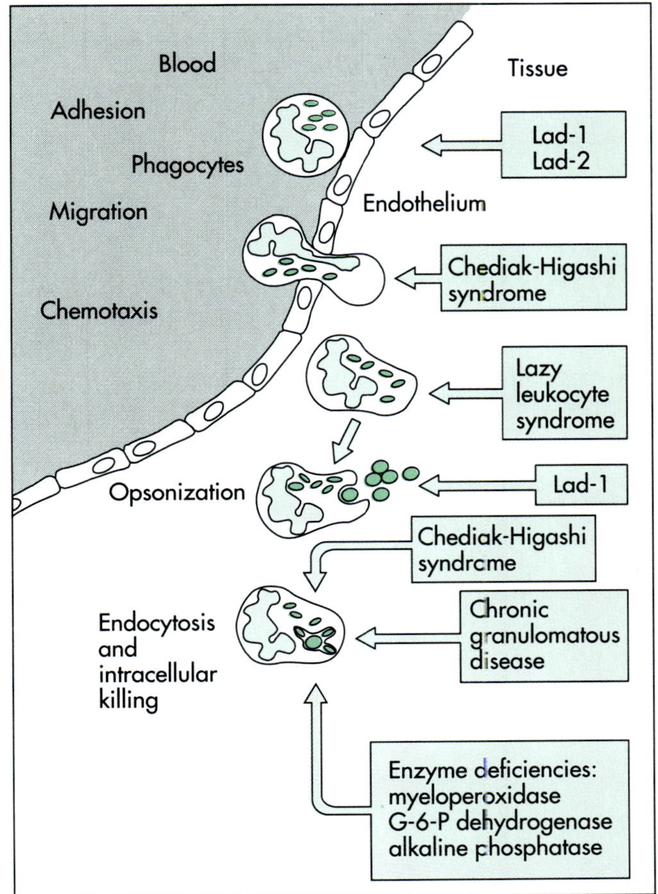

Fig. 1.36 Consequences of phagocyte dysfunction.

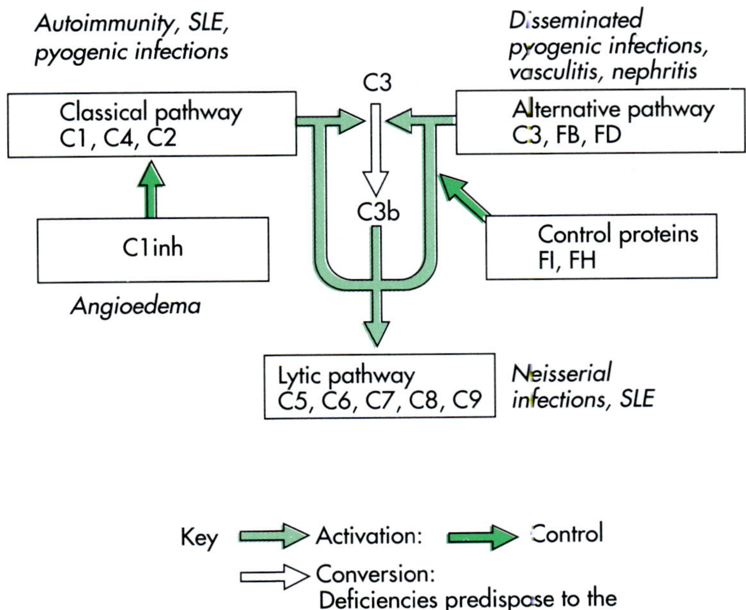

Fig. 1.37 Consequences of deficiencies in the complement pathways.

Box 1.2

MAJOR OPPORTUNISTIC INFECTIONS
Pneumocystis pneumonia
Chronic cryptosporidiosis
Toxoplasma cerebral abscess
Extraintestinal strongyloidiasis
Isosporiasis
Esophageal/bronchial candidiasis
Cryptococcosis
Histoplasmosis
Atypical mycobacterial infection
Cytomegalovirus infection
Herpes simplex ulceration or disseminated herpes
Progressive multifocal leukoencephalopathy

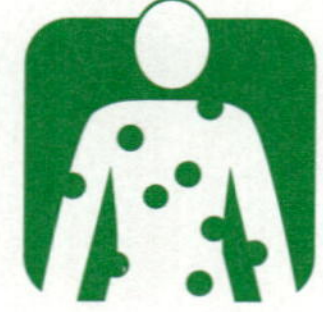

- **Immunodeficiency (Figs. 1.35 to 1.37 and Box 1.2; see also Table 6.2 in Chapter 6)** Lack of specific immune components increases susceptibility to specific infections and tumors.

Multiple Choice Review Questions

1-5. Match the correct item from the list below to each of the following phrases. Each lettered item may be used once, more than once, or not at all.

a. macrophage
b. NK cell
c. neutrophil
d. mast cell
e. $CD4^+$ T lymphocyte
f. $CD8^+$ T lymphocyte
g. B lymphocyte
h. plasma cell

1. interacts with the exogenous pathway of antigen presentation, binds to a peptide presented by MHC class II antigens
2. kills target cell in an MHC unrestricted manner
3. phagocytic non-antigen presenting cell, indicative of bacterial infection
4. releases histamine upon antigen binding to cell surface IgE
5. produces antibody but cannot differentiate or grow

6-10. Match the correct item from the list below to each of the following phrases. Each lettered item may be used once, more than once, or not at all.

a. Agammaglobulinemia
b. Chronic granulomatous disease of childhood
c. Multiple myeloma
d. Agranulocytosis
e. C3 deficiency
f. Systemic lupus erythematosus
g. AIDS

6. increased susceptibility to *Staphylococcus aureus* infections
7. increased recurrences of cytomegalovirus and susceptibility to yeast infections
8. increased levels of anti-DNA antibodies
9. increased susceptibility to *Streptococcus pneumoniae* and *Neisseria meningitidis*
10. increased susceptibility to respiratory infections and chronic diarrhea

11. All of the following statements are correct *except*

a. IgM and IgD can be expressed simultaneously on the cell surface of subpopulations of B cells.
b. The gene for the IgE heavy chain consists of V, D, J, and ϵ gene segments.
c. Addition of the J chain to IgA promotes its secretion.
d. The fragment Fab′ of IgG binds antigen and complement.
e. The RNA transcribed for IgD contains gene sequences for IgM.

12. All of the following statements regarding a bacterial infection are correct *except*

a. Neutrophils are the first cells to arrive at the infected site.
b. Neutrophils die after ingestion and killing of the invading microorganisms.
c. The phagolysosome is formed by the fusion of the phagosome and primary lysosome.
d. Neutrophils are attracted to the site of infection by the C8 and C9 components of complement.
e. Hydrogen peroxide and myeloperoxidase are found in the phagolysosomes.

13. All of the following statements about complement are true *except*

a. Complement is activated by bacterial cell surfaces.
b. Complement is activated by antibody-antigen complexes.
c. C1 binding to antibody promotes cleavage of C2 and C3 and then cleavage of C4 and C5.
d. C5a induces acute inflammation.
e. C9 cleavage causes membrane disruption.

14. A kidney transplant patient is suffering from graft rejection. All of the following statements could be true *except*

a. T lymphocytes in the graft are being activated in a graft-versus-host reaction.
b. T lymphocytes in the host are being activated in a host-versus-graft reaction.
c. Only $CD8^+$ T cells are involved in graft rejection reactions.
d. $CD8^+$ T cells are being activated in an allotypic reaction.
e. Only two of the three of the ideal match of HLA-A, HLA-B, and HLA-DR loci were possible.

15. All of the following statements regarding activation of $CD4^+$ T cells are true *except*

a. Binding of the $CD4^+$ T cells to peptide and MHC class II molecules on an antigen presenting cell is sufficient for activation.
b. Calcium ion mobilization is required for activation.
c. Activation of protein kinases is required.
d. The activation is mediated through the CD3 complex of the T cell receptor.
e. Binding to target cells is facilitated by adhesion proteins.

16-20. Match the correct item from the list below to each of the following phrases. Each lettered item may be used once, more than once, or not at all.

a. IgA
b. IgG
c. IgM
d. IgE
e. IgD

16. secreted in pentameric form
17. found almost exclusively on the cell surface
18. deficiency of this antibody results in increased susceptibility to respiratory infections
19. can cross the placenta
20. promotes Type 1 hypersensitivity reactions

Chapter 2

Bacteriology

Section 2.1 Bacterial Morphology

Knowledge of bacterial morphology is essential for the understanding of bacterial pathogenesis.

Gram-positive and gram-negative bacteria differ in many respects, including pathogenesis, sites of infection, and antibiotic sensitivity.

- **Eukaryotes and Prokaryotes (Table 2.1)** Eukaryotes are "true" cells with nucleii and organelles. Prokaryotes lack these structures. The difference between eukaryotes and prokaryotes is the basis for antimicrobial action.

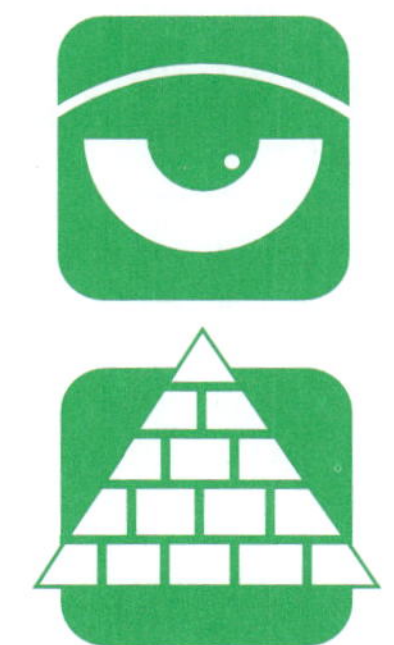

- **Prokaryotic Structure**
  - Bacterial morphology
    1. Size
       - 0.2 µm: Mycoplasma
       - 1 µm: *E. coli*
       - 3 µm: *Bacillus anthracis*
    2. Shape
       - **Coccus:** spherical, e.g., *Streptococcus* spp.
       - **Bacillus:** rod-shaped, e.g., *Escherichia coli*
       - **Spirillium:** snakelike, e.g., treponemes
       - **Filamentous:** Nocardia, Actinomyces
    3. Arrangement
       - **Diploid:** paired cells, e.g., *Neisseria gonorrhoea*
       - **Chains:** streptococci
       - **Grape-like clusters:** staphylococci
    4. Gram stain characteristics
       The Gram stain distinguishes two major classes of bacteria.
       - P . . . Purple . . . Positive
       - Red . . . Negative
       - **Gram staining protocol:**

         Step 1: crystal violet—primary stain
         Step 2: Gram's iodine—precipitates stain
         Step 3: solvent (alcohol or acetone)—decolorizes gram-negative bacteria
         Step 4: safranin—counterstains gram-negative bacteria a red color
       - **Basis of stain:** The thick peptidoglycan cell wall of gram-positive bacteria traps the crystal violet stain. The decolorizer dissolves the

Table 2.1 *Major Characteristics of Eukaryotes and Prokaryotes*

Characteristics	Eukaryotes	Prokaryotes
Major groups	Algae, fungi, protozoa, plants, animals	Bacteria
Size (approximate)	>5 μm	0.5-3 μm
Nuclear structures		
Nucleus	Classic membrane	No nuclear membrane
Chromosomes	Strands of DNA	Single, circular DNA
Cytoplasmic structures		
Mitochondria	Present	Absent
Golgi bodies	Present	Absent
Endoplasmic reticulum	Present	Absent
Ribosomes (sedimentation coefficient)	80S (60S + 40S)	70S (50S + 30S)
Cytoplasmic membrane	Contains sterols	Does not contain sterols*
Cell wall	Absent or composed of cellulose or chitin	Complex structure containing protein, lipids, and peptidoglycans
Reproduction	Sexual and asexual	Asexual (binary fission)
Movement	Flagella, if present, are complex	Flagella, if present, are simple
Respiration	Via mitochondria	Via cytoplasmic membrane

From Holt S. In Slots J, Taubman M, editors: *Contemporary oral microbiology and immunology,* St Louis, 1992, Mosby.
*Except in *Mycoplasma.*

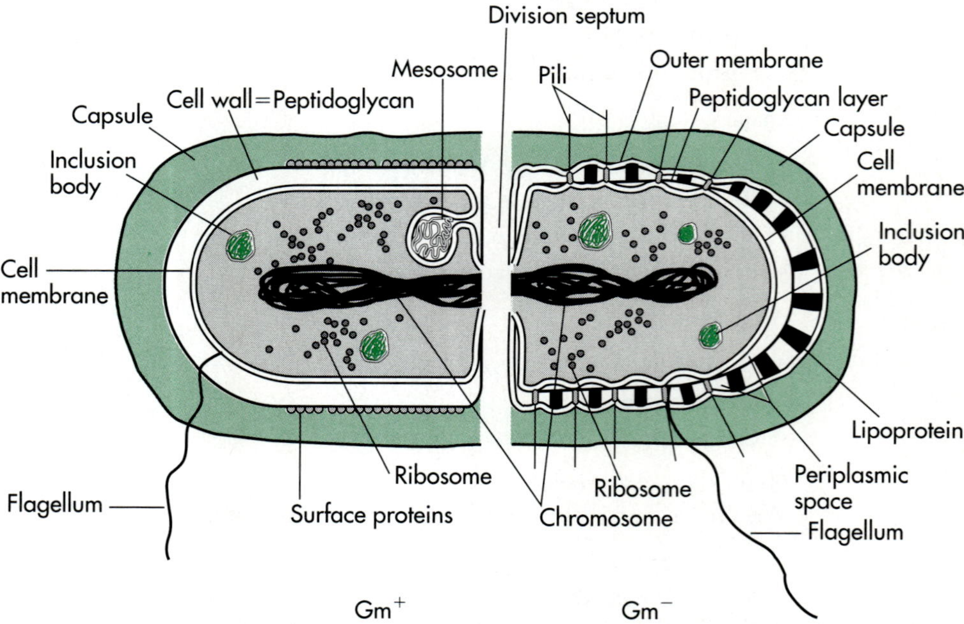

Fig. 2.1 Gram-positive and gram-negative bacteria. Gram-positive bacteria have thick peptidoglycan. Gram-negative bacteria have thin peptidoglycan and an outer membrane.

outer membrane, allowing the stain to be washed out of the thin peptidoglycan of gram-negative bacteria. The red safranin counterstain allows the gram-negative organisms to be visualized.

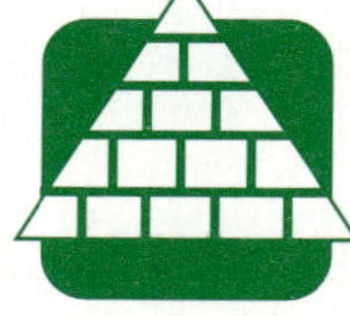

Bacterial Ultrastructure (Fig. 2.1) Gram-positive and gram-negative bacteria have a similar internal structure but a very different external structure.

Internal bacterial structures

— ***The chromosome or the nucleoid*** Unlike eukaryotic DNA, the bacterial chromosome is a **single circle** and lacks **histones. Plasmids,** which are small, circular fragments of extrachromosomal DNA, may also be present.

— ***The cytoplasm***

• No organelles, such as mitochondria, are present in bacteria. The **ribosomes** are **70S in size** and are made up of a 30S and a 50S subunit, unlike eukaryotic ribosomes, which are **80S in size** and consist of a 40S and a 60S subunit.

• There is no nuclear membrane. The functions of transcription and translation are, therefore, coupled (i.e., ribosomes can bind and protein can be synthesized as the mRNA is being transcribed and is still attached to the DNA).

— ***The cytoplasmic membrane***

• The cytoplasmic membrane of bacteria is structurally similar to the eukaryotic membrane but contains no steroids (e.g., cholesterol).

• The membrane is an important site for a number of metabolic activities and contains enzymes related to

- energy production (e.g., electron transport chain, F1 ATPase)
- transport of nutrients
- synthesis of structural components

• *Mesosomes* are coiled-up sections of the membrane that may act as anchors to bind and pull apart duplicated chromosomes during cell division.

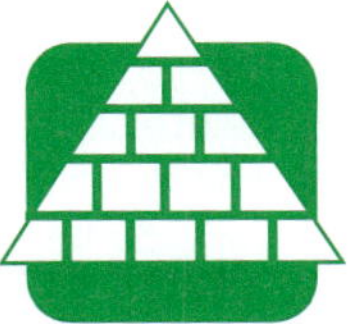

External bacterial structures

— ***The cell envelope (Tables 2.2 and 2.3)***

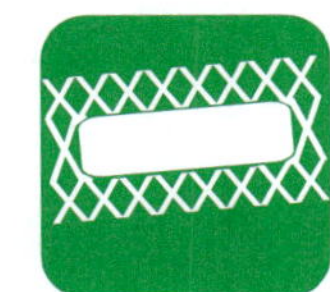

Gram-positive bacteria (Fig. 2.2). Gram-positive bacteria have a **thick, multilayered** cell wall (150 to 500Å in diameter) composed of **peptidoglycan (murein)** surrounding their plasma membrane. The peptidoglycan is an exoskeleton, essential for bacterial structure.

• Teichoic acid, lipoteichoic acids, and other complex polysaccharides (usually called C polysaccharides) are also present in the cell wall. Proteins, such as the M protein of streptococci and the R protein of staphylococci also associate with the peptidoglycan. The teichoic acid and M protein are virulence factors.

• Removal of the peptidoglycan, for example, by degradation with lysozyme, produces a **protoplast,** which does not have a rigid cell-wall structure. The cytoplasm of the protoplast is hyperosmotic and will therefore lyse unless osmotically stabilized.

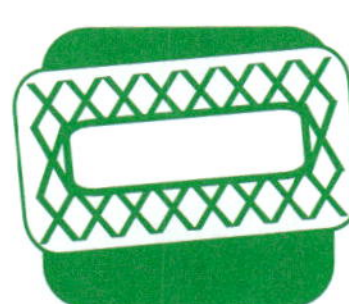

Gram-negative bacteria (Fig. 2.3). The cell wall of gram-negative bacteria has a **thin peptidoglycan layer** (one layer thick) but is surrounded by an **outer membrane.**

• The outer membrane maintains bacterial structure and acts as a permeability barrier to large molecules (e.g., proteins such as lysozyme), and hydrophobic molecules. It protects the enteric bacteria from ad-

Table 2.2 *Bacterial Membrane Structures*

Structure	Chemical Constituents
Plasma Membrane	Phospholipids, proteins, and enzymes involved in generation of energy, membrane potential, and transport
Cell Wall	
Gram-positive Bacteria	
Peptidoglycan	Glycan chains of NAG and NAM, cross-linked by tetrapeptide bridge
Teichoic acid	Polyribitol phosphate or glycerol phosphate cross-linked to peptidoglycan
Lipoteichoic acid	Lipid-linked teichoic acid
Gram-negative Bacteria	
Peptidoglycan	Thinner version of that found in gram-positive bacteria
Periplasmic space	Contains enzymes involved in transport, degradation, and synthesis
Outer membrane	Phospholipids with saturated fatty acids
Proteins	Porins, lipoprotein, transport proteins
Lipopolysaccharide (LPS)	Lipid A, core, O-antigen
Other Structures	
Capsule	Polysaccharides (disaccharides and trisaccharides) and polypeptides
Pili	Pilin, adhesins
Flagella	Motor proteins, flagellin
Proteins	e.g., M protein of streptococci

NAG, N-Acetyl glycosamine; *NAM*, N-acetyl muramic acid.

Table 2.3 *Functions of the Bacterial Envelope*

Function	Component
Structural rigidity	All
Packaging of internal contents	All
Permeability barrier	Outer membrane or plasma membrane
Metabolite uptake	Membrane and periplasmic transport proteins, porins, permeases
Energy production	Plasma membrane
Adhesion to host cells	Pili, proteins, teichoic acid
Immune recognition by host	All outer structures
Escape from host immune recognition	Capsule, M protein
Antibiotic sensitivity	Peptidoglycan synthetic enzymes
Antibiotic resistance	Outer membrane
Motility	Flagella
Mating	Pili
Adhesion	Pili

verse environmental conditions, such as the digestive system of the host.

- The outer membrane contains **lipopolysaccharide (LPS)**, proteins, and phospholipids.
- No teichoic or lipoteichoic acids are present.
- The **periplasmic space** is between the outer membrane and the

A

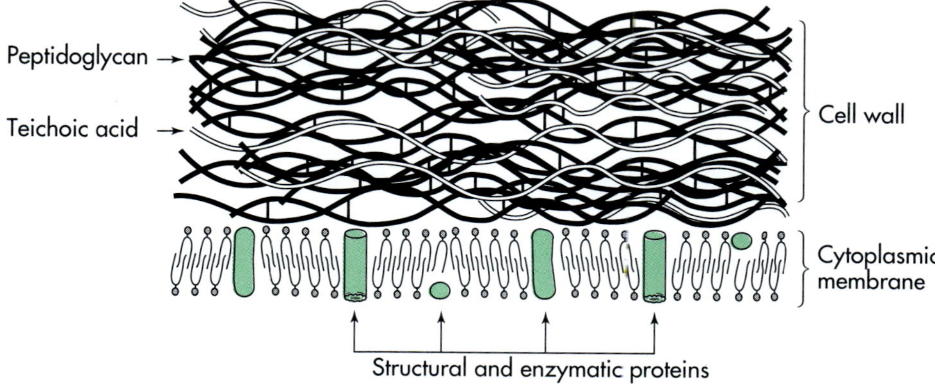

B

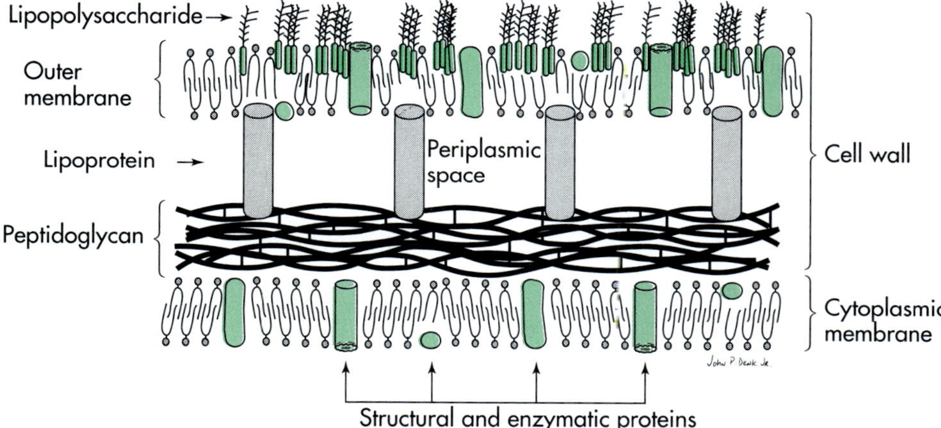

Fig. 2.2 Comparison of the gram-positive and the gram-negative bacterial cell wall. **A,** Gram-positive bacteria have a thick peptidoglycan layer that contains teichoic acid. **B,** Gram-negative bacteria have a thin peptidoglycan (one layer thick) and an outer membrane that contains lipopolysaccharide, phospholipids, and proteins. The periplasmic space between the cytoplasmic and outer membranes contains transport, degradative, and cell wall synthetic proteins. The outer membrane is joined to the cytoplasmic membrane at adhesion points.

cytoplasmic membrane and contains degradative enzymes, including beta-lactamase and transport proteins.

- The outer membrane is held together by divalent cation linkages between phosphates on LPS molecules and by hydrophobic interactions between the LPS and proteins. It can be disrupted by antibiotics (e.g., polymyxin) or by removal of magnesium and calcium ions.
- The outer membrane is connected to the cytoplasmic membrane at adhesion sites and tied to the peptidoglycan by **lipoprotein** (a protein that is covalently linked to the peptidoglycan and inserted into the outer membrane).
- **Porins** produce hydrophilic channels in the outer membrane,

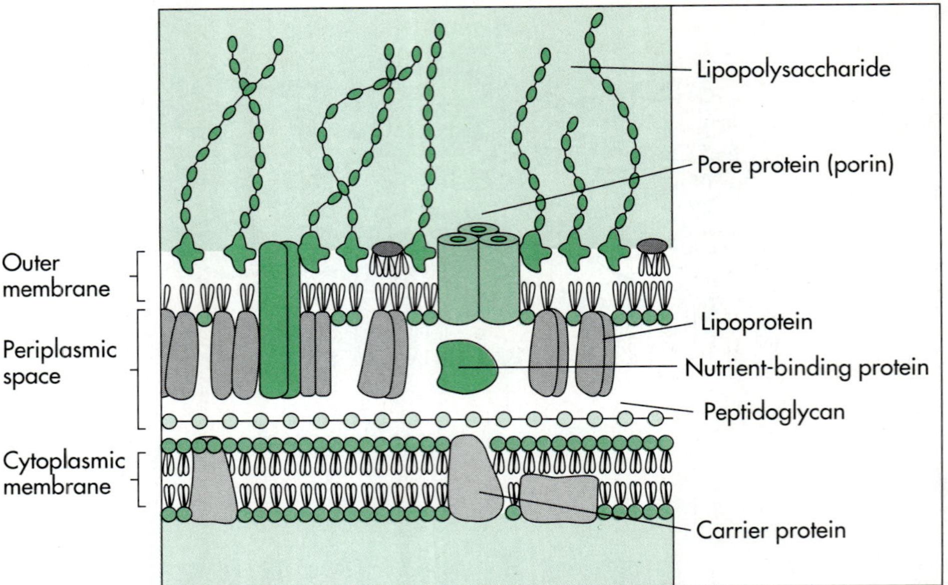

Fig. 2.3 Three-dimensional structure of the gram-negative cell envelope. Outside the cytoplasmic membrane is a thin peptidoglycan layer, the periplasmic space, and an outer membrane. Porin proteins and other membrane proteins in the outer membrane allow entry of small hydrophilic molecules. LPS (endotoxin) is on the outer layer of the outer membrane. *(Modified from Newman NG, Nisengard R:* Oral microbiology and immunology, *Philadelphia, 1988, Saunders.)*

which allow passage of small, charged molecules only. *Porin channels control the passage of antibiotics.*

- Removal of the outer membrane (by removal of divalent cations) and peptidoglycan (by lysozyme) produces a **spheroplast.**
- The differences between gram-positive and gram-negative bacteria are summarized in Table 2.4.

Mycobacteria. The mycobacteria have a peptidoglycan layer (of a slightly different structure), intertwined and covalently attached to an arabinogalactan polymer and surrounded by a waxlike lipid coat consisting of **mycolic acid** (large α-alkyl, branched β-hydroxy fatty acids), **cord factor** (glycolipid consisting of trehalose and two mycolic acids), **wax D** (glycolipid consisting of 15 to 20 mycolic acids and sugar), and sulfolipids. These bacteria are identified by acid-fast staining. The coat is responsible for virulence and is antiphagocytic. *Corynebacterium* and *Nocardia* spp. also produce mycolic acid.

Major Components of the Bacterial Cell Wall

- **Peptidoglycan (mucopeptide, murein) (Fig. 2.4)** The peptidoglycan is a rigid mesh responsible for the structural integrity and shape of the bacterial cell and essential for bacterial viability. The mesh is made up of ropelike linear polysaccharide chains that are crosslinked by peptides. The mesh is relatively porous, especially to antibiotics.

  - The polysaccharide is made up of the repeating disaccharides N-acetyl-glucosamine (NAG) and N-acetylmuramic acid (NAM): –NAG-NAM–NAG-NAM–NAG-NAM–NAG-NAM–

Table 2.4 ***Membrane Characteristics of Gram-positive and Gram-negative Bacteria***

	Gram-positive	Gram-negative
Outer membrane	None	+
Cell wall	Thicker	Thinner
LPS	None	+
Endotoxin	None	+
Teichoic acids	Often present	Absent
Sporulation	Some strains	None
Capsule	Sometimes present	Sometimes present
Lysozyme	Sensitive	Resistant
Antibacterial activity of penicillin	More susceptible	More resistant
Exotoxin production	Sometimes	Sometimes

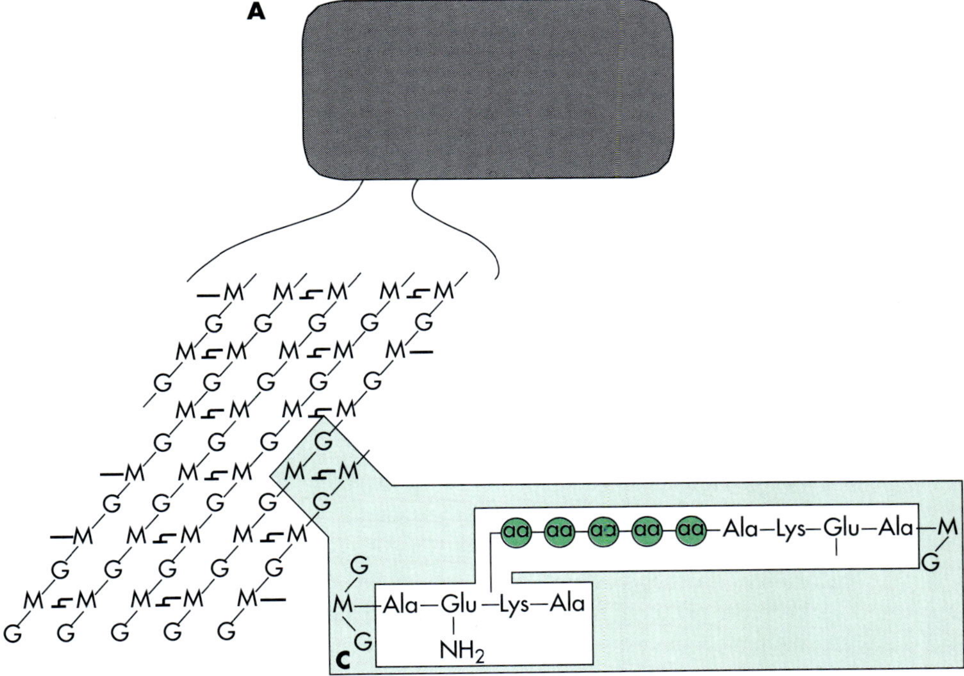

Fig. 2.4 General structure of the peptidoglycan component of the cell wall. **A,** The peptidoglycan forms a meshlike layer around the cell. **B,** The peptidoglycan mesh consists of a polysaccharide polymer that is crosslinked by peptide bonds. **C,** Peptides are crosslinked through a peptide bond between the terminal D-alanine from one chain and a lysine (or other diamino-amino acid) from the other chain. A pentaglycine bridge (aa-aa-aa) expands the crosslink in *S. aureus.* *(Redrawn from Talaro K., Talaro A:* Foundations in microbiology, *Dubuque, Iowa, 1993, Wm. C. Brown.)*

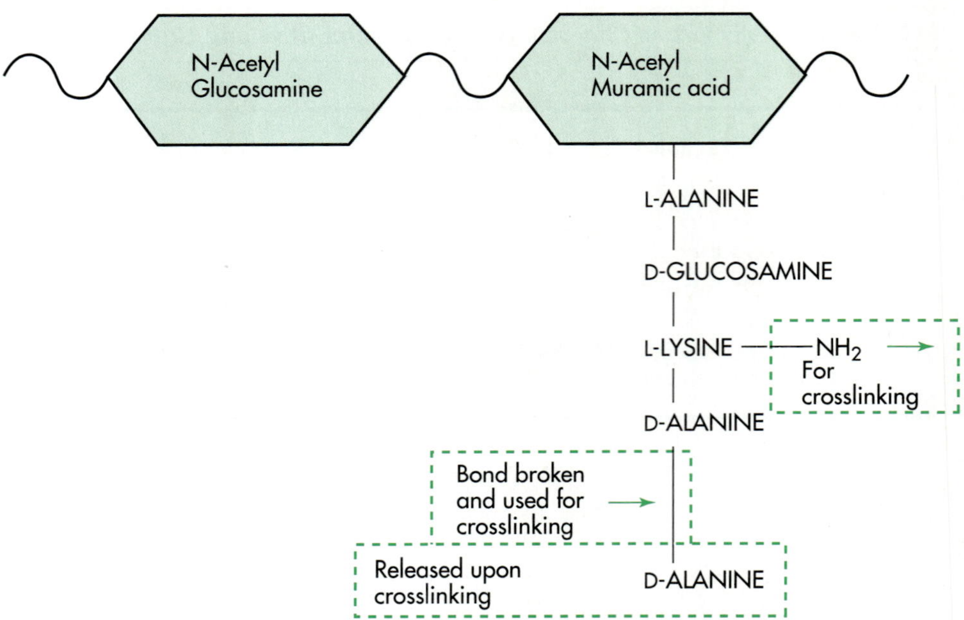

Fig. 2.5 Precursor of peptidoglycan. The peptidoglycan is built from prefabricated units that contain a pentapeptide attached to the N-acetyl muramic acid. The pentapeptide contains a terminal D-alanine-D-alanine. This dipeptide is required for crosslinking the peptidoglycan and is the basis for beta-lactam antibiotic and vancomycin antibiotic action.

- The peptide portion is attached to the N-acetylmuramic acid (NAM). The peptide contains both D and L amino acids (D amino acids are unusual). The basic sequence of the tetrapeptide is NAM–aa1-aa2-diamino-amino acid-D-ala. Examples of diamino-amino acids are lysine, diaminopimelic acid, and diaminobutyric acid. The precursor form of the peptide has an extra D-alanine (Fig. 2.5).
- The **peptide crosslink** is formed between the free, or amino end of the diamino-amino acid in the third position of the peptide and the D-alanine in the fourth position of another chain. *S. aureus* utilizes a $(gly)_5$ bridge between these amino acids to lengthen the crosslink.
- The rigidity of the peptidoglycan mesh is determined by the number of crosslinks and the length of the crosslink.
- The peptidoglycan is constantly being synthesized and degraded. Inhibition of synthesis or crosslinking (e.g., by antibiotics) weakens the mesh, weakens the bacterial structure, and leads to lysis and cell death. **Lysozyme,** an enzyme produced by bacteria and also present in human tears, cleaves the glycan portion of the peptidoglycan molecule.

Teichoic and lipoteichoic acids Teichoic and lipoteichoic acids are polymers of chemically modified ribose or glycerol connected by phosphates (Fig. 2.6). Ribitol teichoic acid is polyribitol phosphate with attached glycosyl moieties. Other structures are possible.

- Teichoic acid is covalently attached to the peptidoglycan and is present in many gram-positive but not in gram-negative bacteria.
- Teichoic acids are antigenic and may determine strain differences.
- Lipoteichoic acid contains a fatty acid molecule and is anchored in the membrane.

A **Ribitol-Teichoic Acid (Staphylococcal)**

B **Glycerol Teichoic Acid (Lactobacillus)**

Fig. 2.6 Teichoic acid. Teichoic acid is a polymer of chemically modified **(A)** ribitol, or **(B)** glycerol phosphate. The nature of the modification (sugars, amino acids, etc.) can define the serotype of the bacteria. Teichoic acid may be covalently attached to the peptidoglycan. Lipoteichoic acid is anchored in the cytoplasmic membrane by a covalently attached fatty acid.

• Lipoteichoic acids are shed into the culture medium and host tissue.

• Teichoic and lipoteichoic acids may promote adherence to host tissue. For example, lipoteichoic acid of group A streptococci promotes adherence to oral epithelial cells.

• Lipoteichoic acid can initiate weak, endotoxin-like activities.

● **Lipopolysaccharide (LPS, endotoxin) (Fig. 2.7)** LPS is found only in gram-negative bacteria and is an essential element of the outer membrane.

It consists of three structural sections: lipid A, the core polysaccharide (rough core), and the O-antigen.

— ***Lipid A (endotoxin)***

• Lipid A is a diphospho, fatty acid-modified glucosamine disaccharide that is essential to the bacterium. The fatty acids anchor the structure in the outer membrane. The phosphates connect LPS units together into aggregates. One carbohydrate chain is attached to the disaccharide backbone and extends away from the bacteria.

• The basic structure of lipid A is similar for all gram-negative bacteria and identical for related bacteria.

• Lipid A provides the endotoxin activity to LPS. It is a powerful

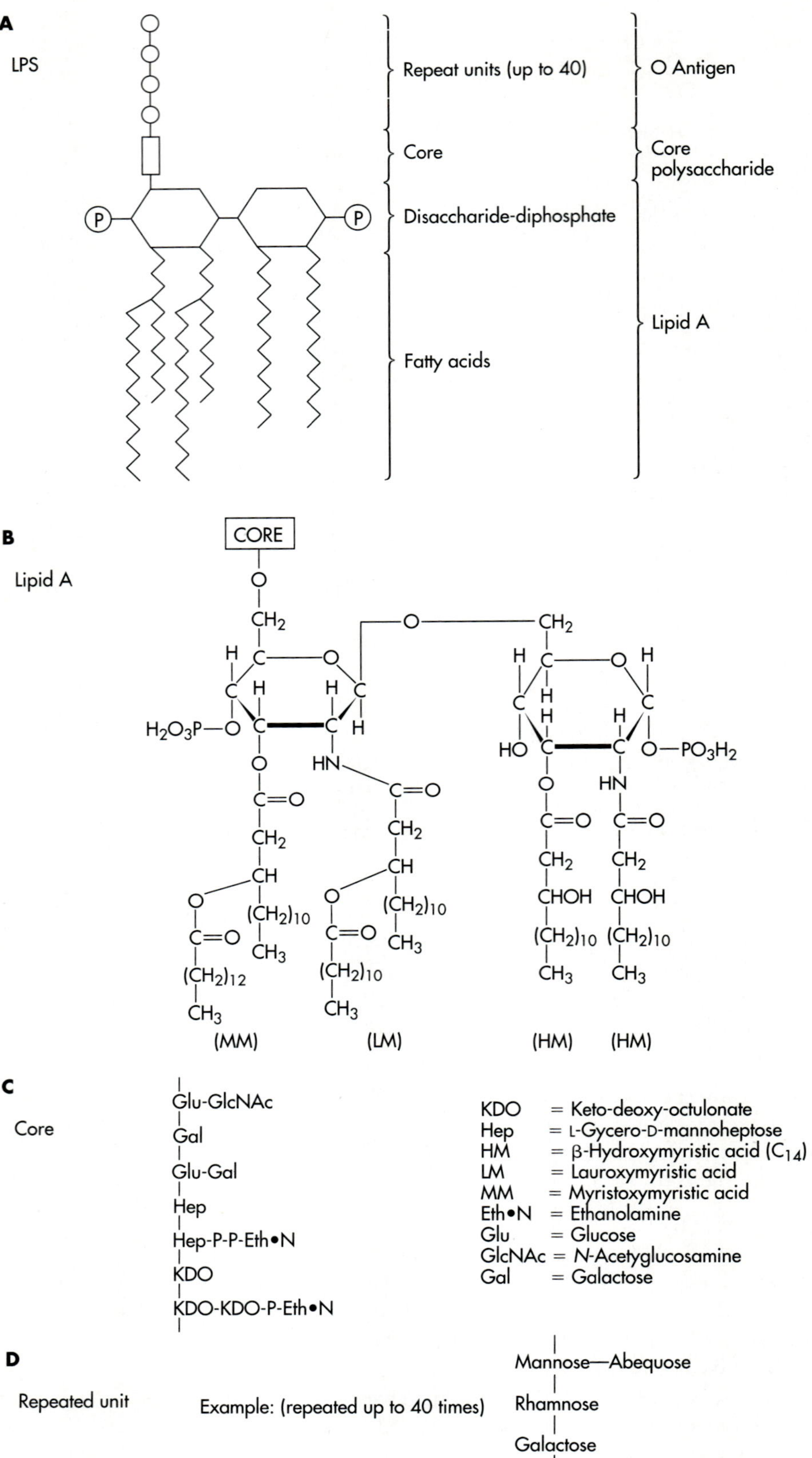

Fig. 2.7 The lipopolysaccharide (LPS) of the gram-negative cell envelope. **A,** Segment of the polymer showing the arrangements of the major constituents. **B,** Structure of lipid A of *Salmonella typhimurium*. **C,** Polysaccharide core. **D,** Typical repeat unit *(Salmonella typhimurium)*. *(Redrawn from Brooks GF, Butel JS, Ornston LN, editors:* Jawetz, Melnick and Adelberg's medical microbiology, *ed 19, Norwalk, Conn, 1991, Appleton & Lange.)*

stimulator of immune cells (B cells and macrophages), and induces macrophages and other cells to release interleukin-1 and interleukin-6, tumor necrosis factor, and other biologically active molecules. It causes fever and can cause shock. The **Shwartzman reaction** (disseminated intravascular coagulation [DIC]) may follow release of large amounts of endotoxin into the bloodstream.

- LPS is shed from the bacteria into culture medium or host tissues. *Neisseria meningitidis* sheds large amounts of LPS, which results in fever and other symptoms.

— *Core polysaccharide*

- The core polysaccharide is a branched polysaccharide of 9 to 12 sugars attached to Lipid A.
- The core structure is species specific (i.e., all *E. coli* have the same core structure).

— *O-antigen*

- The O-antigen is a long, linear polysaccharide that is made up of repeating saccharide units, which is attached to the core.
- It distinguishes serotypes (strains) of a bacterial species.

Biosynthesis of the Cell Wall Synthesis of new cell wall components is essential for the replication of the cell. The cell wall is also a target for antibiotics.

- New peptidoglycan is synthesized in a defined growth zone, usually in a ring around the equator of the cell.
- Bacteria have a specialized mechanism for construction of external membrane-associated structures (e.g., peptidoglycan, LPS, teichoic acids, and capsular material). Component units are prefabricated inside the bacteria, translocated to the outside, and assembled there.

Peptidoglycan synthesis (Figs. 2.8 and 2.9) Peptidoglycan synthesis proceeds in four steps:

1. **In the cytoplasm:** Substrates are activated and assembled into units in the cytoplasm.

    - The uridine diphosphate (UDP)-NAM-pentapeptide unit (UDP-NAM-aa-aa-aa-D-ala-D-ala) is assembled enzymatically.

2. **At the membrane:** The assembled unit is attached to the bactoprenol (undecaprenol, C55 isoprenoid) carrier molecule at the membrane through a pyrophosphate link, releasing uridine monophosphate (UMP). N-acetyl glucosamine is added.

    - Some bacteria (e.g., *S. aureus*) add a pentaglycine or some other chain to the diamino-amino acid at the third position of the peptide chain to lengthen the crosslink.
    - This completes the building block.

3. **On the outside:** The unit is shifted to the outside of the cell and the pyrophosphate link provides the energy for attachment to the growing glycan chain (see Fig. 2.8, *B*).
4. **Outside the cell:** Peptide chains from adjacent glycan chains are crosslinked by a peptide bond exchange (transpeptidation) between the amine of the amino acid in the third position of the pentapeptide (e.g., lysine) or the N-terminus of the pentaglycine chain and the D-alanine at the

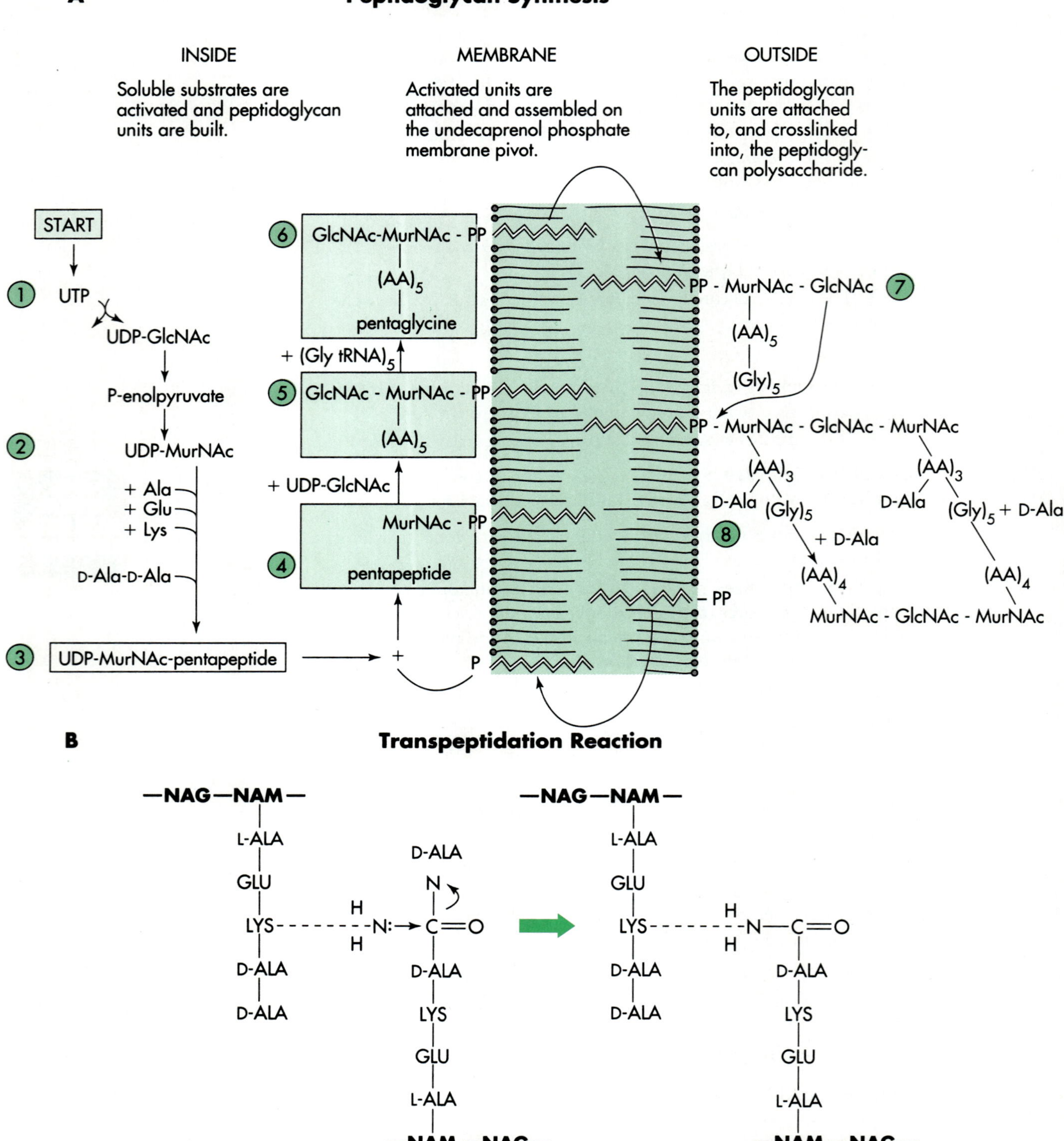

Fig. 2.8 Peptidoglycan synthesis. **A,** Peptidoglycan synthesis occurs in three phases: (1) Peptidoglycan is synthesized from prefabricated units constructed and activated for assembly and transport inside the cell; (2) at the membrane, the units are assembled onto the undecaprenol phosphate conveyor belt, and assembly is completed; (3) the unit is translocated to the outside of the cell where it is attached to the polysaccharide chain, and the peptide is crosslinked to finish the construction. Such a construction job mimics the assembly of a space station. **B,** The cross-linking reaction is a transpeptidation. One peptide bond (produced inside the cell) is traded for another (outside the cell) with the release of D-alanine. The enzymes that catalyze the reaction are called D-alanine, D-alanine transpeptidase-carboxypeptidases. These enzymes are the targets of beta-lactam antibiotics and are called penicillin binding proteins.

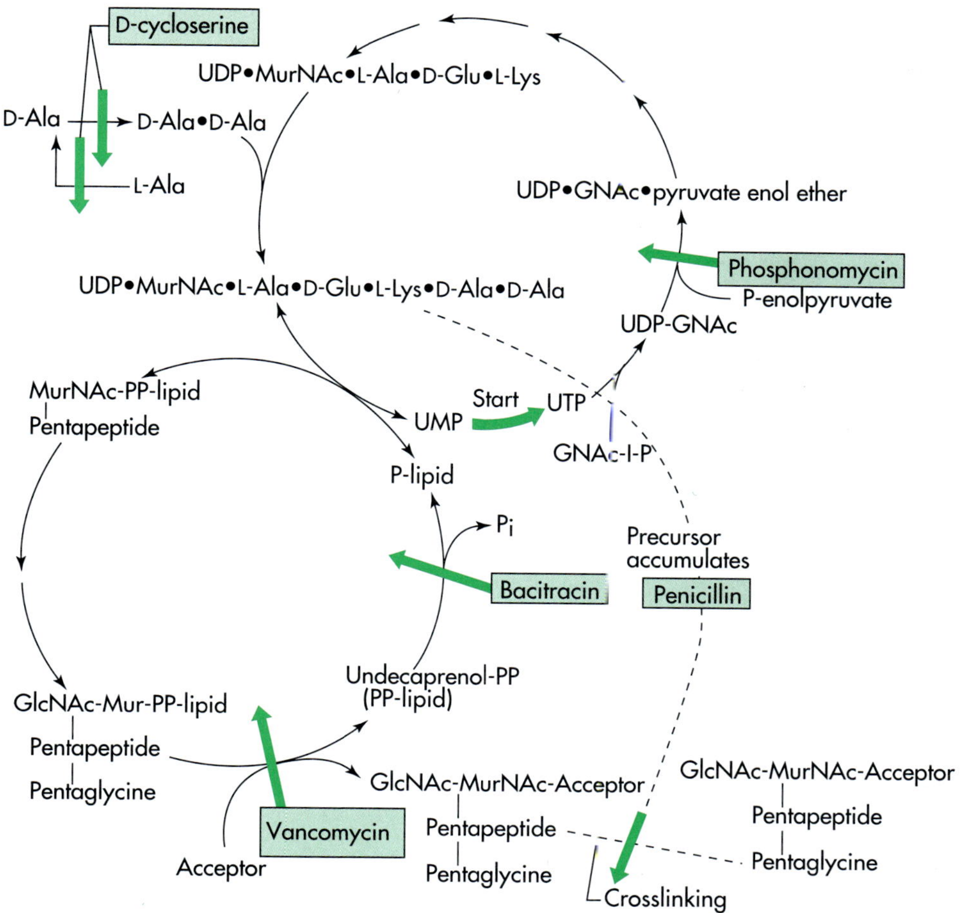

Fig. 2.9 Peptidoglycan synthesis and inhibitors of the process. This figure provides another presentation of the four steps in peptidoglycan synthesis. Step 1, occurring inside the cell, is represented by the top circle. Step 2, occurring on the membrane conveyor belt (bactoprenol), is represented by the bottom circle. Steps 3 and 4, occurring outside the cell, are represented at the bottom right of the figure. The sites of action for the antibiotics *(boxes)* are indicated by the dark arrows. *(Redrawn from Davis, Dulbecco, Eisen, Ginsberg:* Microbiology, *ed 4, Philadelphia, 1990, Lippincott.)*

fourth position, releasing the terminal D-alanine of the precursor. This step requires no additional energy because peptide bonds are "traded."

- The crosslinking reaction is catalyzed by membrane-bound transpeptidases. Related enzymes, such as D,D-carboxypeptidases, remove extra terminal D-alanines, which will limit the extent of crosslinking.
- Penicillin and related beta-lactam antibiotics resemble the "transition state" conformation of the D-ala-D-ala when bound to these enzymes.
- The transpeptidases and the D,D-carboxypeptidases are known as penicillin binding proteins (PBPs). Different PBPs are used for extending the peptidoglycan, creating a septum for cell division and curving the mesh (providing cell shape).

- **Lipopolysaccharide synthesis** The lipid A and core portions are enzymatically synthesized in a sequential manner on the inside surface of the cytoplasmic membrane.

- The O-antigen is made up of 50 to 100 repeat units. Each of these repeat units is assembled on a bactoprenol molecule and then transferred to a growing O-antigen chain.
- The finished O-antigen chain is transferred to the core–lipid A structure.
- The LPS molecule is translocated through adhesion sites to the outer surface of the outer membrane.

- **Teichoic acid and capsule synthesis** Both these structures have building blocks made up of repeating units and utilize the bactoprenol conveyor belt as for LPS synthesis.

— ***The capsule*** Some bacteria (gram-positive and gram-negative) are surrounded by loose layers of polysaccharide or protein. The capsule is hard to see on regular staining but can be visualized by exclusion of India ink particles. The capsule is poorly antigenic, is antiphagocytic, and promotes the virulence of certain organisms (e.g., *Streptococcus pneumoniae*).

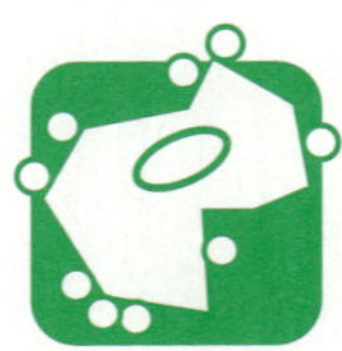

— ***The fimbriae (pili)*** Fimbriae are hairlike structures composed of protein subunits (pilins). They promote adherence of the bacterium to the host (alternate names for pili: adhesins, lectins, evasins, or aggressins). Fimbriae are a virulence factor for *N. gonorrhoea.*

F pili (sex pili) promote the transfer of large segments of bacterial chromosomes between bacteria. Production of the F pilus is encoded by a plasmid (F factor).

— ***The flagella*** The flagella are structures that confer motility. They consist of ropelike propellers composed of protein subunits (flagellin), anchored in the bacterial membranes through hook and basal body structures and driven by membrane potential. The flagella facilitate movement towards food (chemotaxis). Flagella express antigenic determinants that distinguish strains of organisms.

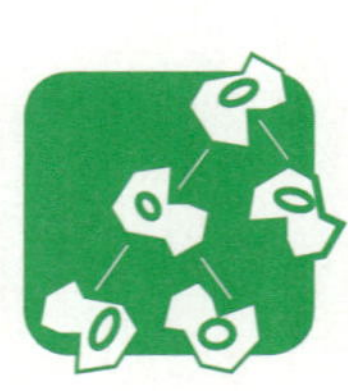

Cell Division

- Bacterial growth proceeds through the following phases:
  - **lag phase:** acclimatizion to the medium and initiation of DNA synthesis
  - **exponential growth phase:** doubling of cells under optimal growth conditions
  - **stationary phase:** no growth; initiated upon depletion of an essential nutrient
- New chromosome synthesis is initiated at the origin of replication.
- Multiple initiations may occur before actual cell division occurs.
- Daughter chromosomes attach to mesosomes in the membrane, which pull them into the daughter cells.
- Septum formation (membrane and new peptidoglycan) occurs in the center of the cell and divides the daughter cells.
- Initiation events may take place two generations before the process is completed.
- Every chromosome initially must be completed despite culture conditions, e.g., starvation.

Spores and Spore Synthesis

Only gram-positive bacteria can make spores. The spore coat is like a double layer of peptidoglycan. The spore is resistant to heating, drying, and harsh conditions.

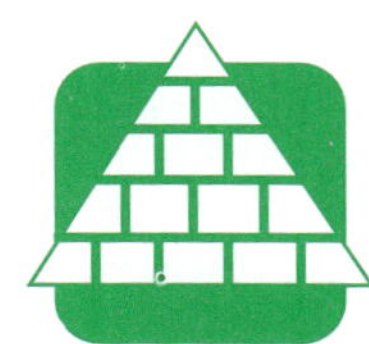

Spore structure

- **Core:** consists of the chromosome, a minimum number of enzymes for energy metabolism, a high concentration of calcium ions, and **dipicolinic acid**—a spore-specific compound that chelates calcium ions and contributes to heat resistance
- **Inner membrane:** consists of the cellular cytoplasmic membrane
- **Cortex:** contains loosely cross-linked peptidoglycan
- **Outer membrane:** membrane faces toward the inside because of the mechanism of spore formation
- **Tough protein coat:** protein similar to keratin with highly cross-linked disulfide bonds (80% of the protein of the spore); forms a major barrier to chemicals
- **Exosporium:** lipoprotein membrane

Spore formation

Spore formation is a variation on cell division.

- **Initiation:** follows decrease in growth rate because of depletion of essential nutrients; there is a switch to spore mRNA and protein synthesis and shut-off of other mRNA synthesis

Production of antibiotics and toxins often occurs prior to sporulation.

- **Germination:** activation is initiated by damage to the coat by trauma, water, or aging; energy is required; protein and DNA are produced; once initiated, germination must proceed to its conclusion

Section 2.2 Bacterial Genetics

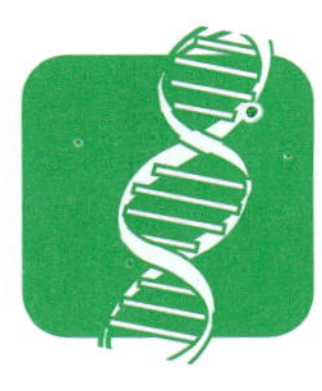

Vocabulary

- **Allele:** An allele is a particular example of a gene. Each variant of a given gene is a different allele of that gene. Genes that are represented by multiple variants in a population are said to be **polymorphic.**
- **Cistron:** A cistron is a structural gene, a complementation unit.
- **Codon:** A codon is a triplet of nucleotides that specifies an amino acid or a translation stop signal.
- **Plasmid:** A plasmid is an extrachromosomal genetic element (an independent replicon). Most plasmids are circular double-stranded DNA molecules, although linear plasmids have been found in a few cases.
- **Promoter:** A promoter is the nucleotide sequence in an operon that is recognized and bound by **RNA polymerase.**
- **Replicon:** A replicon is a replication unit, consisting of a replication origin, a replication terminus, and the intervening sequence.

Organization of Genetic Information

Genome

The genome represents the total collection of genes carried by a bacterium, both on its chromosome and on its extrachromosomal genetic elements, if any. The chromosome of a typical bacterium such as *Escherichia coli* is a single, double-stranded, circular molecule of DNA containing approximately 5 million base pairs (or 5000 kilobase pairs). The smallest bacterial chromosomes (from *Mycoplasma*) are about one quarter this size. Each genome contains many *operons.*

- **Operon or transcription unit** An operon is a group of one or more structural genes expressed from a particular promoter and ending at a transcriptional terminator. Those with multiple structural genes are **polycistronic,** for example, the *E. coli lactose (lac)* operon for lactose utilization (Fig. 2.10) or *tryptophan (trp)* operon for tryptophan biosynthesis (Fig. 2.11).
- **Gene** A gene is a sequence of nucleotides that has a biological function. Examples of genes are protein structural genes (coding genes), ribosomal RNA genes, and genes that are recognition or binding sites for other molecules (promoter genes).

Mechanisms for Genetic Transfer

- **Transformation** Transformation is the process by which bacteria take up fragments of naked DNA and incorporate them into their genomes (Fig. 2.12 on p. 59).
- **Transduction** Transduction is the process by which bacteria take up fragments of DNA that have been packaged into bacteriophage particles and incorporate them into their genomes. Transduction can be classified as **specialized** or **generalized** according to whether the phages transfer specific genes (usually those that are adjacent to their integration sites in the genome) or transfer any gene through random packaging of DNA (Fig. 2.13 on p. 60).
- **Conjugation** Conjugation is the process by which DNA is passed by direct cell-to-cell contact, that is, by mating. Conjugation results in the asymmetrical transfer of DNA from a donor (or male) cell to a recipient (or female) cell. The mating type of the cell depends on the presence (in the male cell) or absence (in the female cell) of a **conjugative plasmid** such as the **F (fertility) plasmid** of *E. coli.* The conjugative plasmid contains genes that convey properties of the donor including the ability to synthesize sex pili and to initiate DNA synthesis at the *transfer origin (OriT)* of the plasmid.

  What DNA gets transferred in a mating depends on the physical state and location of the transfer origin of the conjugative plasmid. As an independent plasmid, the F plasmid transfers itself, converting recipients into F^+ male cells (Fig. 2.14 on p. 61). If the plasmid is associated with a fragment of chromosomal DNA, it is designated an F' plasmid, and when it is transferred, it carries that fragment with it into the recipient, converting it into an F' male cell. If the F plasmid sequence is integrated into the bacterial chromosome, the cell is designated an *Hfr (H*igh *f*requency of *r*ecombination) cell. An Hfr cell transfers chromosomal genes in an order determined by the position and orientation of the integrated *OriT.* It rarely causes recipients to become Hfr males, and then only if conjugation has first transferred the entire bacterial chromosome.

Mobile Genetic Elements

- **Plasmids** Plasmids are extrachromosomal genetic elements that are independent replicons. Most plasmids are circular double-stranded DNA molecules, although linear plasmids have been found in a few cases. Some plasmids, such as the *E. coli* F plasmid, are **episomes** which means they can integrate into the host chromosome. Some carry important genes, such as multiple drug resistance genes or toxin genes (Fig. 2.15 on p. 62).

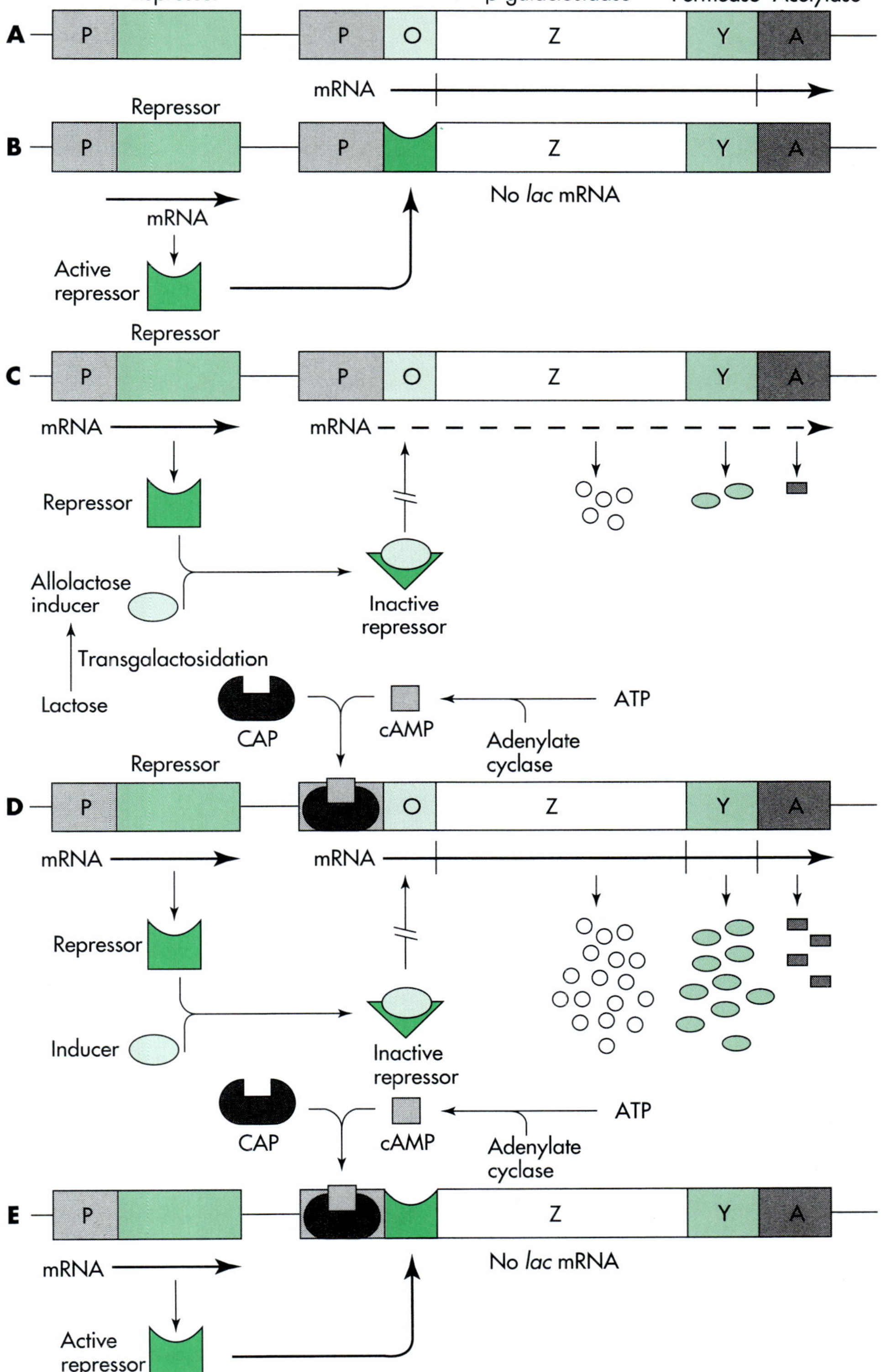

Fig. 2.10 The lactose operon. **A,** The lactose operon is transcribed as a polycistronic mRNA from the promoter *(P)* and translated into three proteins: β-galactosidase *(Z),* permease *(Y),* and acetylase *(A).* The *lacI* gene encodes the repressor protein. **B,** The lactose operon is not transcribed in the absence of an allolactose inducer, as the repressor competes with the RNA polymerase at the operator site *(O).* **C,** The repressor, complexed with the inducer, does not recognize the operator because of a conformation change in the repressor. The *lac* operon is thus transcribed at a low level. **D,** *E. coli* is grown in a poor medium in presence of lactose as the carbon source. Both the inducer and the CAP-cAMP complex are bound to the promoter, which is fully "turned on," and a high level of *lac* mRNA is transcribed and translated. **E,** Growth of *E. coli* in a poor medium without lactose will result in the binding of the CAP-cAMP complex to the promoter region and binding of the active repressor to the operator sequence, as no inducer is available. The result will be that the *lac* operon will not be transcribed.

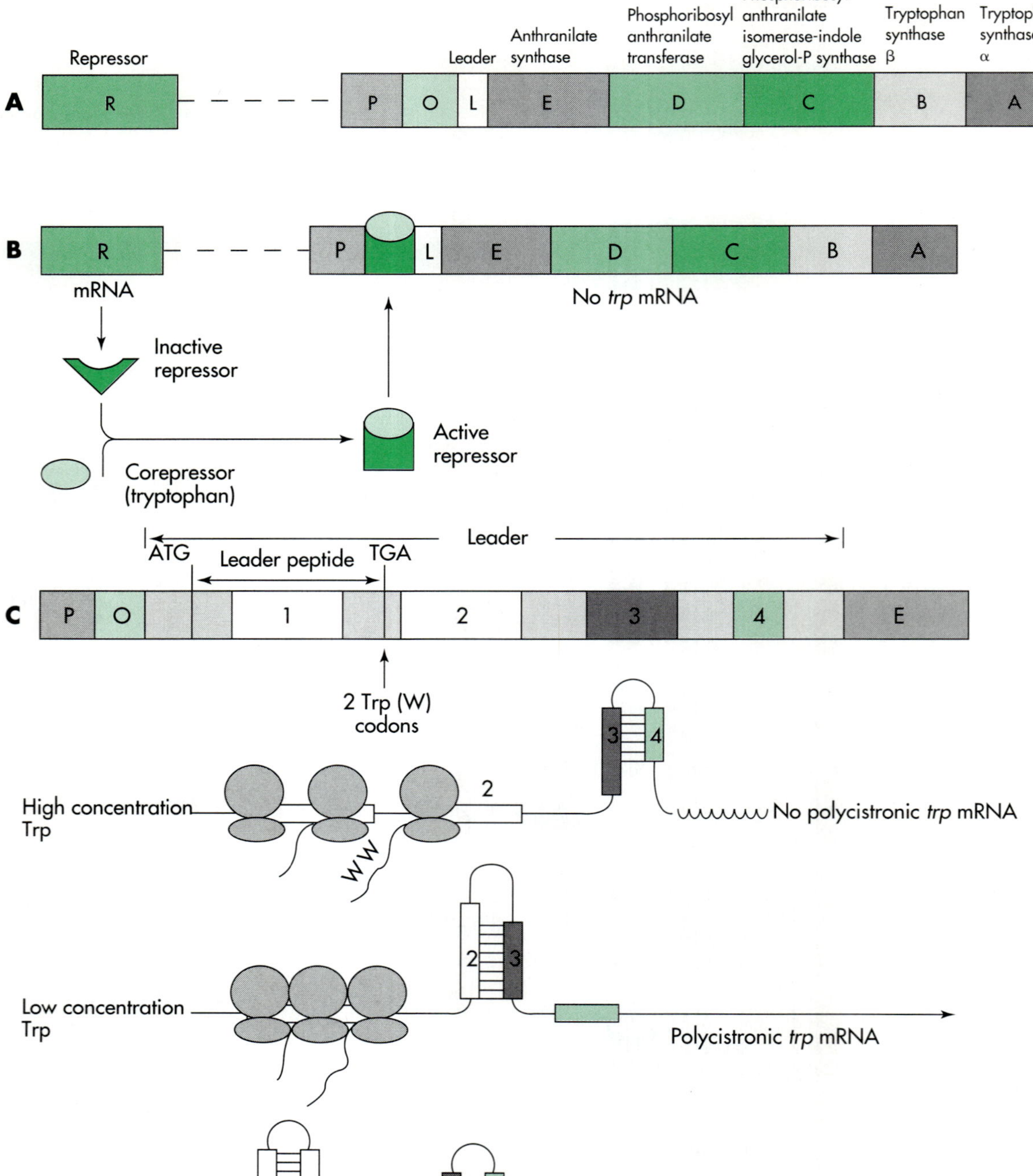

Fig. 2.11 Regulation of the tryptophan operon. **A,** The *trp* operon encodes the five enzymes necessary for tryptophan biosynthesis. The *trp* operon is under dual control. **B,** The conformation of the inactive repressor protein is changed following its binding by the corepressor, tryptophan. The resulting active repressor binds to the operator *(O),* blocking any transcription of the *trp* mRNA by the RNA polymerase. **C,** The *trp* operon is also under the control of an attenuation-antitermination mechanism. Upstream the structural genes are the promoter *(P),* the operator, and a leader *(L)* that can be transcribed into a short peptide containing two tryptophans *(W)* near its distal end. The leader mRNA possesses four repeats (1, 2, 3, and 4), which can pair differently according to the tryptophan availability, leading to an early termination of transcription of the operon or its full transcription. In the presence of a high concentration of tryptophan, regions 3 and 4 of the leader mRNA can pair, forming a terminator hairpin, and no transcription of the *trp* operon occurs. However, in the presence of little or no tryptophan, the ribosomes stall in region 1 when translating the leader peptide because of the tandem of tryptophan codons. Then regions 2 and 3 can pair, forming the antiterminator hairpin, and leading to transcription of the *trp* genes. Finally, the regions 1:2 and 3:4 of the free leader mRNA can pair, also leading to a stop of transcription before the first structural gene *trpE.*

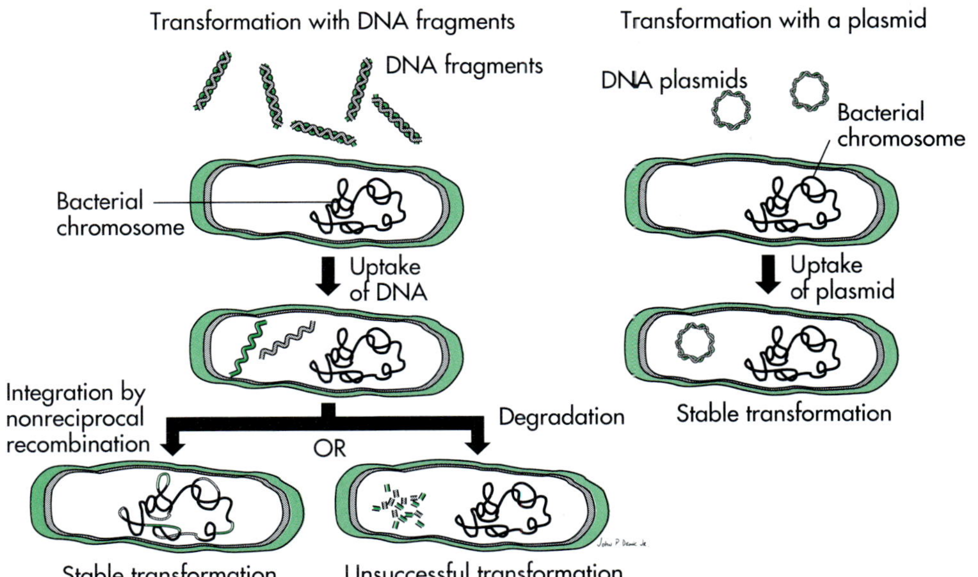

Fig. 2.12 Bacterial transformation. Foreign DNA can be taken up or forced into bacteria and either incorporated into the chromosome or maintained as a plasmid. This "transforms" the bacterium into a new organism.

- **Bacteriophages or bacterial viruses** Bacteriophages are extrachromosomal genetic elements that can survive outside a host cell because the nucleic acid genome (which may be DNA or RNA, single- or double-stranded, circular or linear), is protected by a protein coat. Bacteriophages that can integrate into the host genome without killing the host, such as the *E. coli bacteriophage lambda (λ)* (Fig. 2.16 on p. 62), are termed **lysogenic** phages. Some lysogenic bacteriophages carry toxin genes. For example, *Corynephage* β carries the gene for diphtheria toxin.
- **Transposons** Transposons are mobile genetic elements that are dependent replicons. They can move from one position to another in the genome, or between different molecules of DNA. The simplest transposons are called *insertion sequences.* Complex transposons carry other genes, such as genes that provide resistance against antibiotics (see Fig. 2.15).

Recombination

- **Homologous (legitimate) recombination** This refers to recombination between closely related DNA sequences that generally substitute one sequence for another and require a set of enzymes (in *E. coli* these are produced by the rec genes).
- **Nonhomologous (illegitimate) recombination** This is recombination between dissimilar DNA sequences that generally produce insertions or deletions and usually require specialized (sometimes site-specific) recombination enzymes, such as those produced by many transposons and lysogenic bacteriophages.

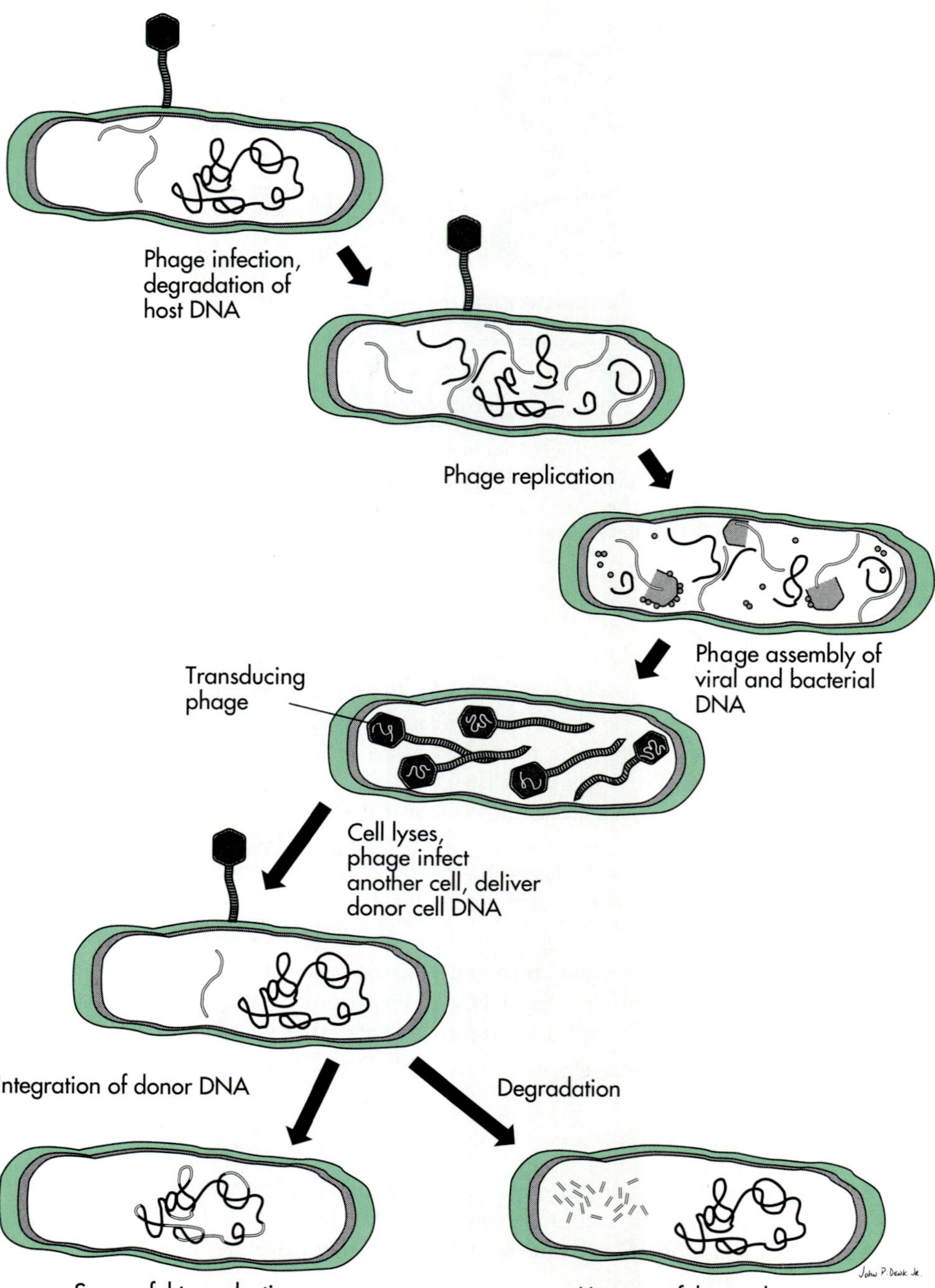

Fig. 2.13 Transduction by bacteriophages. Bacteriophage infection can deliver genes into the target cell providing the cell survives.

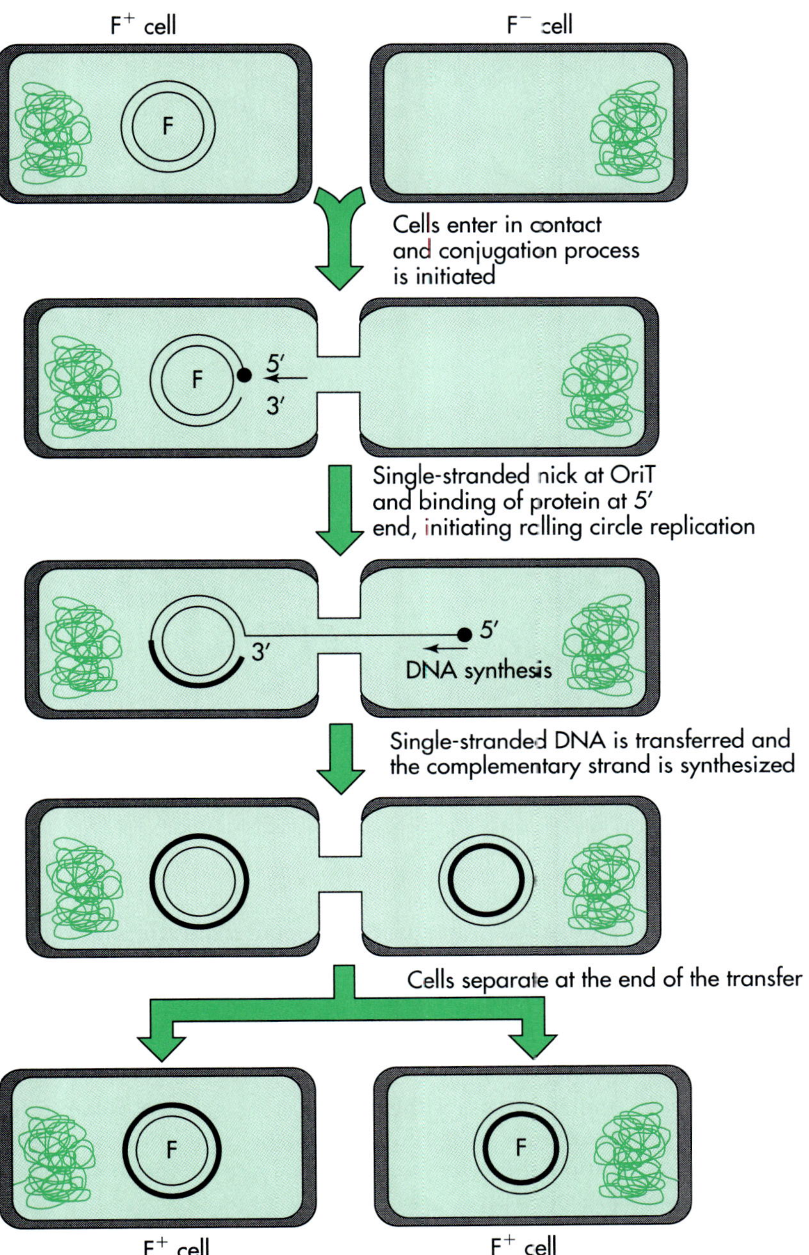

Fig. 2.14 Genetic transfer of the F plasmid by conjugation.

Section 2.3 Bacterial Virulence Factors and Pathogenesis

Generalizations

- Virulent bacteria cause disease upon infection of readily accessible, non-sterile sites, as well as other tissues.
- Normal microbial flora can cause disease when they invade or are inserted into normally sterile sites.
- Disease results when tissue is destroyed, the function of an organ is com-

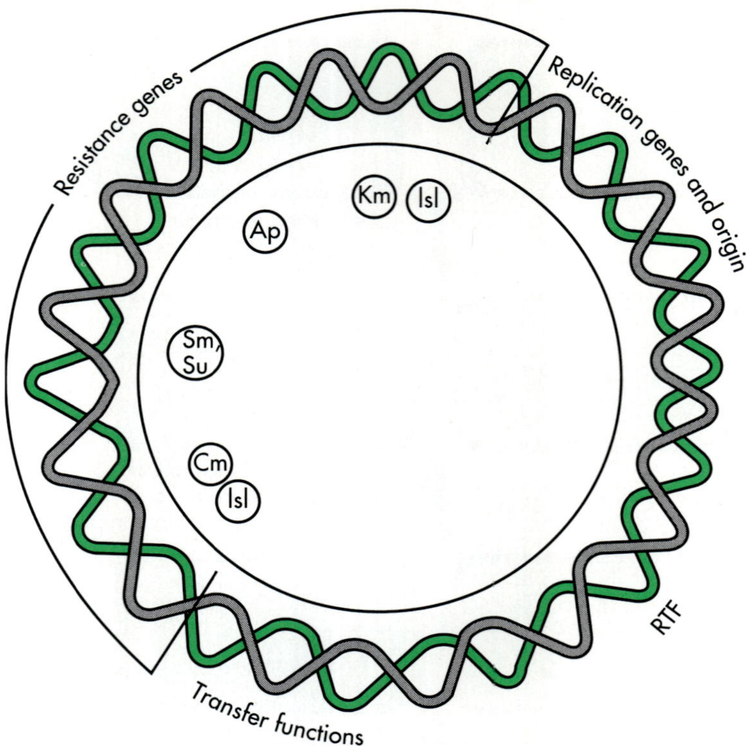

Fig. 2.15 Example of a resistance plasmid. This plasmid encodes genes required for its replication (RTF) and for antibiotic resistance: *Cm,* Chloramphenicol; *Sm,* streptomycin; *Su,* sulfonamide; *Ap,* ampicillin; and *Km,* kanamycin.

promised, or the immune and inflammatory responses are stimulated to produce systemic symptoms (e.g., fever, runny nose, headache, tiredness).

- Bacteria that spread from the primary site of infection are more virulent.
- The blood is an excellent route for spreading bacteria throughout the body.
- The longer a bacterium is in the host the more damage it can do.
- The host immune response is the best weapon against a bacterial infection and therefore, any mechanism that allows for escape from immune attack (e.g., avoidance or inactivation of phagocytosis, antibody, or complement action) enhances bacterial pathogenicity.

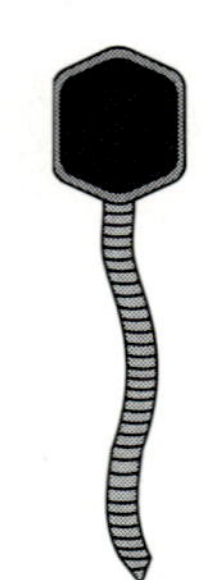

Fig. 2.16 Bacteriophage lambda.

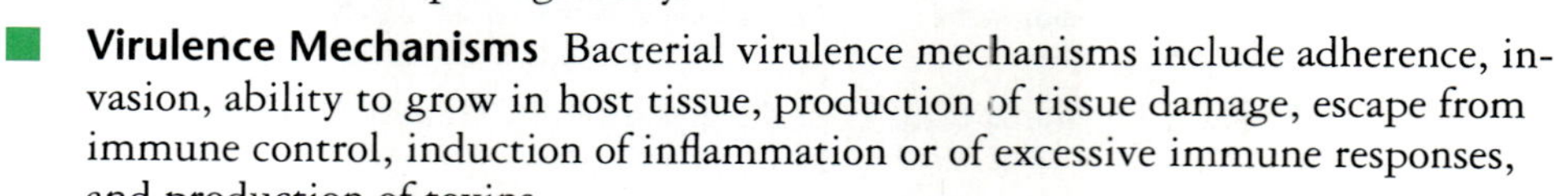

Virulence Mechanisms Bacterial virulence mechanisms include adherence, invasion, ability to grow in host tissue, production of tissue damage, escape from immune control, induction of inflammation or of excessive immune responses, and production of toxins.

The mnemonic, EAT RICE, may serve to recall the various virulence mechanisms.

E nzymes (tissue damaging)
A dhesion
T oxin (exotoxin)

R esistance mechanisms to antibiotics and immune response
I nvasion
C apsule
E ndotoxin

Table 2.5 *Examples of Microbial Adherence Mechanisms*

Microbe	Adhesin	Receptor
Bacteria		
Staphylococcus aureus	Lipoteichoic acid	Unknown
Staphylococcus spp.	Slime	Unknown
Streptococcus, group A	LTA-M protein complex	Unknown
Streptococcus, group B	Protein	N-acetyl-D-glucosamine
Escherichia coli	Type 1 fimbriae	D-mannose
	CFA/1 fimbriae	GM ganglioside
	P fimbriae	P blood group glycolipid
Other Enterobacteriaceae	Type 1 fimbriae	D-mannose
Neisseria gonorrhoeae	Fimbriae	GD_1 ganglioside
Treponema pallidum	P_1, P_2, P_3	Fibronectin
Chlamydia	Cell surface lectin	*N*-acetyl-D-glucosamine
Mycoplasma pneumoniae	Protein P1	Sialic acid

- **Adherence** Adherence to the epithelial or the endothelial cell linings of the bladder, the intestine, blood vessels, and other tissues allows the bacteria to colonize and prevents the bacteria from being washed away.

  The fimbriae (pili) are the major structures involved in bacterial adherence. Table 2.5 lists some microbial adherence mechanisms.
- **Invasion** The ability to break through tissue barriers provides access to sterile sites and susceptible tissue. For example, *Shigella* species break through the mucosa of the colon, causing ulceration and bacteremia.
- **Growth** Some bacteria have very defined growth requirements. For example, *Legionella* organisms grow in the lung and do not readily spread since they cannot tolerate higher temperatures (>35° C).

  Bacteria are part of the normal flora in many sites. Growth in normally sterile sites can cause problems.

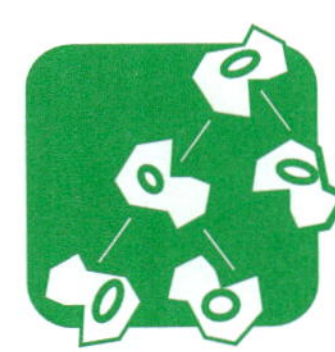

Sterile sites	**Nonsterile sites**
Blood	Urine
Cerebrospinal fluid	Mouth
Brain	Saliva
Organs	Pharynx
Lower lung	Nares

- **Tissue damage**
  - Bacterial growth produces acids, gas, and other byproducts that are toxic to tissue. An example is *Clostridium perfringens,* an organism that causes gas gangrene.
  - Many bacteria release enzymes that degrade tissue. Among these are
    - *Clostridium perfringens:* lecithinase
    - *Streptococci:* hemolysin, streptokinase
    - *Staphylococci:* hyaluronidase, fibrinolysin, lipases
  - Toxins (see discussion later in this section) are released by many bacteria and can cause tissue breakdown.
  - Tissue destruction promotes the spread of bacteria, especially if blood vessels are involved.

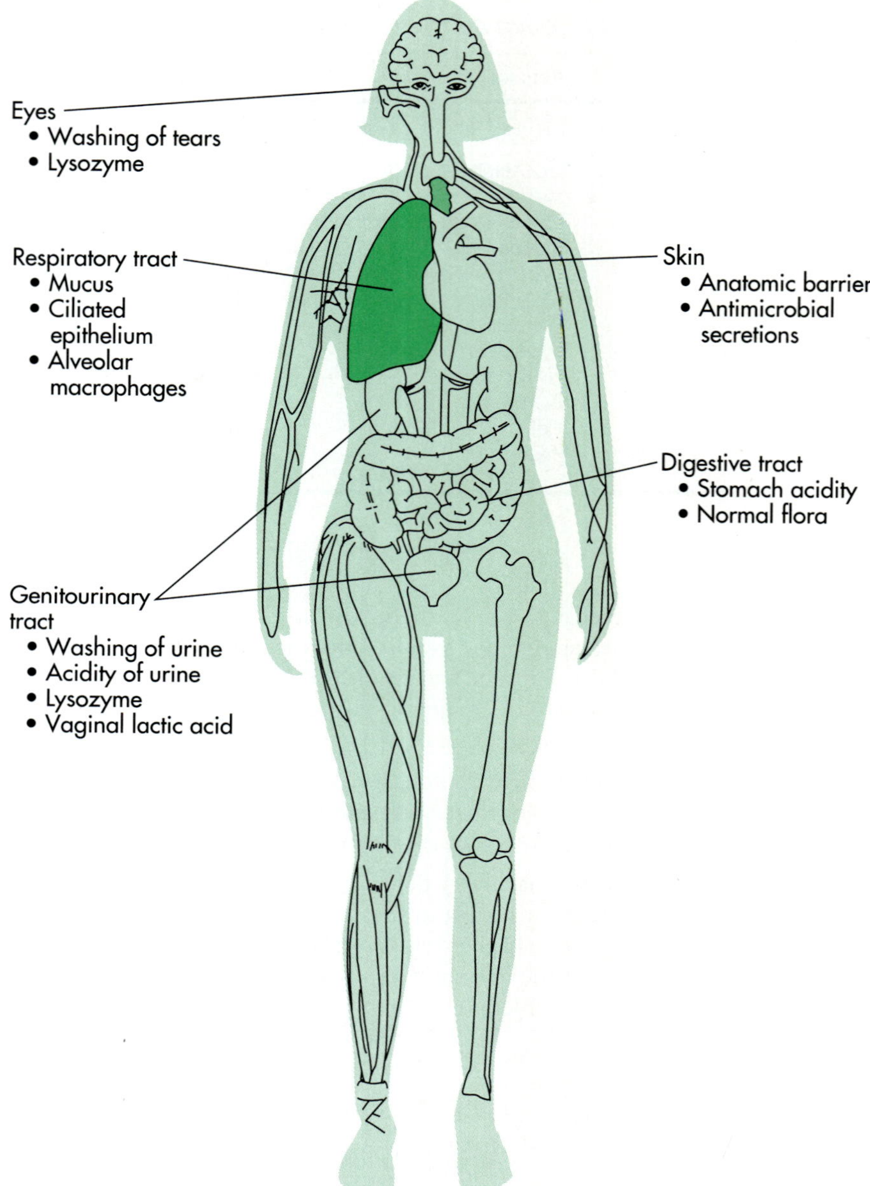

Fig. 2.17 External defense barriers of the human body.

Host defenses Several components comprise the host defense mechanism.

1. Natural barriers (Fig. 2.17)
   Lysozyme in tears and mucus is effective against gram-positive bacteria.
2. Nonspecific immune response
   A. Cellular response:

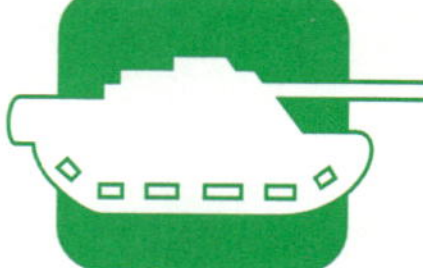

- Neutrophils or polymorphonuclear (PMN) phagocytes engulf and kill by means of peroxides, superoxide anions, hypochlorous acid, and cationic proteins for gram-negative bacteria (cathepsin G).

Deficiencies in the production of antibacterial products by PMNs

Box 2.1

EXAMPLES OF ENCAPSULATED MICROORGANISMS

Staphylococcus aureus
Streptococcus pneumoniae
Streptococcus pyogenes (group A)
Streptococcus agalactiae (group B)
Bacillus anthracis
Bacillus subtilis
Neisseria gonorrhoeae
Neisseria meningitidis
Hemophilus influenzae
Escherichia coli
Klebsiella pneumoniae
Salmonella
Yersinia pestis
Campylobacter fetus
Pseudomonas aeruginosa
Bacteroides fragilis
Cryptococcus neoformans (Yeast)

increases the risk for infection. For example, in Chediak Higashi Syndrome there is a cationic protein deficiency resulting in chronic skin infections. In chronic granulomatous disease (CGD) there is a deficiency in myeloperoxidase or glucose-6-phosphate dehydrogenase that decreases the production of toxic oxygen species.

Bacterial infection is often indicated by the presence of PMNs in a normally sterile site or fluid and by a left shift indicative of recruitment of immature neutrophils (bands) from the bone marrow.

- Macrophages and monocytes engulf and kill bacteria, produce lymphokines and interferon, and present antigens to $CD4^+$ T cells.

B. Complement activation:

C3 is generated by the alternative (properdin) pathway, which is activated by capsular material and other bacterial polysaccharides.

Activated complement components opsonize the bacteria and puncture the cell membrane.

3. Specific immune responses

- Antibody is the major antibacterial immune response.
- Antibody opsonizes bacteria for phagocytic uptake.
- Antibody (IgG and IgM) activates the complement cascade.
- T cells may respond to intracellular bacterial infections, for example, *mycobacteria* and *Listeria monocytogenes.*

Escape from immune control

1. Production of a capsule

The capsule is probably one of the most important virulence factors of bacteria (Box 2.1).

Capsules (slime layers)

- are composed of polysaccharides or proteins
- are poorly antigenic (Hyaluronic acid capsule of *Streptococcus pyogenes* mimics human connective tissue, thereby preventing an immune response.)

Table 2.6 ***Methods Developed to Circumvent Phagocytic Killing***

Method	Example
Inhibition of phagolysosome fusion	*Legionella, Mycobacterium tuberculosis, Chlamydia*
Resistance to lysosomal enzymes	*Salmonella typhimurium, Coxiella, Ehrlichia, Mycobacterium leprae, Leishmania*
Adaptation to cytoplasmic replication	*Listeria, Francisella, Rickettsia*

- deter phagocytosis
- protect against degradation in phagosomes of macrophages and neutrophils

The virulence of certain organisms is correlated with the presence of a capsule (e.g., *Streptococcus pneumoniae, Neisseria meningitidis*).

2. Evasion of the immune response by intracellular growth without inactivation (especially in macrophages)

Some of the strategies that certain bacterial species have developed to bypass intracellular killing are listed in Table 2.6.

3. Inactivation of phagocytic cell function

Some of the mechanisms that bacteria use to inactivate phagocytes are:

- inhibition of phagocytosis (e.g., M protein of *S. pyogenes* is antiphagocytic)
- prevention of intracellular killing by capsules
- production of catalase to reduce the effectiveness of phagolysosomal killing by the myeloperoxidase system (e.g., *Staphylococcus* spp.)
- killing of cells (e.g., streptolysins of *Streptococcus pyogenes* and the alpha-toxin of *Clostridium perfringens*)

4. Inactivation of antibody

- *N. gonorrhoeae* synthesizes a protease that breaks down IgA.
- *S. aureus* produces an IgG-binding protein called Protein A.

- **Induction of inflammatory responses or excessive immune responses**
  In many cases, the immune response to the bacterium is responsible for tissue damage. (This, however, is more true for viruses than for bacteria.) Examples of such organisms are *chlamydia, treponemes,* and *borrelia.*

  Rheumatic fever, which is a sequela to streptococcal infections is caused by antibodies to the Streptococcal M protein that cross-react with and initiate damage to the heart. *Poststreptococcal glomerulonephritis* is caused by formation of immune complexes that deposit in the glomeruli of the kidneys and cause nephritis.

- **Superantigens (Fig. 2.18)**

  • Superantigens are toxinlike molecules that activate T cells by binding to both the T cell receptor and an MHC class II molecule on another cell without requiring antigen.

  • This nonspecific means of activating T cells can stimulate

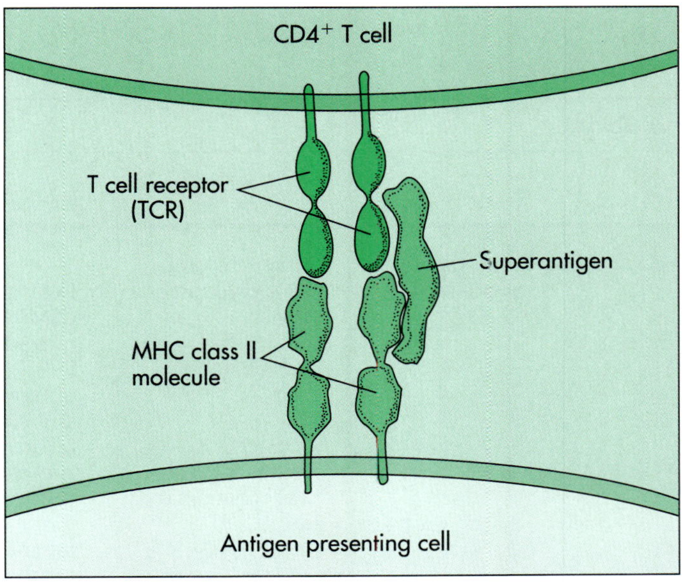

Fig. 2.18 Superantigen binding to external regions of the T-cell receptor and of the major histocompatibility complex (MHC) class II molecules.

life-threatening autoimmune responses by stimulating the release of large amounts of interleukins, for example, IL-1 and IL-2.

- Superantigen stimulation of T cells can lead to death of the T cells and loss of immune responsiveness.
- Examples of superantigens are the following:
  - Toxic shock syndrome toxin (TSST) of *S. aureus*
  - Staphylococcal enterotoxins
  - Erythrogenic toxin A or C of *S. pyogenes*

Toxins

— *Endotoxin*

- Endotoxin causes fever and shock.
- *All gram-negative bacteria make endotoxin, which is the lipid A portion of lipopolysaccharide.*
- Endotoxin is released from gram-negative bacteria and binds and activates B lymphocytes and macrophages.
- Responses to endotoxin:
  - Induction of endogenous pyrogens: IL-1, TNF, IL-6, prostaglandins
  - Initiation of complement and blood coagulation cascades
  - Activation of B lymphocytes
  - Fever, hypotension, shock, and possibly death
  - **Schwartzman Reaction**—a shocklike response to endotoxin

— ***Exotoxin*** Some bacteria produce protein toxins that inactivate or alter cellular properties. Many bacterial toxins are dimeric with an A and a B subunit. The B subunit binds to the host cell surface and the A subunit enters the cell and exerts its biologic effects. The characteristics of some A-B types of exotoxins are presented in Table 2.7.

***Note:* Endotoxin is not the same as exotoxin.**

Table 2.7 *Properties of A-B Type Bacterial Toxins*

Toxin	Organism	Genetic Control	Subunit Structure	Target Cell Receptor	Biologic Effects
Anthrax toxins	*B. anthracis*	Plasmid	Three separate proteins (EF, LF, PA)	Unknown, probably glycoprotein	EF + PA: increase in target cell cAMP level, localized edema; LF + PA: death of target cells and experimental animals
Bordetella adenylate cyclase toxin	*Bordetella* species	Chromosomal	A-B	Unknown, probably glycolipid	Increase in target cell cAMP level; modified cell function or cell death
Botulinum toxin	*C. botulinum*	Phage	A-B	Possibly ganglioside (GD_{1b})	Decrease in peripheral presynaptic acetylcholine release; flaccid paralysis
Cholera toxin	*V. cholerae*	Chromosomal	A-5B	Ganglioside (GM_1)	Activation of adenylate cyclase, increase in cAMP level; secretory diarrhea
Diphtheria toxin	*C. diphtheriae*	Phage	A-B	Probably glycoprotein	Inhibition of protein synthesis; cell death
Heat-labile enterotoxins	*E. coli*	Plasmid	Similar or identical to cholera toxin		
Pertussis toxin	*B. pertussis*	Chromosomal	A-5B	Unknown, probably glycoprotein	Block of signal transduction mediated by target G proteins
Pseudomonas exotoxin A	*P. aeruginosa*	Chromosomal	A-B	Unknown, but different from diphtheria toxin	Similar or identical to diphtheria toxin
Shiga toxin	*S. dysenteriae*	Chromosomal	A-5B	Glycoprotein or glycolipid	Inhibition of protein synthesis, cell death
Shiga-like toxins	*Shigella* species, *E. coli*	Phage	Similar or identical to shiga toxin		
Tetanus toxin	*C. tetani*	Plasmid	A-B	Ganglioside (GT_1) and/or GD_{1b}	Decrease in neurotransmitter release from inhibitory neurons; spastic paralysis

Modified from Mandell G, Douglas G, Bennett J: *Principles and practice of infectious disease,* ed 3, New York, 1990, Churchill Livingstone.

Section 2.4 Laboratory Diagnosis of Bacterial Diseases

Bacteria can be identified by growth and colony characteristics, morphology, gram stain reaction, biochemical tests, and immunologic tests (Fig. 2.19).

Staining Reactions

Gram stain

- Bacteria are heat fixed onto a slide and stained first with crystal violet, then with Gram's iodine, which precipitates the stain.
- The decolorization step removes untrapped stain, and the safranin counterstains gram-negative bacteria red.
- The thick gram-positive peptidoglycan cell wall traps the stain and resists decolorization, thus causing gram-positive organisms to appear purple.
- The gram stain does not work on old cultures or on cultures treated with beta-lactam antibiotics.
- The organisms appear gram variable because the peptidoglycan is weakened.

Acid-fast stain

- This stain is used to identify mycobacteria and nocardia, which have a waxlike outer layer.

Bacterial Growth and Isolation Bacterial growth, isolation, and preliminary identification can be performed using appropriate media (Tables 2.8 and 2.9). Appropriate procedures for obtaining samples are provided in Table 2.10. Some bacteria have special growth requirements, for example, special metabolites, anaerobic culture conditions, or a higher carbon dioxide tension.

Biochemical Tests Analysis of basic biochemical capabilities (for example, the use of certain metabolites such as sugars and the formation of certain end-products) helps to distinguish different bacteria.

Examples of biochemical tests:

- Catalase test: distinguishes staphylococci from streptococci
- Coagulase test: differentiates pathogenic *S. aureus* from *S. epidermidis*
- Oxidase test: positive reaction identifies *Pseudomonas, Neisseria,* and *Moraxella* spp.

Immunologic Tests Antigens can be useful in identifying bacteria and in distinguishing between different strains of bacteria. For example, serotypes of *E. coli* are distinguished by possessing different O-antigens (lipopolysaccharide). Enterohemorrhagic strains of *E. coli* are of the serotype O157:H7.

Agglutination reactions

- Ouchterlony test: diffusion of antigen and antibody in agar, with precipitation at the equivalence point (see Fig. 1.10).
- Latex agglutination: agglutination of latex beads coated with antibody by antigen or bacteria.

Direct antigen visualization

- Immunofluorescence: e.g., *Treponema pallidum*
- EIA: enzyme immunoassay on tissue sections

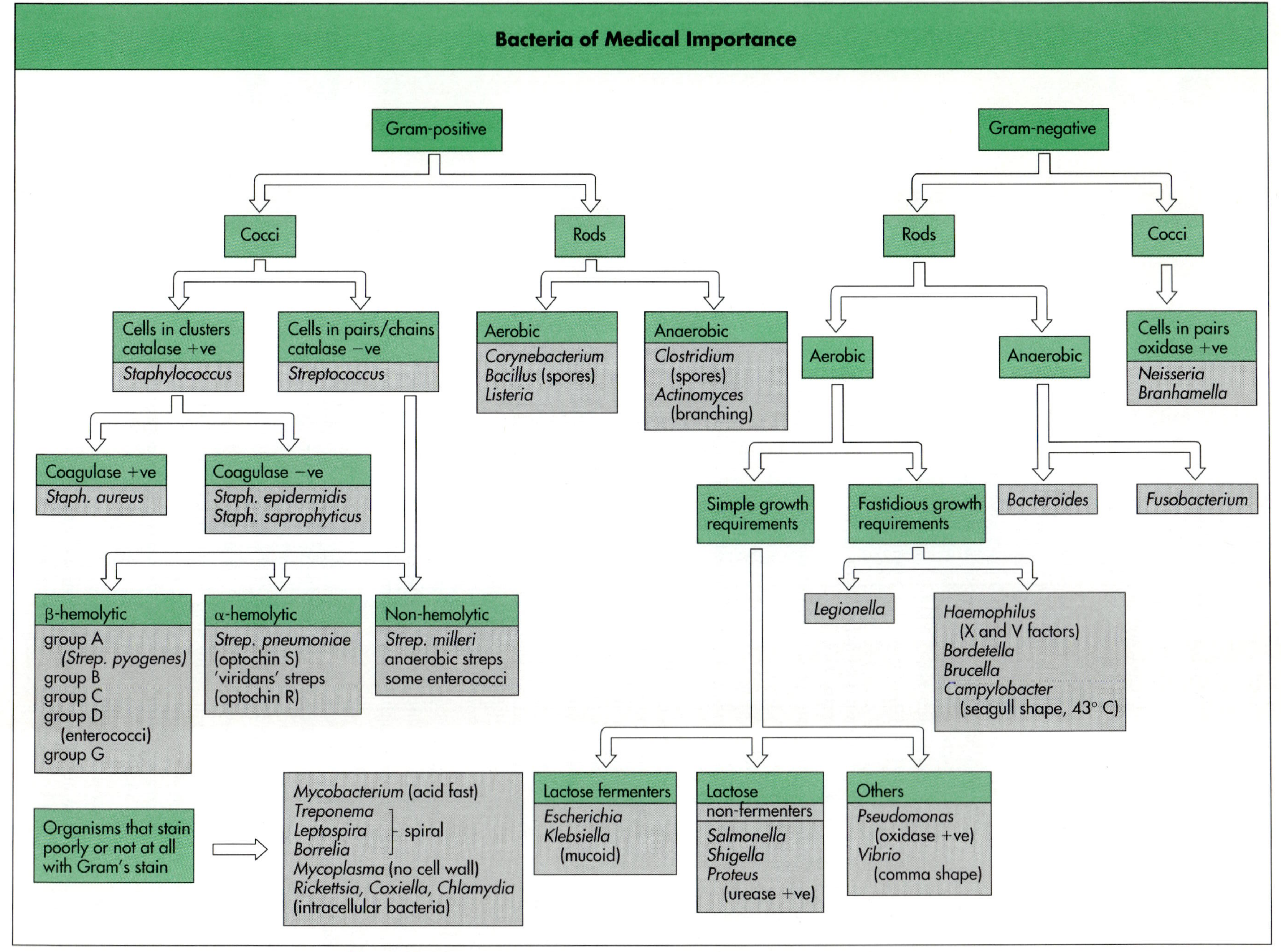

Fig. 2.19 Characteristic laboratory properties of medically important bacteria.

Table 2.8 *Bacterial Culture Media*

Medium	Bacteria Isolated or Identified
Non-selective	
Blood agar	All bacteria
Selective and Differential	
Mannitol salt agar	*Staphylococcus aureus*
MacConkey's agar	Gram-negative enteric bacilli (colonies of lactose-positive bacteria are red)
Eosin methylene blue (EMB) agar	Gram-negative enteric bacilli
Hektoen enteric (HE) agar	Gram-negative enteric bacilli (colonies of H_2S producers are black; colonies of sucrose fermenters are yellow-red)
Special Media	
Chocolate agar (blood heated to release factors X and V)	*Neisseria* and *Hemophilus* spp.
Thayer-Martin medium (selective chocolate agar)	*Neisseria gonorrhoeae*
Lowenstein-Jensen medium	Mycobacteria

Table 2.9 *Significant Colony Characteristics*

Characteristic	Bacteria Identified
Hemolysis in Blood Agar	
Alpha (green zone around colony)	*Streptococcus viridans*
Beta (clear zone around colony)	*Streptococcus pyogenes* Staphylococci
Swarming	*Proteus mirabilis* *Proteus vulgaris*

- Antigen detection
  - ELISA: enzyme linked immunosorbent assay
  - RIA: radioimmunoassay

Antibiotic Sensitivity Testing

- **Minimal inhibitory concentration (MIC)** The MIC is the lowest concentration of drug that inhibits bacterial growth and can be determined by testing serial dilutions of antibiotic on the organism isolated from the patient.
- **Minimal biocidal concentration (MBC)** The MBC is the lowest concentration of drug that *kills* the bacteria. It can be determined by plating the bacteria tested for MIC. Certain antibiotics and lower concentrations of other antibiotics may only be *bacteriostatic* (i.e., they do not kill, but only inhibit growth).
- **Kirby-Bauer disk diffusion assay** Antibiotic-impregnated disks are placed on top of a freshly plated bacterial isolate. The antibiotic diffuses from the disk into the agar medium. The diameters of the zones of inhibition for the various antibiotics (the zone is different for each antibiotic) have

Table 2.10 *Specimens For Bacterial Analysis*

Specimen	Collection	Comments
Blood, for routine culture	Use blood culture bottles with enriched nutrients.	Performed on patients suspected to have bacteremia; bacteremia may be continuous or intermittent.
	Number of samples: two to three separate samplings are ideal.	Collecting more than three samples over a 24 hour period provides little advantage; a single blood culture may be positive because of contamination, intermittent bacteremia, or a low bacterial count.
	Volume of blood: 20 ml/culture in adults; 5-10 ml/culture in children; 1-2 ml/culture in neonates.	A large volume of blood per sampling is preferred because more than half the patients have fewer than one organism/ml of blood; there is a greater than 40% increase in yield when the culture volume is increased from 10 to 20 ml.
Blood, for intracellular organisms	Collect by lysis centrifugation.	Same principle in collection as for routine blood culture; intracellular bacteria are released by lysis of cells and concentrated.
Cerebrospinal fluid	Use sterile screw-capped tube; inoculate on appropriate culture media.	Bacterial meningitis is an emergency because of rapid progression and high mortality. Specimen should be transported to the laboratory and processed immediately for gram staining, culture, antigen detection, etc. Specimen should not be refrigerated or heated.
Catheter (venous or arterial)	Use sterile container for transport.	Catheter should be removed aseptically. The catheter should be rolled across a blood agar plate and a semiquantitative culture should be performed.
Throat swab	Place in transport medium.	Contact with saliva should be avoided (growth of *Streptococcus pyogenes* may be inhibited).
Ear aspirate (otitis media)	Use sterile container.	Specimen should be aspirated with a needle and syringe and sent to laboratory for culture. Culture of external ear has no predictive value for otitis media.
Sputum	Use sterile container.	Expectorated sputum is frequently contaminated with oral flora. Sputum culture should be interpreted with a good knowledge of gram-stain results. Sputum specimens with more than 25 squamous epithelial cells per low power microscopic field and with no predominant bacteria should not be accepted for processing.
Tissue specimen	Use sterile screw-capped tube and sterile anaerobic tube or vial.	Representative sample from the border and the center of the lesion should be obtained.
Exudates (transudates, wound drainage, ulcers) or pus (abscess, wound)	Immerse swab into transport medium; aspirate into sterile container. If the aspirate is from an abscess or a closed cavity, use anaerobic transport system.	Avoid contamination with surfaces. If aspirated from an abscess or a closed cavity, consider culture for aerobes and anaerobes.

Continued.

Table 2.10 ***Specimens For Bacterial Analysis—cont'd***

Specimen	Collection	Comments
Specimen from sterile sites (e.g., synovium, peritoneum, chest)	Use sterile container.	Injection of air into the culture bottle should be avoided because this will inhibit growth of anaerobes.
Urine, midstream Urine, catheterized	Use sterile container.	Specimen must be transported immediately to the laboratory.
Genital or urethral cultures	Immerse swab in transport medium.	Some genital pathogens are extremely labile. Only the area of inflammation should be sampled.
Feces	Transport in a screw-capped container.	Specimen should be transported to laboratory rapidly to prevent production of acid by normal fecal flora.

been correlated with the achievable blood levels of those antibiotics to indicate sensitivity and resistance. The Kirby-Bauer method is *not useful* for all infections because it only reflects levels in blood. For example, it cannot be used for infections of the central nervous system (CNS) or bone.

Section 2.5 Antibacterial Drugs and Vaccines

Antimicrobial Drugs

- An antimicrobial drug is a drug that kills (**bacteriocidal**) or stops the growth (**bacteriostatic**) of a bacterium or fungus.
- Most antimicrobials are **inhibitors of essential enzymes** or **disrupters of membranes.**
- Good targets for antimicrobial drugs are microbial structures or enzymes that have no mammalian counterpart or that differ from their mammalian counterpart, for example, **peptidoglycan and 70S ribosomal units.**

Determinants of Sensitivity or Resistance to Antimicrobial Drugs

1. The ability to inhibit an essential enzyme (e.g., D-ala-D-ala transpeptidase is inhibited by penicillin) is influenced by the following factors:

   - The binding efficiency to the target enzyme (if the drug is too bulky to fit into the active site or if a mutation altered the active site, the effectiveness of the drug will be decreased).
   - The amount of target enzyme in the bacteria (more enzyme would require more inhibitor).
   - Importance of the enzyme target. The enzyme or the pathway has to be an essential one for the antibiotic to be useful.

2. The ability of the drug to be sufficiently concentrated at its site of action in the bacterial cell is an important consideration.

   - The outer membrane of gram-negative bacteria is a barrier to large-sized and hydrophobic drugs.

Box 2.2

BASIC MECHANISMS OF ANTIBIOTIC ACTION

Inhibition of Cell Wall Synthesis

Penicillins
Cephalosporins
Cephamycins
Carbapenems
Monobactams
β-lactamase inhibitors
Vancomycin
Bacitracin
Isoniazid
Cycloserine
Ethionamide

Disruption of Cell Membranes

Polymyxins

Inhibition of Protein Synthesis

Aminoglycosides
Tetracyclines
Chloramphenicol
Macrolides
Clindamycin

Inhibition of Nucleic Acid Synthesis

Rifampin
Quinolones
Metronidazole

Antimetabolites

Sulfonamides
Trimethoprim
Dapsone

- The porin channels in the gram-negative outer membrane provide entry for only *small hydrophilic* drugs.
- An active transport mechanism may be required to concentrate the drug. For example, tetracycline is actively transported into cells. Resistance can occur if tetracycline is also actively pumped out of cells.

3. Some bacteria synthesize enzymes that inactivate antibiotics. These enzymes may be encoded on the chromosome or on a plasmid.

- Degradative enzymes break down the antibiotic (e.g., beta-lactamase cleaves the beta-lactam ring of penicillins).
- Enzymes may cause drug modifications (e.g., acetylation or phosphorylation of aminoglycosides) that prevent their action.

4. The pharmacologic properties of a drug may determine its effectiveness. Some of these are

- acid stability (for orally administered drugs)
- tissue distribution
- biological half-life (stability and retention in the body)

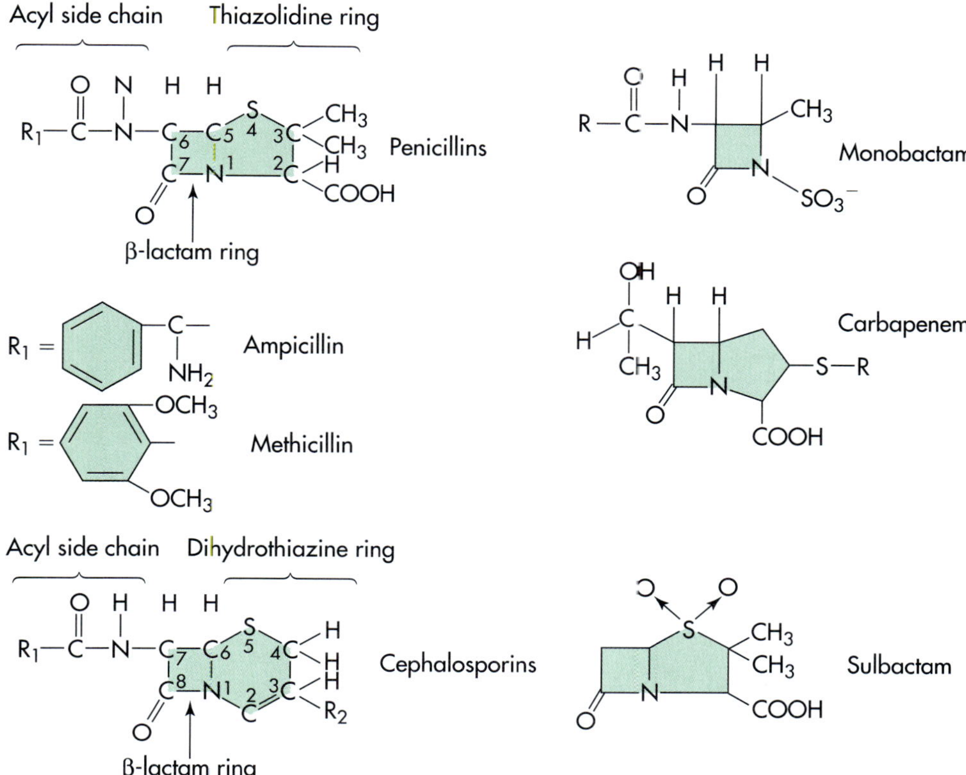

Fig. 2.20 General structures of the main classes of β-lactam antibiotics. Addition of a hydrophilic unit for R_1 increases activity to gram-negative bacteria; a bulky unit increases resistance to β-lactamases. Additional variations are possible at some of the non-R group positions. For example, the cephamycins and cephalosporins differ by replacing the sulfur molecule at the 5 position with oxygen. The arrow points to the bond that is broken during β-lactamase catalyzed hydrolysis. *(Modified from Wingard LB, Brody TM, Larner J, et al., editors:* Human pharmacology: molecular to clinical, *St Louis, 1991, Mosby.)*

Mechanisms of Action of Antibacterial Drugs and Resistance to Antibacterial Drugs (Box 2.2)

Inhibitors of peptidoglycan synthesis (see Fig. 2.9)

— *Beta-lactam antibiotics (penicillins, cephalosporins, monobactams, and carbapenems) (Fig. 2.20)*

- The **beta-lactam ring** is essential for the activity of these antibiotics. Penicillins look like the backbone of the terminal D-ala-D-ala of the peptide precursor used for cross-linking of the peptidoglycan.
- The target enzymes for beta-lactam antibiotics are transpeptidases and D,D carboxypeptidases (also known as **penicillin binding proteins [PBPs]**), enzymes responsible for cross-linking the peptidoglycan.
- Inhibition of cross-linking weakens the peptidoglycan and allows degradative processes to further weaken the structure. This leads to cell lysis.
- Beta-lactam antibiotics are **bacteriocidal.**
- For a beta-lactam antibiotic to be effective, the drug must reach

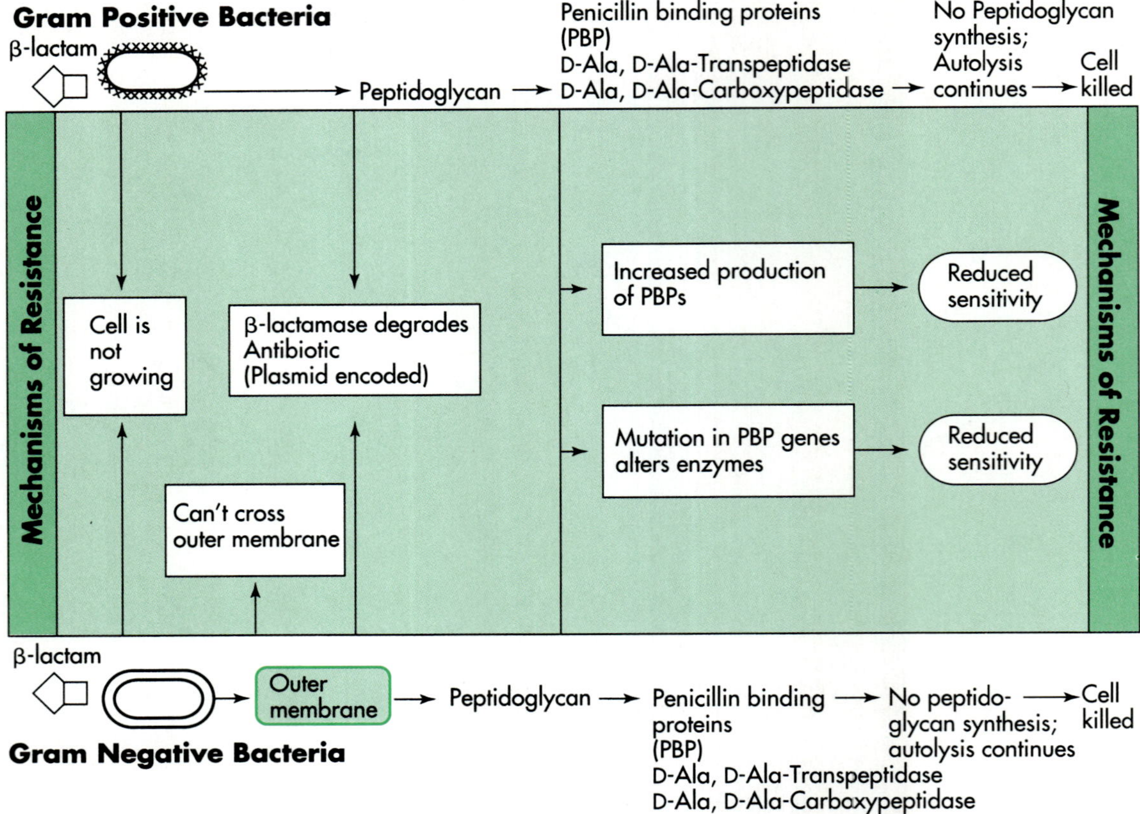

Fig. 2.21 Mechanisms of resistance to beta-lactam antibiotics. Beta-lactam antibiotics must reach the penicillin binding protein target enzymes in a growing cell before being degraded, in order to kill the cell. *(Figure modified from Wingard LB, Brody TM, Larner J, and Schwartz:* Human pharmacology: molecular to clinical, *St Louis, 1991, Mosby.)*

its target at the surface of the cytoplasmic membrane and bind a sufficient concentration of the enzyme.

- Beta-lactam antibiotics **act only on growing cells.**

Mechanisms of resistance to beta-lactam antibiotics (Fig. 2.21)

1. The gram-negative bacterial outer membrane limits uptake of the more hydrophobic and bulky beta-lactam antibiotics.
2. Many strains of bacteria make beta-lactamase, an enzyme that cleaves the beta-lactam ring, inactivating the drug.
3. The beta-lactamase gene is encoded on plasmids, allowing for easy spread of resistance through a bacterial population and even to related strains.
4. A chromosomal mutation may change the active site of the target enzymes so that the drug can no longer bind.
5. A bacterium may synthesize high levels of enzyme, requiring more inhibitor (more drug).
6. A mutation in the porin proteins can alter the permeability of the drug (e.g., imipenems).

Derivatives and analogs

- Smaller drugs with increased hydrophilicity (e.g., ampicillin) pass through the porins of the outer membrane of gram-negative bacteria.

- Bulkier derivatives are generally more resistant to beta-lactamases.
- Analogs of penicillin (clavulanic acid, sulbactam) administered with beta-lactam antibiotics, inhibit the beta-lactamase.

— ***Vancomycin***

- Vancomycin is a complex glycopeptide that is used **only for gram-positive** bacteria.
- Vancomycin is too bulky to pass through the outer membrane of gram-negative bacteria.
- Vancomycin **inhibits the translocation of precursors and, therefore, elongation of the peptidoglycan** carbohydrate chain.
- Resistance to vancomycin among gram-positive bacteria is not common.
- Vancomycin is the drug of choice for many infections caused by beta-lactam resistant organisms (especially staphylococcal infections).

— ***Bacitracin and cycloserine***

- Bacitracin prevents reuse of the lipid carrier that translocates the peptidoglycan precursors from the cytoplasm across the membrane.
- Bacitracin is used in most **topical antibiotic ointments.**
- Cycloserine inhibits the enzymes that make the D-alanine and the D-ala-D-ala dipeptide portion of the peptide chain of the peptidoglycan precursor.
- Cycloserine is sometimes used for treatment of tuberculosis.

Disruption of microbial membranes

— ***Polymyxins***

- Polymyxins are peptide antibiotics that are especially active against gram-negative bacteria.
- Polymyxins can disrupt the outer membrane and the cytoplasmic membrane of gram-negative bacteria.
- The selectivity for bacteria is based on differences in lipid composition of prokaryotic and eukaryotic cell membranes.
- Polymyxins are used in most **topical antibiotic ointments.**

— ***Amphotericin and nystatin***

- Amphotericin and nystatin are **antifungal compounds.**
- These drugs interact with **cholesterol** in fungal membranes, disrupt their structure, and create pores in the membranes, increasing their permeability.
- The toxicity of these drugs limits their use to severe cases only.

Inhibitors of DNA replication

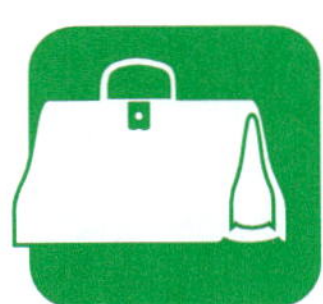

— ***Topoisomerase inhibitors:***

- Topoisomerases are essential for maintaining proper DNA structure for transcription and replication of the chromosome.
- Gyrase is one of the topoisomerases.

Quinolones

- Quinolones inhibit bacterial gyrase activity.

Table 2.11 ***Inhibitors of Bacterial Ribosome Function***

Drug	Target	Action	Result	Resistance
Aminoglycosides (streptomycin, gentamycin, tobramycin, amikacin, kanamycin)	30S ribosomal subunit	Misreads, blocks initiation	C	(1) Mutation of ribosomal binding site; (2) decreased antibiotic uptake; or (3) enzymatic modification of drug, e.g., acetylation or phosphorylation (plasmid encoded)
Tetracyclines	30S/tRNA complex	Block tRNA binding	S	Increased efflux from cell (plasmid-encoded)
Chloramphenicol	50S/tRNA complex	Blocks peptidyl transfer	C	Enzymatic modification of drug (plasmid-encoded)
Macrolides (erythromycin)	50S subunit	Blocks chain extension	S	Methylation of ribosomal target blocks the binding of drug (plasmid-encoded)

C, Bacteriocidal; *S*, bacteriostatic.

- Resistance to quinolones arises upon mutation or impermeability of the gyrase enzyme.
- They are broad-spectrum antibiotics.
- Examples of quinolone antibiotics are ciprofloxacin, norfloxacin, and nalidixic acid.

- **Inhibitors of mRNA transcription**

  — ***Rifampin***

  - Rifampin binds to the bacterial **RNA polymerase** and prevents initiation of mRNA synthesis.
  - Resistance occurs readily because of mutations in RNA polymerase.

- **Inhibitors of protein synthesis (Table 2.11)**

  - Bacterial protein synthesis is a prime target for antibiotics. The bacterial ribosome is 70S in size and all the ribosomal proteins are different from those in the 80S eukaryotic ribosome.
  - Antibiotics either prevent initiation of protein synthesis, peptide bond formation or chain elongation, or cause misreading of the mRNA.
  - Resistance results from enzymatic inactivation of the antibiotic or its target site, mutation of the target site, or altered transport of the drug.

- **Inhibition of nucleotide biosynthesis** Sulfa drugs and trimethoprim inhibit the synthesis of folic acid, which is required for production of nucleic acids (Fig. 2.22).

- **Other mechanisms** Antituberculosis drugs, such as isoniazid, ethionamide, and pyrazinamide exert their action by inhibiting the synthesis of mycolic acid and other waxy components of the mycobacterial cell wall.

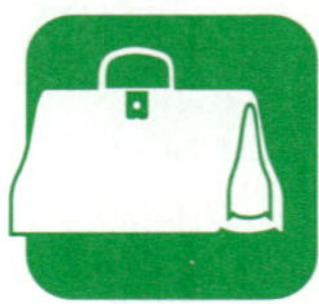

Vaccines

- Types of immunization

  1. **Passive immunization:** Treatment with immune serum globulin (gamma globulin). The most commonly treated diseases and the source of the immune serum are listed on page 79.

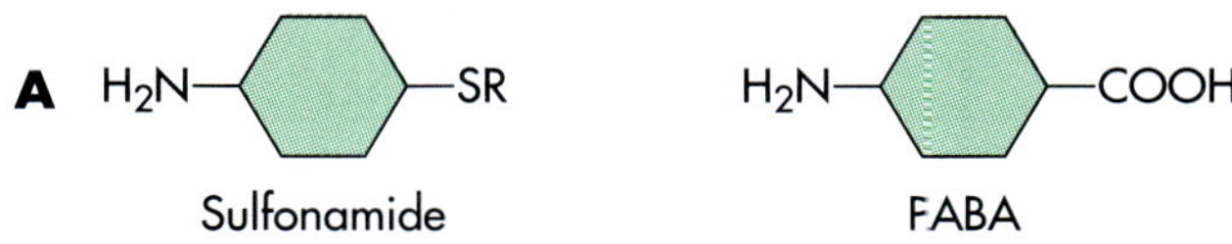

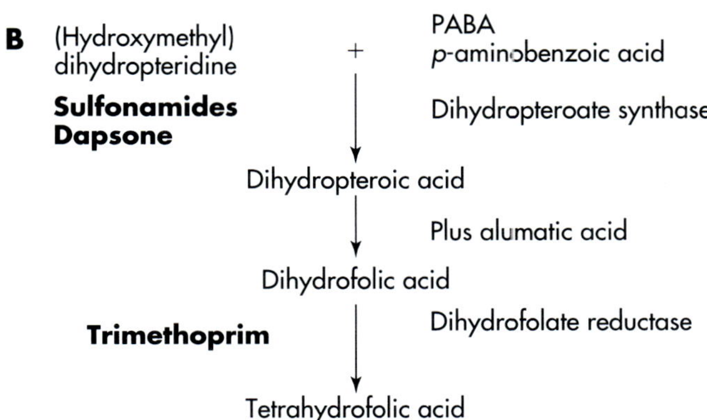

Fig. 2.22 Antimetabolic activity. **A,** Sulfonamides, which resemble PABA, and dapsone competitively inhibit dihydropteroate synthase. **B,** Trimethoprim inhibits enzymatic action of dihydrofolate reductase. Both steps interfere with synthesis of folic acid, which is required by bacteria.

Disease	Source
tetanus	human or equine
botulism	equine
diphtheria	equine

2. **Active immunization:** Induction of an immune response with inactivated or live vaccines.

- **Bacterial vaccines (Table 2.12)**
  - Vaccines for bacterial disease use inactivated organisms except for *M. tuberculosis* (BCG) vaccine.
  - Many antibacterial vaccines are toxoids (i.e., inactivated toxins).
  - The *hemophilus influenza B* (Hib) vaccine consists of the capsular polysaccharide conjugated to protein.
  - For a further discussion of vaccines, see Section 3.4.

Section 2.6 Staphylococci

- **General features** Staphylococci are gram-positive cocci.
- **Laboratory identification** Laboratory identification of the staphylococci is based on the following characteristics:
  - They grow in gram-positive grapelike clusters.
  - They are **catalase positive.**
  - They grow in 7.5% salt.
  - They ferment mannitol.

Table 2.12 *Common Bacterial Vaccines**

Bacteria (Disease)	Vaccine Components	Indications
Corynebacterium diphtheriae (diphtheria)	Toxoid	Children and adults
Clostridium tetani (tetanus)	Toxoid	Children and adults
Bordetella pertussis (pertussis)	Killed cell	Children
Hemophilus influenzae B (Hib; Hemophilus disease)	Capsule polysaccharide; capsule polysaccharide-protein conjugate	Children
Streptococcal pneumoniae (Pneumococcus)	Capsule polysaccharide	Children and adults

*Listed in order of frequency of use.

- *Staphylococcus aureus* is **coagulase positive**; *Staphylococcus epidermidis* and other staphylococci are **coagulase negative.**

Staphylococcus aureus

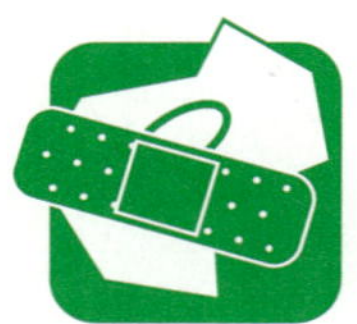

- **Pathogenesis** *S. aureus* can be part of the normal skin flora or carried in the nasopharynx, without causing disease. Infection can cause tissue destruction by invasive toxins or degradative enzymes (Tables 2.13 and 2.14).

  S. aureus adheres to fibronectin on mucosal surfaces by lipoteichoic acid. Virulence factors promote

  - tissue destruction, which provides metabolites and facilitates spread within the host
  - escape from phagocytic killing and immune control

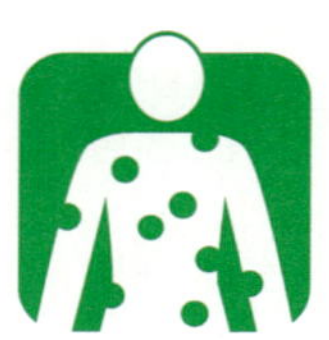

- **Diseases** Staphylococci can cause infections of the skin and internal organs, which can lead to bacteremia. The severity ranges from benign skin lesions to life-threatening systemic tissue destroying infections.

  The diseases associated with *S. aureus* are the following:

  - Toxin-mediated diseases
    - Staphylococcal toxic shock syndrome (TSST is a superantigen)
    - Staphylococcal scalded skin syndrome
    - Staphylococcal food poisoning
  - Cutaneous infections
    - Folliculitis
    - Furuncles
    - Carbuncles
    - Wound infections
  - Bacteremia, endocarditis
  - Pneumonia, empyema
  - Osteomyelitis
  - Septic arthritis

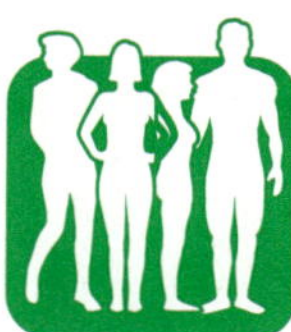

- **Epidemiology**

  Mode of spread: *Infection* can arise from the normal flora of the skin, the nasopharynx, the gastrointestinal (GI) tract, and the urinary tract. Infection is spread by contact or by fomites.

  Toxemia (food poisoning) results from the ingestion of the preformed

Table 2.13 *Mechanisms of Staphylococcal Pathogenesis: Toxins*

Toxin	Comments
Exfoliative toxin: exfoliative toxin A and B (also known as exfoliatin or epidermolytic toxin)	Breaks down intercellular bridges (desmosomes) in the stratum granulosum of the epithelium; toxin is responsible for scalded skin syndrome
Toxic shock syndrome toxin 1 (TSST 1) (formerly known as pyrogenic exotoxin C or enterotoxin F)	Acts as a superantigen; responsible for toxic shock syndrome
Enterotoxins (A-E)	Found in both *S. aureus* and *S. epidermidis*; acts as a superantigen; responsible for symptoms of gastroenteritis in food poisoning
Cytolytic toxins	
Alpha-toxin	Cytotoxic for erythrocytes, leukocytes, hepatocytes, platelets, human diploid fibroblasts, HeLa cells, and Ehrlich ascites carcinoma cells; causes necrosis when given subcutaneously
Beta-toxin (also known as sphingomyelinase C)	Toxic for erythrocytes, leukocytes, macrophages, and fibroblasts; together with alpha-toxin, beta-toxin is responsible for tissue destruction and abscess formation
Delta-toxin	Toxic to a wide variety of cells because of disruption of the cellular membrane
Gamma-toxin	Toxic to a wide variety of cells; mechanism of action unknown
Leukocidin	Kills macrophages and neutrophils by increasing leukocyte cell membrane permeability; confers resistance to phagocytosis

Table 2.14 *Mechanisms of Staphylococcal Pathogenesis: Enzymes and Proteins*

Enzyme	Action
Catalase	Prevents intracellular killing
Coagulase	Causes coagulation of fibrin
Hyaluronidase	Promotes tissue destruction and spread of bacteria
Fibrinolysin	Promotes tissue destruction and spread of bacteria
Lipase	Promotes tissue destruction and spread of bacteria
Nuclease	Promotes tissue destruction and spread of bacteria
Penicillinase	Confers antibiotic resistance on organisms
Protein A	Binds Fc portion of IgG
Teichoic and lipoteichoic acids	Promotes adherence
Other substances	
Capsular material	Prevents intracellular killing

toxin in foods, especially picnic and party foods, such as meat (cold cuts) and salad (potato or egg).

Populations affected: Staphylococci pose a risk for the following groups of people:

- Babies—staphylococcal scalded skin syndrome
- Young children—impetigo
- Trauma victims—wound infections, bacteremia
- Patients with intravascular catheters—bacteremia, endocarditis
- Patients of all ages with compromised pulmonary function—pneumonia

- Menstruating women—toxic shock syndrome

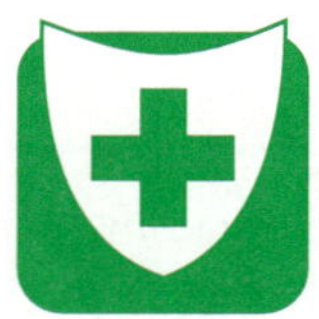

Occurrence: Staphylococci are ubiquitous and disseminated worldwide. Food poisoning is more common in summer.

- **Prevention** Preventive measures include handwashing, proper cleansing of wounds, refrigerating foods, and preparing foods properly.
- **Treatment**

- Most strains of *Staphylococcus* are resistant to penicillins because they produce beta-lactamase.
- Penicillinase-resistant beta-lactam antibiotics, such as nafcillin, oxacillin, and first-generation cephalosporins should be used.
- Methicillin-resistant *Staphylococcus* spp. have a modified target enzyme and therefore are resistant to other beta-lactam antibiotics. Vancomycin is used for severe infections. These organisms are frequently susceptible to minocycline.

Coagulase-Negative Staphylococci (*S. epidermidis* and *S. saprophyticies*)

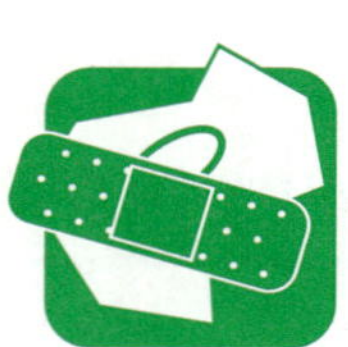

- **Pathogenesis**
  - These organisms normally are benign colonizers of the skin.
  - They can adhere to congenitally (or otherwise) defective heart valves, artificial heart valves, catheters, shunts, and prosthetic joints. Adherence may lead to colonization and destruction of tissue by degradative enzymes.

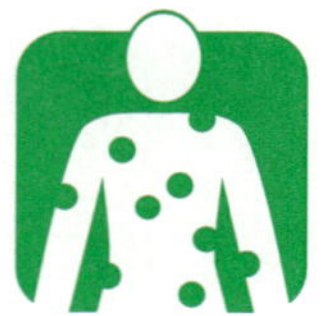

- **Diseases**
  - *S. epidermidis* is associated with persistent bacteremia following the implantation of artificial heart valves, vascular catheters, shunts, and prosthetic joints.
  - *S. saprophyticus* causes urinary infections in sexually active women.

Section 2.7 Streptococci

- **General features**
  - Streptococci are gram-positive cocci, spherical or football-shaped, and occurring as diplococci or in chains.
  - They are **catalase-negative.**
  - They produce species-dependent hemolysis in blood agar.

- **Laboratory identification**

Serologic: Lancefield groups (A through H and K through V) are based on serologic identification of group-specific cell wall carbohydrate (C-carbohydrate).

Hemolysis: Streptococci can be identified by their reaction in blood agar (Table 2.15).

Group A: *Streptococcus pyogenes*

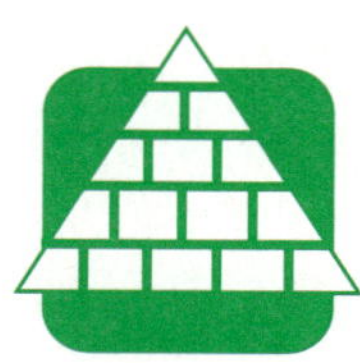

- **Structure** The **capsule** contains hyaluronic acid with a chemical structure identical to that of the hyaluronic acid in the human host. The capsule is **nonimmunogenic and antiphagocytic.**

The **cell wall components** of importance are

- group A carbohydrate (N-acetylglucosamine-rhamnose)
- lipoteichoic acid associated with fimbriae—helps in adherence

Table 2.15 ***Streptococcal Hemolysis***

Alpha (incomplete hemolysis—greenish zone around colony)	*Viridans* group, *Enterococcus* spp.
Beta (complete hemolysis—clear zone around colony)	*S. pyogenes* (Group A), *S. anginosus*
Gamma (no hemolysis)	*S. viridans, Enterococcus* spp.

The **proteins:**

- M protein—antigenic, antiphagocytic, helps in adherence
- T protein (trypsin resistant protein)
- R protein
- F protein—fibronectin-binding protein (helps in adherence)

- **Laboratory identification** *S. pyogenes* can be identified by the following tests:
  - beta hemolysis in blood agar
  - bacitracin (A disk) sensitivity (A disk for group A)
  - serology for group A specific carbohydrates
  - ASO (anti-streptolysin O) titer—antibodies to streptolysin O appear 3 to 4 weeks after primary infection; useful in diagnosis of glomerulonephritis or rheumatic fever

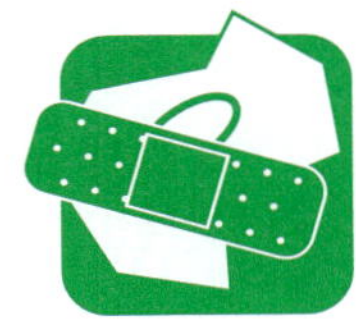

- **Pathogenesis** The pathogenesis of *S. pyogenes* can be ascribed to the following (Table 2.16):
  - resistance to phagocytosis because of M protein and capsule
  - adherence to mucoepithelium because of F protein and lipoteichoic acid
  - destruction of tissue by release of toxins and enzymes

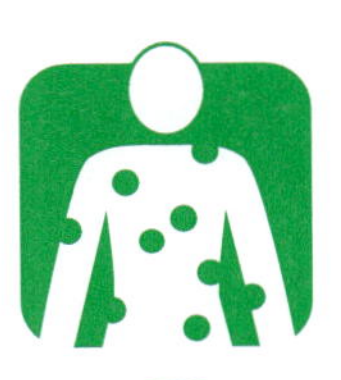

- **Diseases**

— ***Suppurative (pus forming) diseases***

1. Pharyngitis (strep throat)
   - primarily a disease of children
   - sore throat, fever, general malaise, headache within 2 to 4 days of exposure
   - red throat with possible exudate or cervical lymphadenopathy
   - often indistinguishable from viral infection

2. Scarlet fever
   - sequela (complication) of pharyngitis
   - diffuse erythematous rash on upper chest within 1 to 2 days of development of pharyngitis, which then spreads to extremities; areas around mouth, palms, and soles are excluded
   - strawberry tongue
   - rash disappears in 5 to 7 days with desquamation

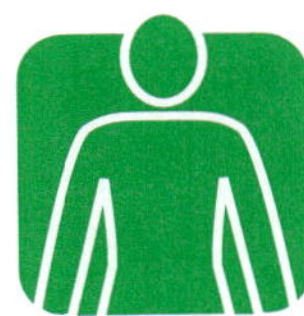

3. Streptococcal toxic shock syndrome

Table 2.16 ***Pathogenic Mechanisms of Group A Streptococci***

Mechanism	Comments
Adherence	
F protein	Binds to fibronectin on mucoepithelium
Lipoteichoic acid	Binds to mucoepithelium
Antiphagocytic Structures	
Capsule	Is nonimmunogenic
M protein	Prevents opsonization
Toxins	
Pyrogenic or erythrogenic toxins A, B, and C	Encoded by a bacteriophage; act as superantigens; enhance delayed-type hypersensitivity reactions; cause rash in scarlet fever
Enzymes	
Streptolysin S	Lyses leukocytes, erythrocytes, and platelets
Streptolysin O	Lyses leukocytes, erythrocytes, and platelets
Streptokinases	Liquefies blood clots and facilitates spread of bacteria into tissue
DNase	Degrades host DNA
Hyaluronidase ("spreading factor")	Promotes tissue destruction and bacterial spread

- production of exotoxin A by *S. pyogenes*
- usually associated with severe tissue infection: cellulitis, necrotizing fasciitis, multisystem toxicity, and multiorgan failure

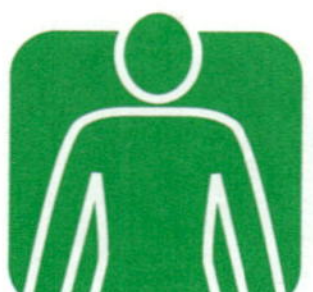

4. Pyoderma
   - colonization and infection of skin following direct contact with a fomite, an infected child, insect vector, or a cut or a break in the skin
   - most often seen in young children, 2 to 5 years of age
   - related to poor hygeine
5. Erysipelas deep skin infections, cellulitis
   - an acute superficial cellulitis with clear borders
   - common in young children or older adults
   - face is most commonly involved
   - lymphatic involvement
6. Other suppurative diseases
   - pneumonia
   - puerperal sepsis

— ***Nonsuppurative diseases*** These are complications of the primary disease.

Rheumatic fever is an inflammation of the heart, joints, blood vessels, and subcutaneous tissues, accompanied by polyarthritis and rash. The Jones criteria for diagnosis of rheumatic fever are given in Box 2.3.

Acute glomerular nephritis is an acute inflammation of renal glomeruli, with edema, hypertension, hematuria, and proteinuria.

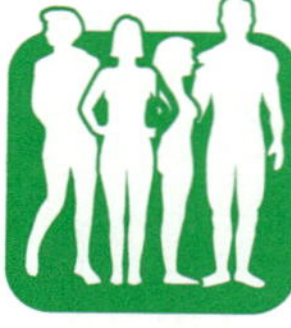

● **Epidemiology**

Mode of spread: Pharyngitis is spread by respiratory droplets. Pyo-

Box 2.3

1992 REVISED JONES CRITERIA FOR THE DIAGNOSIS OF RHEUMATIC FEVER

The diagnosis of rheumatic fever is highly likely if supported by evidence of a preceding group A streptococcal infection and the presence of two major manifestations or one major and two minor manifestations.

Supporting Evidence of Antecedent Group A Streptococcal Infection

Positive throat culture
Positive streptococcal antigen test
Elevated or rising streptococcal antibody titer

Major Manifestations

Carditis
Polyarthritis
Chorea
Erythema marginatum
Subcutaneous nodules

Minor Manifestations

Clinical findings: arthralgia, fever
Laboratory findings
Elevated acute phase reactants (erythrocyte sedimentation rate, C-reactive protein)
Prolonged PR interval on electrocardiography

From *JAMA* 268:2069-2073, 1992.

derma occurs when breaks in the skin come in contact with an infected person, a fomite, or an insect vector. Other diseases are complications of the primary disease.

Populations affected: Children 5 to 15 years of age are primarily affected. Pyoderma occurs in children with poor hygeine.

Occurrence: Pharyngitis is more common in winter and fall. Pyoderma is more common in warm, wet environments, and in summer.

- **Prevention** Practicing good hygiene can lead to a decrease of streptococcal infections.
- **Treatment** Group A pharyngitis is treated in order to prevent potential sequelae, such as rheumatic fever and glomerulonephritis. *S. pyogenes* is sensitive to Penicillin G.

Group B: *Streptococcus agalactiae*

- **Structure** *S. agalactiae* occur as gram-positive cocci in chains.
- **Laboratory identification** Laboratory identification is based on the following reactions:
  - beta-hemolysis in blood agar
  - bacitracin resistance
  - CAMP factor-enhanced beta-hemolysis of *S. aureus*
  - serologic detection of group B-specific polysaccharide

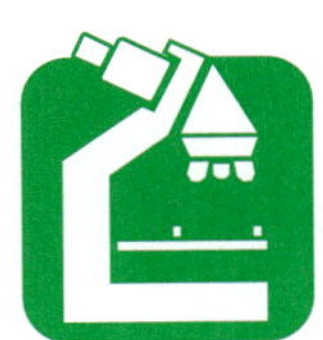

- **Pathogenesis**
  - The capsule is antiphagocytic.
  - Protection against *S. agalactiae* requires anticapsule antibodies.
  - Degradative enzymes produced by the organisms include deoxyribonucleases, hyaluronidase, neuraminidase, proteases, hippurase, and hemolysins.

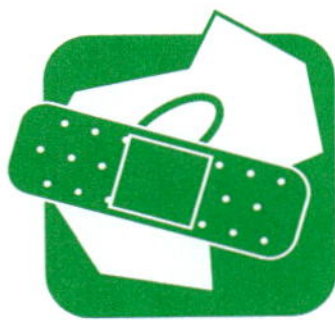

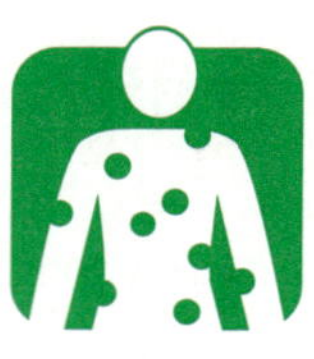

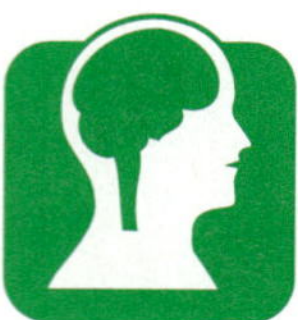

- **Diseases**
  1. Early-onset neonatal disease
     - age of onset: less than 7 days
     - acquisition: in utero or at delivery
     - symptoms: bacteremia, pneumonia, meningitis
     - mortality: high
  2. Late-onset neonatal disease
     - age of onset: 1 week to 3 months
     - acquisition: postpartum
     - symptoms: bacteremia, meningitis, osteomyelitis
     - mortality: low (<20%)
  3. Postpartum sepsis
     - patients: women (postpartum)
     - acquisition: wound infection after birth
     - symptoms: endometritis, wound infection

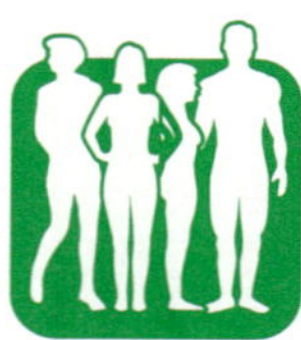

- **Epidemiology**

  Mode of spread: Infection is acquired during the birthing process.

  Populations affected: **Neonates** and **postpartum women** are the individuals most at risk. Neonates may be less able to eliminate a capsulated organism.

  Occurrence: *S. agalactiae* is ubiquitous.

- **Treatment** *S. agalactiae* infections are treated with penicillin G alone or in combination with aminoglycosides.

  Serious cases may require passive immunization.

Other Beta-Hemolytic Streptococci (Groups C, F, and G)

S. pyogenes-like *Streptococcus anginosus* (or *S. milleri*) is part of the normal flora of the pharynx, GI tract, and genitourinary tract. It causes pharyngitis, epiglottitis, sinusitis, meningitis, tissue and bone infections, intraabdominal abscesses, pericarditis, and endocarditis.

S. equi, S. zooepidemicus, S. equisimilis are other streptococci belonging to these groups.

Viridans Streptococci *(Streptococcus mutans, Streptococcus sanguis, Streptococcus anginosus)*

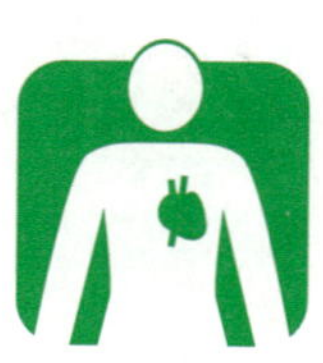

- **Laboratory identification** No hemolysis (γ) viridans streptococci may be nonhemolytic or alpha-hemolytic. They must be grown in blood cultures.
- **Pathogenesis** Viridans streptococci are part of the normal flora of the mouth and teeth. They adhere to tooth enamel and damaged heart valves.
- **Diseases**
  1. Bacteremia
  2. Endocarditis
  3. Dental caries
- **Epidemiology**

  Populations affected: People with **damaged heart valves** are at risk.

  Mode of spread: Being part of the normal flora, bacteria can enter the bloodstream during dental work or after oral trauma.
- **Treatment** Penicillin is the drug of choice.

- **Prevention** Antibiotic prophylaxis of the at-risk population can help reduce the incidence of infection.

Streptococcus pneumoniae

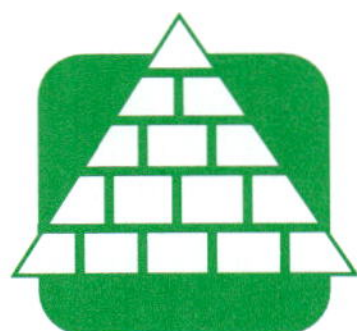

- **Structure** *S. pneumoniae* is **encapsulated.** The C substance, a surface-exposed teichoic acid, reacts and precipitates serum protein (C-reactive protein) in the presence of calcium.
- **Laboratory identification** *S. pneumoniae* is identified by
  - alpha hemolysis on blood agar
  - inhibition by **optochin (P disk for Pneumonia)**

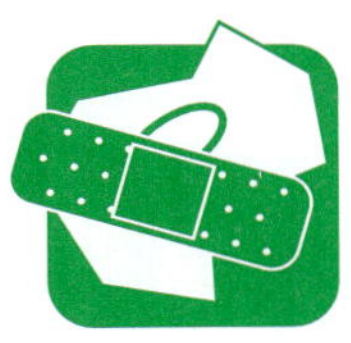

- **Pathogenesis** The factors contributing to pathogenesis of *S. pneumoniae* are the following:
  - capsule: antiphagocytic; required for virulence
  - pneumolysin: similar to streptolysin O; lyses cells
  - purpura-production principle: causes skin hemorrhage in animal models
  - neuraminidase (spreading factor): promotes spreading in tissue
  - organism colonizes the oropharynx
  - disease often follows a viral infection
  - disruption of ciliated epithelium (e.g., after influenza or by smoking) prevents clearance of airways and allows aspiration of nasopharyngeal secretions into lower airways; leads to rapid growth in alveolar spaces, tissue destruction, and disease

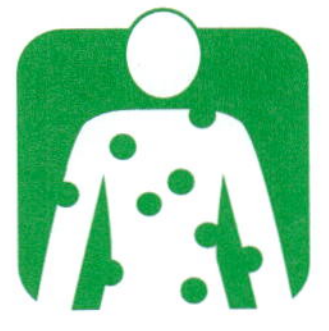

- **Diseases**
  1. Pneumonia
     - most common cause of bacterial pneumonia (500,000 cases per year)
     - abrupt onset, chills, high fever (102° F to 105° F), productive cough with blood-tinged sputum, chest pain
     - generally localized in lower lobes of lungs (lobar pneumonia)
     - good response to antibiotic therapy
     - children and elderly may develop a generalized bronchopneumonia

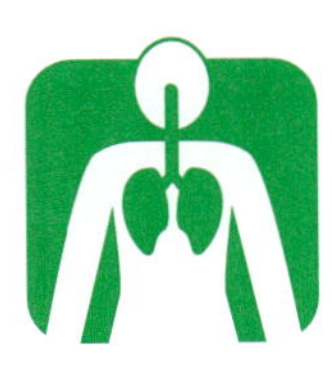

  2. Otitis media (ear aches)
  3. Sinusitis
  4. Bacteremia (in 25% to 30% of pneumonia patients)
  5. Pneumococcal meningitis following bacteremia
     - accounts for 15% of meningitis in children and 30% to 50% of meningitis in adults

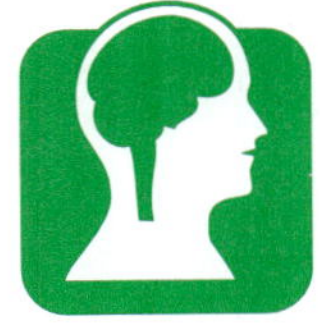

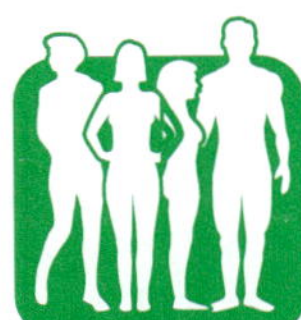

- **Epidemiology**

  Mode of spread: *S. pneumoniae* spreads in aerosol droplets and colonizes the oropharynx. Disruption of normal mucosal and ciliary defenses allows aspiration of bacteria into lungs.

  Populations affected: smokers, children, the elderly, people lacking a spleen, renal transplant recipients, persons with hematologic disorders; sequelae to influenza.

  Occurrence: *S. pneumoniae* is ubiquitous. Infection is most common in winter and spring.

- **Prevention** A **capsular antigen-based vaccine** is immunogenic, but not helpful for the at-risk population (children, the elderly, asplenic patients).
- **Treatment**
  - Infections with *S. pneumoniae* are treated with penicillin, cephalosporins, erythromycin, and chloramphenicol (for meningitis).
  - Penicillin resistance is on the rise.

Enterococci *(Enterococcus faecalis, E. faecium)*

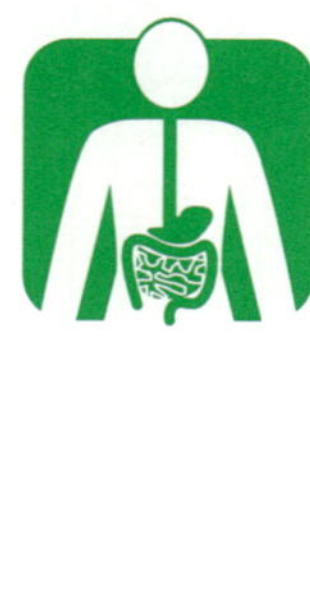

- **Laboratory identification** Enterococci were previously classified as group D streptococci. They grow in media containing bile or high concentrations of salts (similar to their normal growth environment).
- **Pathogenesis** Enterococci are part of the normal flora of the large bowel and are present in feces.
- **Disease**
  - Enterococci are a common cause of urinary tract infections in hospitalized patients.
  - Catheterization and administration of broad-spectrum antibiotics are risk factors for enterococcal disease.
- **Treatment**
  - The organisms are resistant to many antibiotics.
  - A combination of an aminoglycoside and vancomycin or some other cell-wall-active antibiotic is used.

Section 2.8 Bacillus

General Features Organisms of the genus *Bacillus* are gram-positive, **spore forming rods.**

Bacillus anthracis

- **Structure** The organisms occur as single or paired bacilli. Chains or clumps may be seen in culture. They have a capsule containing glutamic acid.
- **Laboratory identification** Large, gram-positive rods.
- **Pathogenesis** Virulence factors of *B. anthracis* include a **capsule** that prevents phagocytosis and an **exotoxin** that produces edema and is very lethal.

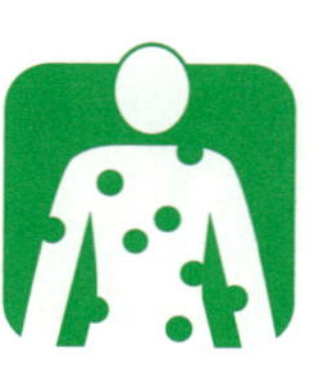

- **Diseases**
  1. Cutaneous anthrax
     - papule at innoculation site; ulcer with vesicles can lead to necrosis with massive edema and systemic problems
     - mortality—20%, unless treated in time
  2. Inhalation anthrax
     - viruslike respiratory illness
     - lung involvement leads to respiratory failure
     - high mortality
  3. Gastrointestinal anthrax
     - rare
     - mesenteric adenopathy, hemorrhages, ascites
     - high mortality

Table 2.17 Bacillus *Species and Their Diseases*

ORGANISM	DISEASE
Bacillus anthracis	Anthrax
Bacillus cereus	Gastroenteritis
	Emetic form
	Diarrheal form
	Panophthalmitis
	Opportunistic infections
Bacillus subtilis	Opportunistic infections
Other *Bacillus* species	Opportunistic infections

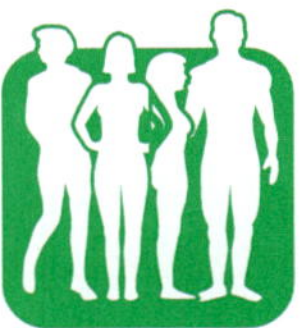

- **Epidemiology** *B. anthracis* was and perhaps still is, a major agent of biological warfare. An outbreak in Russia in 1979 was traced to an accidental release from the military.

  Mode of spread: The spores of *B. anthracis* can survive many years in the soil. Spread of disease occurs by one of the following mechanisms:

  - Inoculation: of a cut or exposed skin by bacteria or spores
  - Inhalation: of spores from contaminated fur, for example, during processing of goat hair (Woolsorter's Disease)
  - Ingestion: rare for humans, common for herbivores, such as sheep, cattle, and goats

  Populations affected: Farmers, sheep or goat handlers, and furriers are at risk.

  Occurrence: Anthrax is rare in the United States.

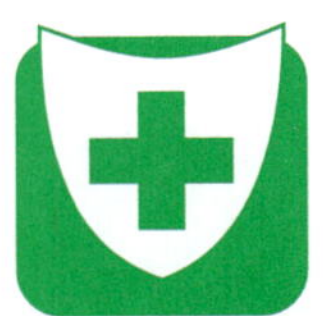

- **Prevention** Anthrax can be controlled by preventing the disease in animals by **vaccination** of animal herds and proper disposal of infected animals. Individuals at risk can be vaccinated.

- **Treatment** Treatment must be started early in the course of disease. Penicillin, or alternatively, tetracycline or chloramphenicol are effective.

Bacillus cereus

- **Pathogenesis**
  - The nature of the enterotoxins secreted determines the type of disease that will occur.
  - The **heat-stable enterotoxin** causes vomiting, whereas the heat-labile enterotoxin causes diarrhea.
  - The toxin is similar to that of *E. coli* or *Vibrio cholera* and acts through the adenylate cyclase–cyclic AMP system.
  - Cereolysin (a hemolysin) and phospholipase C are released in panophthalmitis.

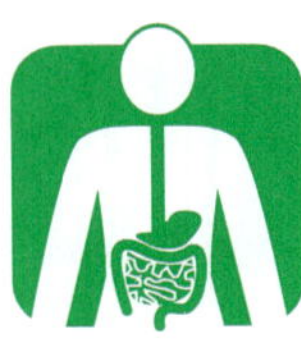

- **Diseases (Table 2.17)**
  1. Food poisoning (diarrhea)
  2. Panophthalmitis
- **Epidemiology**

  Mode of spread: Ingestion of contaminated rice (unrefrigerated) causes emetic disease, and ingestion of contaminated meat or vegetables causes diarrheal disease.

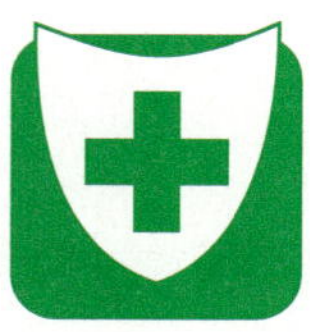

Populations affected: Any person consuming contaminated food is at risk.

Occurrence: *B. cereus* is a ubiquitous soil bacterium.

- **Prevention** Refrigeration of foods after cooking can prevent germination of spores and release of toxins.

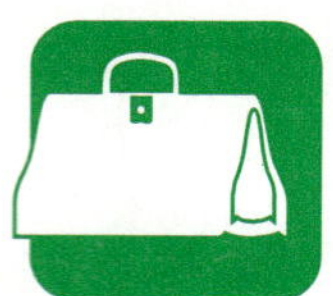

- **Treatment** Supportive therapy is indicated for food poisoning.

■ **Other *Bacillus* Species** Other species of *Bacillus* can act as opportunistic pathogens in compromised patients.

Section 2.9 *Corynebacterium* and *Listeria*

■ Corynebacteria: *Corynebacterium diphtheriae* and Other Less Common Family Members

- **General features**
  - The tox gene for toxin is carried by a lysogenic bacteriophage.
  - The toxin has the **A-B form.**
  - A fragment: enzyme portion—inactivates elongation factor 2 (EF-2), blocks protein synthesis in mammalian cells (the mechanism is similar to that of *Pseudomonas aeroginosa* exotoxin A).
  - B fragment: binds to the cell surface.
- **Laboratory identification**
  - *C. diphtheriae* is a small pleomorphic gram-positive bacillus non-motile and non–spore former.
  - The **Shick test** is used to determine immunity.
- **Pathogenesis** The disease is mediated by an exotoxin.

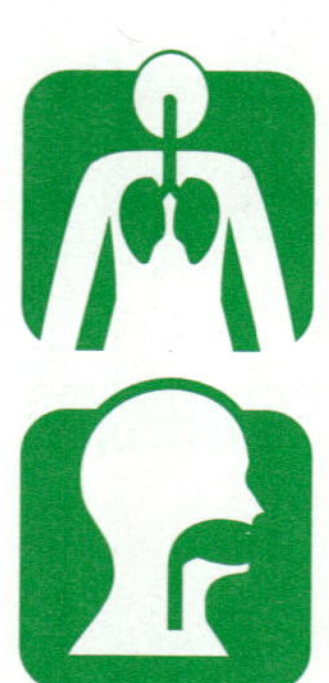

- **Diseases**
  1. Respiratory diphtheria
     - may be a mild respiratory disease with sore throat, low-grade fever, and pseudomembrane or a potentially fatal respiratory disease with tissue destruction and blocked airways.
     - there is sudden onset of malaise and a sore throat, with a thick **pseudomembrane** (consisting of dead cells, bacteria, and fibrin) forming on tonsils, uvula, and palate and extending into the respiratory tract. This pseudomembrane can block breathing and cause death. Attempts to dislodge the pseudomembrane cause bleeding.
  2. Cutaneous diphtheria
  3. Myocarditis, neuropathy, or renal tubular necrosis
     - result from damage to distant organs by exotoxin

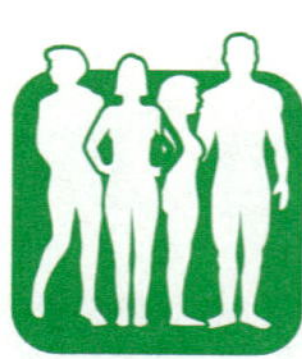

- **Epidemiology**

  Mode of spread: *C. diphtheriae* is spread by respiratory droplets from asymptomatic, nonimmunized carriers and by skin contact.

  Population affected: Unimmunized individuals, children.

  Occurrence: The disease occurs worldwide, especially in crowded cities and in places where vaccination programs are absent or poor.

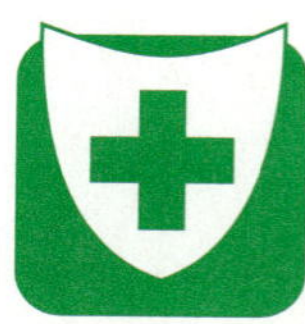

- **Prevention** Diphtheria can be prevented by **vaccination** with **toxoid**

Table 2.18 *Other Corynebacteria and Diphtheroids*

Microorganism	Disease Manifestations
Arcanobacterium haemolyticum	Pharyngitis, skin ulcers
C. urealyticum (group D-2)	Urinary tract infection
C. jeikeium (group JK)	Phlebitis and bacteremia, wound infection
C. minutissimum	Erythrasma

(killed toxin) during childhood as part of the mixed DPT vaccine. Boosters should be given every 10 years.

- **Treatment** Antitoxin should be administered early in the course of the disease. Penicillin or erythromycin should be given to patients, carriers, and close contacts.

- **Other corynebacteria** Table 2.18 lists other corynebacteria that have been implicated in human disease.

Listeria (Listeria monocytogenes)

- **Structure** *Listeria* organisms are small gram-positive coccobacilli that do not form spores.
- **Laboratory identification** *Listeria* is beta hemolytic, catalase positive, and motile.
- **Pathogenesis** *Listeria* is an intracellular pathogen. It secretes listeriolysin O (a beta-hemolysin similar to streptolysin).
- **Diseases**

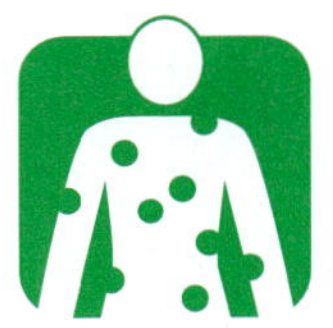

  - The diseases caused by *L. monocytogenes* are described in Table 2.19.
  - Listerial infection is usually asymptomatic, except in immune-deficient individuals.
  - Neonatal disease is of two types:

  1. early onset disease: granulomatosis infantiseptica—high mortality with disseminated abscesses and granulomas in multiple organs
  2. late onset disease: occurs 2 to 3 weeks after birth—meningitis or meningoencephalitis with septicemia

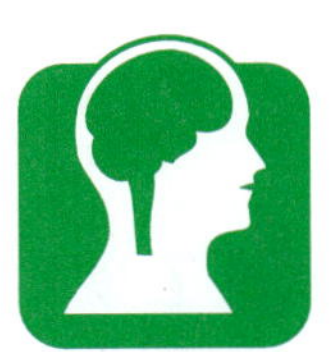

   - Adult disease takes the form of meningitis in individuals with suppressed cell-mediated immunity or sepsis with fever in pregnant women.

- **Epidemiology**

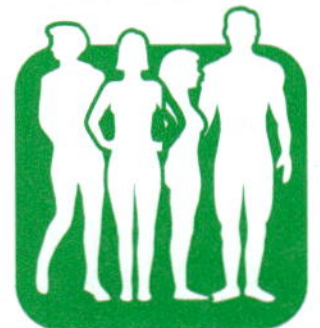

  Mode of spread: Listeriosis is spread by contaminated food, especially dairy products, or is acquired transplacentally.

  Populations affected: Neonates and immune-deficient individuals are most at risk.

  Occurrence: Sporadic outbreaks of the disease occur. The organism is ubiquitous and disease occurs worldwide.

- **Prevention** Pregnant women should avoid partially or uncooked foods of animal origin, unwashed vegetables, and *nonpasteurized dairy products.*

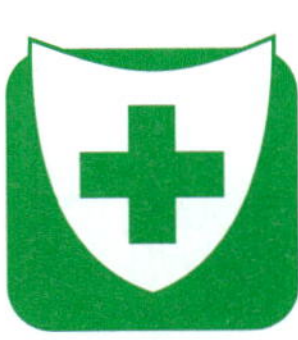

- **Treatment** Ampicillin is the antibiotic of choice for treating listerial infections.

Table 2.19 *Diseases of* **Listeria monocytogenes**

Type of Infection	Comments
Bacteremia in pregnancy	The disease can be transmitted transplacentally
Granulomatosis infantiseptica	In utero transmission resulting in neonatal infection
Sepsis	Neonatal: probably acquired perinatally; in adults: usually occurs in immunosuppressed individuals
CNS infection	Meningitis in neonates and adults
Focal infection	Endocarditis, lymphadenitis, osteomyelitis, hepatitis, cholecystitis, peritonitis, and infections of the skin, eyes, and joints

Section 2.10 Anaerobic Bacteria

Gram-positive Non-Sporeforming Bacteria

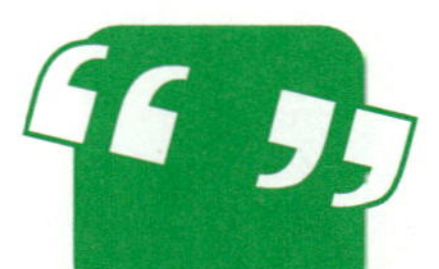

- **Cocci *Peptostreptococcus* and *Peptococcus***
  - These organisms are part of the normal flora in the oral cavity, the female genitourinary tract, and the skin.
  - They cause diseases such as pleuropulmonary infection, sinusitis, brain abscesses, intraabdominal sepsis, pelvic infections, soft tissue infections, endocarditis, and osteomyelitis.
  - Laboratory identification of these organisms is complicated by the requirement for anaerobic conditions.
  - Infections are treated with penicillin or other beta-lactam antibiotics.

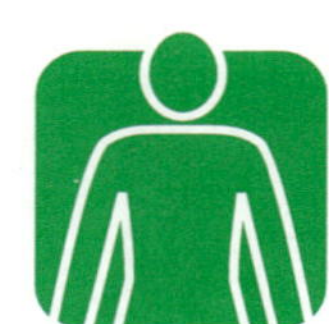

- **Bacilli *(Propionibacterium)***
  - Propionibacteria are small gram-positive bacteria.
  - They are common on the skin surface, conjunctiva, external ear, oropharynx, and the female genital tract.
  - They cause **acne,** which is an infection of sebaceous glands that stimulates an inflammatory response. They also infect prosthetic devices.
- **Treatment** Infections with *Propionibacterium* are treated with benzoyl peroxide (acne creams), erythromycin, and clindamycin.
- **Other organisms** Other organisms in this category that can cause disease belong to the genera *Lactobacillus, Bifidobacterium, Eubacterium, Mobiluncus,* and *Actinomyces* (see Section 2.19).

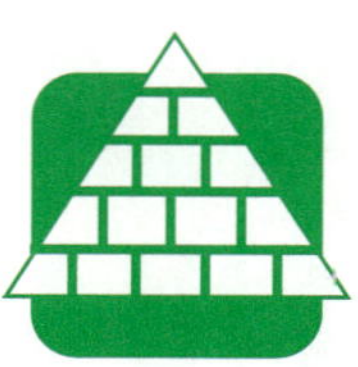

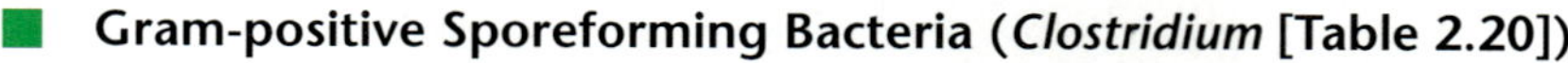

Gram-positive Sporeforming Bacteria (*Clostridium* [Table 2.20])

- ***Clostridium perfringens***

  — ***Structure*** *C. perfringens* is a large boxcar-shaped bacillus. It is subdivided into 5 types, A to E.

  — ***Laboratory identification***
  - It is easily cultured in the laboratory.
  - It is aerotolerant and grows very rapidly.
  - Colonies show characteristic **double zones of hemolysis on blood agar** and have a typical appearance on egg-yolk agar.

  — ***Pathogenesis*** Toxins and degradative enzymes cause extensive tissue damage. A few of these are listed below:

Table 2.20 *Common Clostridial Diseases*

Organism	Disease
C. perfringens	Bacteremia; myonecrosis (gas gangrene); soft tissue infections (e.g., cellulitis, fasciitis); food poisoning; enteritis necroticans
C. tetani	Tetanus
C. botulinum	Food-borne botulism, infant botulism, wound botulism
C. difficile	Antibiotic-associated diarrhea, pseudomembranous colitis
Other *Clostridium* species (e.g., *C. septicum, C. ramosum, C. novyi, C. bifermentans*)	Bacteremia, myonecrosis, soft tissue infections

- Alpha toxin (phospholipase C): *most important toxin*—causes lysis of cells, bleeding, and tissue destruction.
- Beta toxin: necrotizing toxin; causes necrotizing enterocolitis
- Epsilon toxin: increases permeability of gastrointestinal wall
- Iota toxin: necrotizing activity and increased vascular permeability
- Enterotoxin: disrupts ion transport in the ileum by permeabilizing membranes
- Other toxins: enzymes that cause tissue destruction, for example, collagenase, protease, hyaluronidase, DNase, and neuraminidase

Diseases

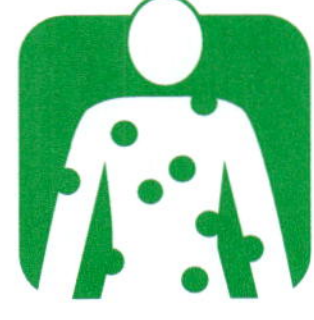

1. Bacteremia
2. **Gas gangrene** (myonecrosisis)
   - disease progresses rapidly from intense pain to extensive muscle necrosis with shock, renal failure, and finally death within 2 days
   - necrotic tissue, gas from bacterial growth, and abundant bacteria are present in muscle
   - prognosis is poor: mortality is greater than 40%
3. Cellulitis, fasciitis, other soft tissue infections
   - destruction of skin tissue similar to that seen in gas gangrene
4. **Food poisoning**
   - common cause of food poisoning
   - results from contaminated meat containing enterotoxinproducing *C. perfringens* type A
   - moderately rapid onset—8 to 24 hours from ingestion of toxin
   - symptoms consist of abdominal cramps and watery diarrhea but no fever, nausea, or vomiting; disease is self-limiting

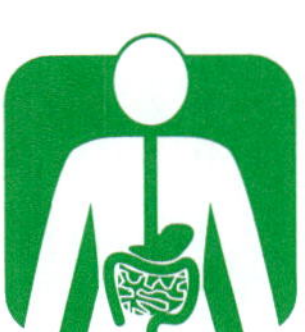

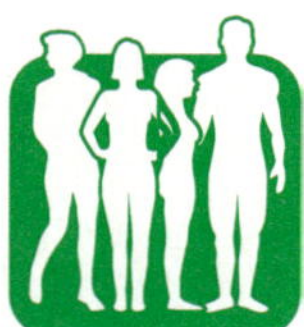

— ***Epidemiology***

Mode of spread: *C. perfringens* is present in soil, water, and sewage. Spore formation allows survival under harsh conditions. It is part of the normal flora of the GI tract.

Populations affected: Surgical and trauma patients may develop a C. perfringens infection. **Diabetics** and persons with poor circulation are at high risk. Persons eating contaminated meat may contract clostridial food poisoning.

Occurrence: The organism is found worldwide.

— ***Prevention*** Proper wound care and appropriate use of antibiotics.

— ***Treatment***

- For bacteremia, treatment consists of antimicrobial therapy (penicillin) and removal of source of bacteremia, such as infected and necrotic materials.
- Gas gangrene is treated with surgical debridement and amputation and high-dose penicillin therapy. Hyperbaric oxygen is used supplementally to stop toxin production.
- Supportive therapy is used for clostridial food poisoning.

● ***Clostridium tetani***

— ***Structure*** *C. tetani* has a "tennis racquet" appearance because of a terminal spore.

— ***Laboratory identification*** *C. tetani* cannot be cultured. It is difficult to grow because of sensitivity to oxygen.

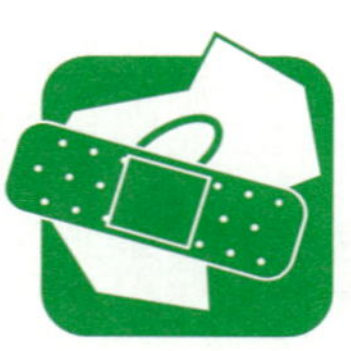

— ***Pathogenesis***

- *C. tetani* secretes **Tetanospasmin,** which is a **neurotoxin** (Fig. 2.23).
- Subunit A **blocks release of neurotransmitters**, resulting in unregulated excitatory synaptic activity and spastic paralysis.
- Subunit B binds to gangliosides on neuronal membranes to promote uptake.
- The toxin must travel from the site of infection to the CNS in order to cause symptoms.

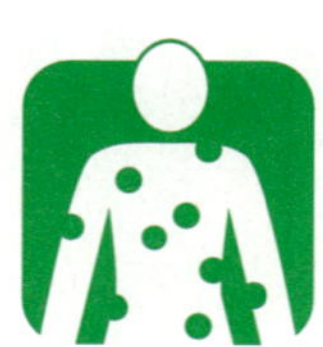

— ***Disease*** Tetanus (Lockjaw or trismus)

- Symptoms include risus sardonicus (a sardonic smile caused by sustained trismus), drooling, sweating, irritability, and persistent back spasms.
- Localized tetanus can occur in a group of muscles.
- The timecourse depends on the site of infection.
- It has a high mortality rate.

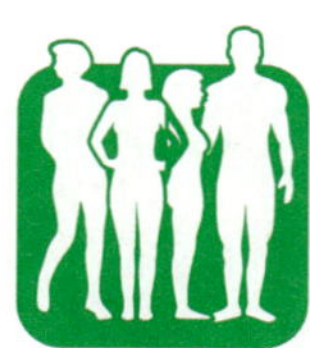

— ***Epidemiology***

Mode of spread:

- Bacteria are present in soil, water, sewage, and are part of the normal flora of many animals.
- Organisms infect cuts and stabwounds from contaminated materials.

Populations affected: Unvaccinated individuals and drug abusers who inject drugs subcutaneously ("skin poppers") are at risk.

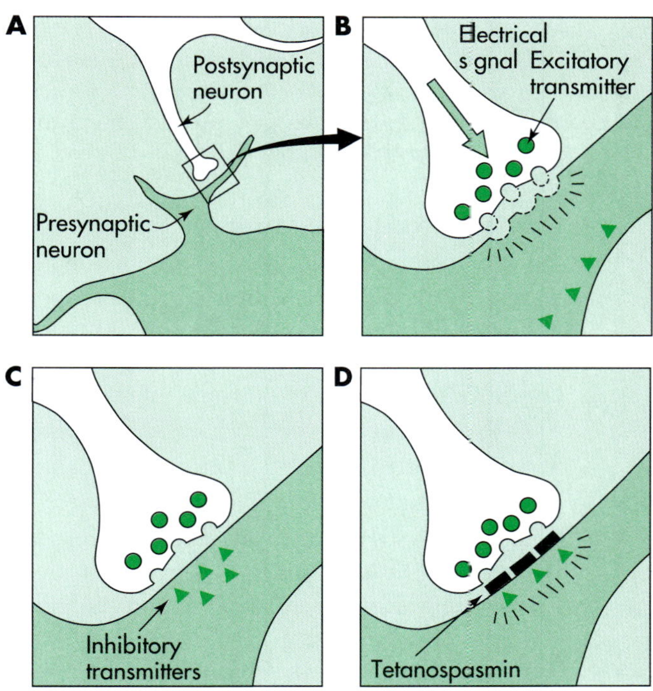

Fig. 2.23 Mechanism of tetanospasmin activity. **A,** Neurotransmission is controlled by the balance between excitatory and inhibitory neurotransmitters. **B,** The inhibitory neurotransmitters (e.g., GABA, glycine) prevent depolarization of the postsynaptic membrane and conduction of the electrical signal. **C,** Tetanospasmin does not interfere with production or storage of GABA or glycine but rather with their release (presynaptic activity). **D,** In the blockage of inhibitory neurotransmitters, excitation of the neuroaxon is unrestrained.

Occurrence: The disease is more prevalent in underdeveloped countries where people are unvaccinated.

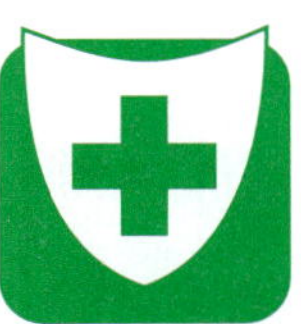

— ***Prevention*** Tetanus can be prevented by routine **vaccination** with **tetanus toxoid** (formaldehyde-inactivated toxin), which is administered as part of the DPT or DT shot. Booster shots are required every 10 years.

— ***Treatment*** Treatment of tetanus involves the following measures:

- debridement of the primary wound
- penicillin therapy
- passive immunization with human tetanus immunoglobulin
- vaccination with toxoid
- isolation of the patient in an environment where exposure to visual or auditory stimuli is at a minimum

● ***Clostridium botulinum***

— ***Laboratory identification*** Demonstration of botulinum toxin in patient specimens or food by immunoassay establishes the diagnosis.

— ***Pathogenesis*** Botulism is mediated by the **botulinum toxin**, which can be ingested (preformed) or *produced in the host.*

The A chain of the toxin is a neurotoxin; the B chain binds to cells. Botulinum toxin **targets cholinergic nerves and blocks neurotransmission** at peripheral cholinergic synapses, preventing release of acetylcholine. Recovery requires regeneration of nerve endings. Spores are heat resistant, but the toxin and bacteria are not.

— *Diseases*

1. Classical or **food-borne botulism** (intoxication)
    - symptoms appear after a 2 day incubation period
    - weakness and dizziness; blurred vision, fixed and dilated pupils; dry mouth; flaccid paralysis; death from respiratory paralysis
2. **Infant botulism** (gastrointestinal infection)
    - most common form of botulism in the United States
    - bacteria colonizing the GI tract release neurotoxin
    - infants less than 1 year of age are at risk
    - initial symptoms are nonspecific, for example, failure to thrive and constipation
    - may progress to flaccid paralysis and respiratory arrest (in 1% to 2% of patients)
    - associated with **honey** fed to newborns
3. Wound botulism
    - Rare—local production of toxin leading to disease

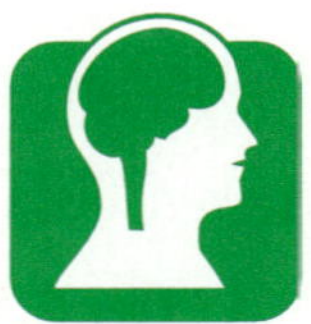

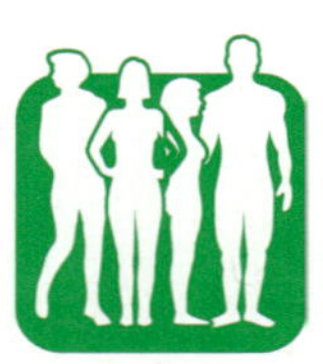

— *Epidemiology*

Mode of spread: Disease occurs by ingestion of preformed toxin, ingestion of bacteria (infants), or by skin inoculation.

Populations affected: Persons eating contaminated foods (particularly home-canned items) and infants (particularly those fed honey) are at risk.

Occurrence: The disease is relatively rare in the United States.

— *Prevention* Adequate heating of home canned food is essential. Heating destroys the toxin.

— *Treatment* Antitoxin should be administered as early as possible. Penicillin and supportive therapy can reduce mortality following intoxication but not infection.

Clostridium difficile

— *Laboratory identification* *C. difficile* infections are identified by testing for toxin in stool by cytotoxicity (to tissue culture cells) or immunoassay. Fecal specimens are cultured on highly selective media to isolate organisms. (The presence of *C. difficile* in culture does not imply disease; the disease is caused by toxins.)

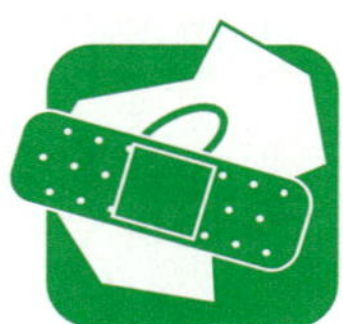

— *Pathogenesis* *C. difficile* may be part of the normal intestinal flora. **Excessive use of antibiotics may permit overgrowth** or acquisition of *C. difficile* which are resistant bacteria.

Other virulence factors are the following:

- toxins
    - enterotoxin (toxin A): promotes fluid secretion and intestinal hemorrhage
    - cytotoxin (toxin B): depolymerizes cellular cytoskeleton

Box 2.4

DISTINCTION OF POTENTIAL ENTERIC PATHOGENS BY LACTOSE FERMENTATION

Lactose-positive Bacteria	Lactose-negative Bacteria
Escherichia coli	*Salmonella**
Klebsiella	*Shigella*
Enterobacter	*Yersinia*
Citrobacter	*Proteus*
Serratia	

*H_2S production

- adhesion factor: binds to human colon cells
- hyaluronidase: has hydrolytic activity

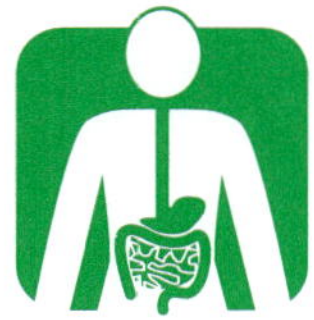

— ***Disease*** Pseudomembranous colitis

- diarrhea that may be bloody; stool may contain leukocytes
- disease may relapse because of presence of spores that are insensitive to oxygen and to antibiotic treatment

— ***Epidemiology***

Mode of spread: The bacteria may be part of the normal flora or may be ingested. Spores allow *C. difficile* to exist in the environment (including hospital). Disease may be transmitted by person-to-person spread.

Populations affected: Patients receiving antibiotics are at risk. Antibiotic exposure permits overgrowth of *C. difficile.*

— ***Treatment*** Antibiotic therapy should be discontinued. If necessary, treatment with metronidazole or vancomycin should be instituted.

Section 2.11 Enterobacteriaceae

● General features

- The Enterobacteriaceae is the largest group of medically important gram-negative bacteria.
- In order to live in the GI tract (enteric environment) they must be facultative anaerobes.

● Structure

- As gram-negative bacteria, Enterobacteriaciae have somatic (O) and capsular (K) polysaccharide antigens, and an outer membrane containing lipopolysaccharide (endotoxin).
- Most of the bacteria have flagella.
- Some have capsules *(Klebsiella* spp. and *Salmonella typhi).*

● Laboratory identification

- All Enterobacteriaciae are *gram-negative rods,* ferment glucose, are catalase positive, and are *oxidase negative.*
- *Lactose fermentation* distinguishes the more benign from the more pathogenic bacteria (Box 2.4).
- (*Hint:* For each member of the Enterobacteriaceae, it is useful to know the following association: gram-negative; oxidase negative; lactose [+ or −].

Box 2.5

ENDOTOXIN-MEDIATED TOXICITY
Fever
Leukopenia followed by leukocytosis
Activation of complement
Thrombocytopenia
Disseminated intravascular coagulation
Decreased peripheral circulation and perfusion to major organs
Shock
Death

For example, *E. coli:* gram-negative, oxidase negative, lactose positive)

— ***Growth media for Enterobacteriaceae***

- MacConkey agar: inhibits gram-positive organisms; lactose fermenters produce red colonies
- Eosin methylene blue (EMB) agar: *E. coli* colonies are green, colonies of pathogens are colorless
- Hektoen enteric agar: non–lactose fermenters produce green colonies; H_2S producers appear black
- *Yersinia* may not grow in the above media

- **Pathogenesis** Many of the mechanisms of virulence are shared by different species of Enterobacteriaceae.

1. Endotoxin: *All organisms produce endotoxin* (Box 2.5).
2. Exotoxins: Some members produce exotoxins.
   - Heat labile enterotoxin: produced by *E. coli;* causes diarrhea; the B subunit binds to cells, whereas the A subunit promotes ADP ribosylation of G proteins, leading to increased levels of cAMP, altered electrolyte transport, and diarrhea
   - Heat stabile enterotoxin: activates cGMP production, promotes fluid loss
   - Shiga toxin: produced by *Shigella dysenteriae;* inhibits protein synthesis
   - Shiga-like toxin (verotoxin): may be associated with hemorrhagic colitis
3. Adhesion: Many of the Enterobacteriaceae produce adhesins on fimbriae (the P fimbriae and the S fimbriae) to promote adhesion to tissue (e.g., to the bladder, leading to urinary tract infection).
4. Intracellular growth: *Shigella, Salmonella, Yersinia,* and enteroinvasive *E. coli* are capable of intracellular growth.
5. Antibiotic resistance: Antibiotic resistance genes on plasmids can be transferred to related bacteria.
6. Capsule: Some organisms such as *Klebsiella* spp. or *Salmonella* spp. have capsules that are antiphagocytic.

Escherichia coli

- **Laboratory identification** *E. coli* can be differentiated from other enteric organisms by the following biochemical characteristics:

Table 2.21 *Gastroenteritis Caused by* Escherichia coli

Organism	Site of Action	Disease	Pathogenesis
Enterotoxigenic *E. coli* (ETEC)	Small intestine	Traveler's diarrhea; infant diarrhea in underdeveloped countries; watery diarrhea, cramps, nausea, low-grade fever	Heat-stable and/or heat-labile enterotoxins; stimulate guanylate or adenylate cyclase activity with fluid and electrolyte loss
Enteroinvasive *E. coli* (EIEC)	Large intestine	Fever, cramping, watery diarrhea followed by development of dysentery with scant, bloody stools	Plasmid-mediated invasion and destruction of epithelial cells lining colon
Enteropathogenic *E. coli* (EPEC)	Small intestine	Infant diarrhea with fever, nausea, vomiting, nonbloody stools	Plasmid-mediated adherence and destruction of epithelial cells
Enterohemorrhagic *E. coli* (EHEC) e.g., O157:H7	Large intestine	Hemorrhagic colitis with severe abdominal cramps, watery diarrhea initially, followed by grossly bloody diarrhea, little or no fever; hemolytic uremic syndrome (HUS)	Mediated by cytotoxic "verotoxin"
Enteroaggregative *E. coli* (EAggEC)	Small intestine	Persistent infant diarrhea, sometimes with gross blood, low-grade fever	Aggregative adherence mediated by plasmid

- it is a lactose fermenter (colonies are pink-purple on MacConkey agar, colorless on Hektoen-Enteric agar, and pink on *Salmonella-Shigella* agar)
- it produces indole, is methyl-red test positive, is Voges-Proskauer reaction negative, and is unable to use citrate

Pathogenesis

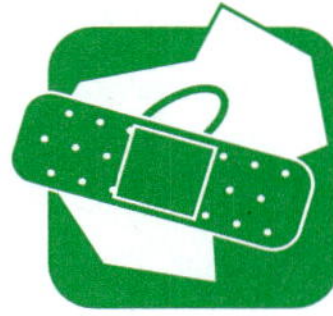

- *E. coli* is part of the normal flora of the bowel.
- All strains produce endotoxin.
- Some strains produce an exotoxin, which may be heat labile or heat stable.
- Some strains are invasive (similar to *Shigella*).
- Some strains are adherent.
- The type of enteric disease caused by *E. coli* is strain-dependent (Table 2.21).

Diseases

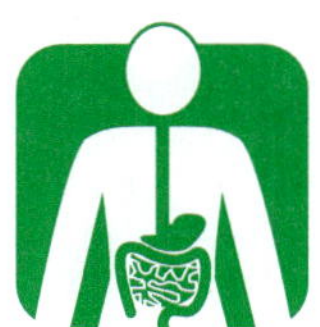

1. Gastroenteritis (see Table 2.21)
2. Septicemia
   - most common gram-negative bacterial agent of septicemia
   - enters from the urinary or the GI tract
3. Urinary tract infection (UTI):

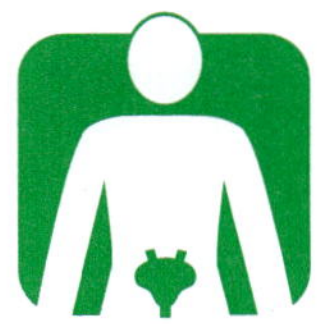

   - *E. coli* is a primary cause of UTIs
   - Gastroenteritis (see Table 2.21)
4. Hemolytic uremic syndrome
   - caused by enterohemorrhagic strains of *E. coli,* e.g., strain O157:H7

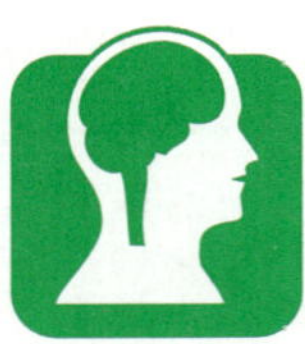

- associated with ingestion of contaminated hamburgers
- strain O157:H7 can be readily identified by growth on sorbitol plates

5. Neonatal meningitis

- *E. coli* and group B streptococci are the most common causes
- most organisms have a capsule (KI antigen)

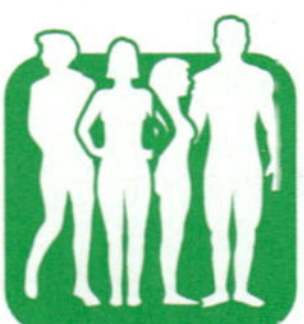

- **Epidemiology**

Mode of spread: Infection with *E. coli* may arise by endogenous spread of normal flora, may be acquired nosocomially, or may be the result of ingestion of contaminated food or water.

Populations affected: The risk of diarrhea is increased in travelers; nosocomial infections are acquired by hospitalized patients (nosocomial infection), and individuals with intestinal perforation are at risk for endogenous infection.

Occurrence: *E. coli* infections occur worldwide.

- **Prevention** Improved hygiene, chlorination of water, and proper cooking of meat (to destroy enterohemorrhagic *E. coli* O157:H7) can help prevent *E. coli* infections.
- **Treatment** The choice of antibiotic depends on the site of infection and on the susceptibility of the organism.

Salmonella

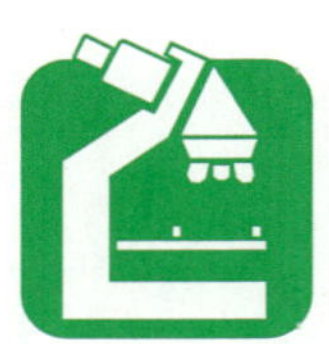

- **Laboratory identification**

• *Salmonella* are gram-negative, oxidase negative, produce H_2S, and are non–lactose fermenting bacilli.

• They form colorless colonies on MacConkey agar, green colonies on Hektoen-Enteric agar, and are colorless with a black center on *Salmonella-Shigella* agar.

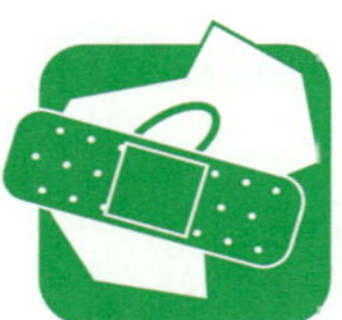

- **Pathogenesis**
  - *Salmonella* are not part of the normal human flora but they can be found in the GI tract of many warm- and cold-blooded animals.
  - The **capsule** is antiphagocytic.
  - *Salmonella* are capable of **intracellular growth.**

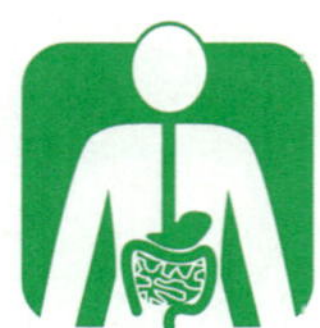

- **Diseases**

1. Enteritis or gastroenteritis

- most common form of salmonellosis
- incubation period of 6 to 48 hours after ingestion of contaminated food
- symptoms include nausea, vomiting, and diarrhea that is not bloody
- symptoms can persist for 2 to 7 days
- may result in a carrier state

2. Typhoid fever (also known as enteric fever)

- incubation period is 10 to 14 days
- etiologic agents are *S. typhi* and other *Salmonella* spp.

- symptoms include fever, headache, myalgia, malaise, and anorexia
- involvement of the Peyer's patches results in gastrointestinal problems (necrosis, hemorrhage, and perforation of intestinal wall) after the second week of illness

3. Paratyphoid fever
   - a milder form of typhoid fever
4. Septicemia
   - commonly associated with salmonella infections of another site
5. Localized infections
   - osteomyelitis (in patients with sickle cell disease)
   - enteritis
   - arthritis
   - meningitis

Asymptomatic *Salmonella* infections can occur in convalescent carriers and chronic carriers.

● **Epidemiology**

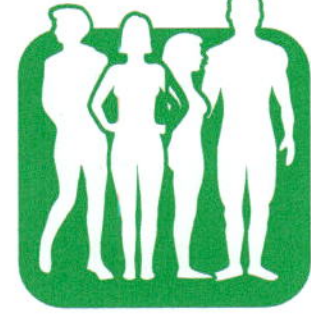

— ***Salmonella gastroenteritis***

Mode of spread: *Salmonella* are spread by the fecal-oral route and by ingestion of large numbers of *Salmonella* in contaminated water and food (especially dairy and poultry products, e.g., raw eggs, improperly cooked chicken, and turkey).

Populations affected: Children less than 1 year of age, the elderly, and AIDS patients are more at risk.

Occurrence: Gastroenteritis can occur year-round.

● **Prevention** Improved hygiene together with proper refrigeration and food preparation can limit *Salmonella* enteritis.

● **Treatment** Gastroenteritis is treated symptomatically.

— ***Typhoid fever***

Mode of spread: Typhoid is spread by the fecal-oral route and by ingestion of contaminated food or water.

Populations affected: Travelers to endemic areas are affected.

Occurrence: It is more prevalent during the warmer months.

● **Prevention** Improvement of hygiene, use of proper food preparation methods, and **immunization.**

● **Treatment** Typhoid is treated with chloramphenicol, quinolones, and broad-spectrum cephalosporins.

■ *Shigella* (*Shigella dysenteriae, S. flexneri, S. boydii, S. sonnei*)

● **Laboratory identification** *Shigella* are gram-negative, oxidase negative, and lactose negative. They form colorless colonies on MacConkeys agar, green on Hektoen-Enteric agar, and colorless on *Salmonella-Shigella* agar.

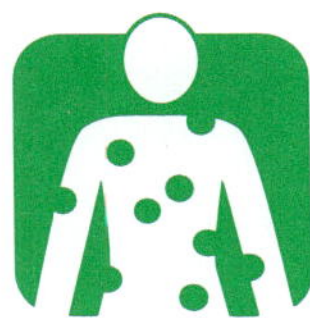

● **Pathogenesis** *Shigella* enterotoxin is responsible for the watery diarrhea. The bacteria **invade** the colonic mucosa; bacteremia is rare.

● **Disease** Shigellosis (bacillary dysentery)

- incubation period is 1 to 3 days

- symptoms consist of abdominal cramps, profuse watery diarrhea, followed by fever and bloody diarrhea

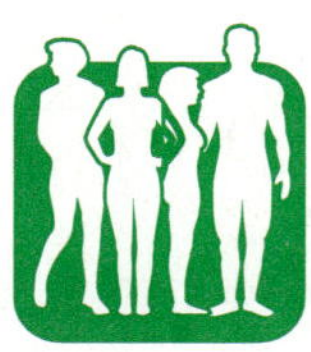

- **Epidemiology**
  Mode of spread: *Shigella* are spread by the fecal-oral route via hands (this is the most common route). The organisms can also be spread by contaminated food or water (less common route).
  Populations affected: Young children in day-care centers and nurseries, patients in long-term care facilities, and homosexual men are at risk.
  Occurrence: Shigellosis is more frequent during the warmer months.

- **Prevention** The disease can be prevented by using good hygiene.

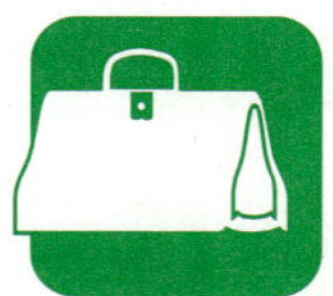

- **Treatment** Patients require supportive care. Antimicrobial therapy may be necessary.

Yersinia (Yersinia pestis, Y. enterocolitica, Y. pseudotuberculosis)

- ***Yersinia pestis***

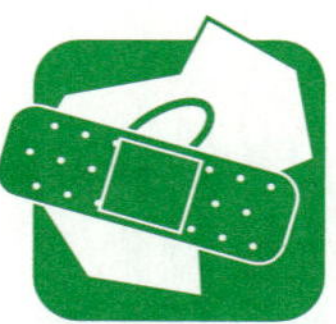

— ***Pathogenesis***
The pathogenesis of *Y. pestis* is based on the following mechanisms:

- antiphagocytic capsule
- intracellular growth
- exotoxin
- disseminated infection
- ability to grow in animals, fleas, and humans

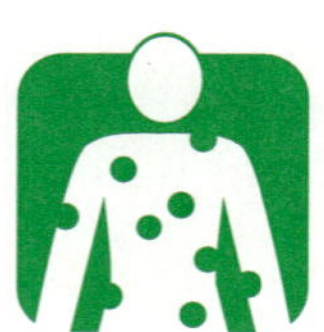

— ***Diseases***

1. Bubonic plague
   - results from a flea bite
   - incubation period of 7 days
   - high fever; painful *bubo* (inflamed, swollen lymph node) in groin or axilla; bacteremia; death
2. Pneumonic plague
   - results from inhalation
   - incubation period of 2 to 3 days
   - fever and malaise, followed 1 day later by respiratory problems that lead to death (fatality is greater than 90% if disease is untreated)

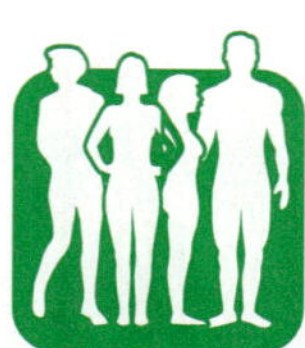

— ***Epidemiology***
Mode of spread: Fleas spread the infection from a mammalian reservoir (rats, dogs, mice, or rabbits). Bacteria are also acquired by contact with contaminated material.
Occurrence: Plague occurs primarily in Asia and Africa. It is endemic among wild animals in the southwestern and western United States. The disease is cyclical, depending on the animal reservoir.

— ***Prevention*** Pest control, improved hygiene, and vaccination (with formalin-killed vaccine) are used to control the disease.

— ***Treatment*** Streptomycin and chloramphenicol are satisfactory treatments.

- ***Yersinia enterocolitica***
  - ***Diseases***
    1. Enterocolitis (most common)
       - diarrhea, fever, and abdominal pain lasting 1 to 2 weeks
       - may lead to a chronic condition lasting more than 1 year
    2. Transfusion-related septicemia

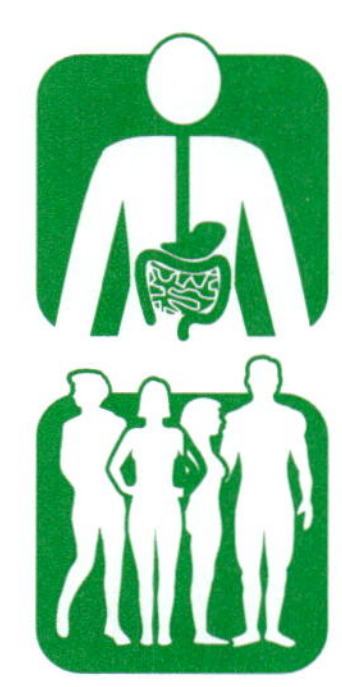

  - ***Epidemiology***
    Mode of spread: The organism is spread via contaminated food products and contaminated blood products.
  - ***Prevention*** The disease can be prevented by using proper food preparation methods.
  - ***Treatment*** Aminoglycosides and trimethoprim-sulfamethoxazole are the antibiotics of choice for treatment of *Y. enterocolitica* infections.

Other Enterobacteriaceae

- ***Klebsiella (Klebsiella pneumoniae)***
  - *K. pneumoniae* has a prominent *capsule,* which is important for virulence.
  - Organisms can be aspirated into the lungs and cause primary lobar pneumonia.
  - Alcoholics and individuals with compromised pulmonary function are at highest risk for developing *Klebsiella* infection.
- ***Proteus (Proteus mirabilis)***
  - *Motility* is a key identifying characteristic of *Proteus.*
  - The organisms cause urinary tract infections.
  - Bacterial urease breaks down urea, increases pH, promotes formation of renal stones, and is toxic to uroepithelium.
- ***Enterobacter, Citrobacter, Serratia,* and *Providencia***
  - Infections with these organisms are usually hospital acquired, with immunocompromised individuals being at risk.
  - *Enterobacter* organisms are resistant to several antibiotics.

SECTION 2.12 *NEISSERIA*

General Features (Box 2.6)

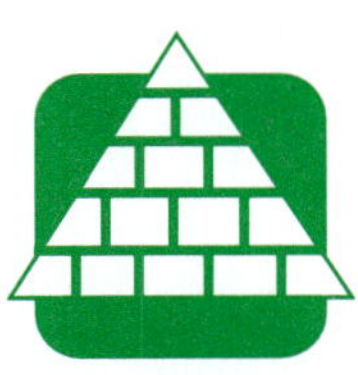

- Structure
  - *Neisseria* are gram-negative diplococci.
  - The outer membrane is loosely attached and readily shed contributing to pathogenesis by releasing lipopolysaccharide (endotoxin) into the host.
  - Pili (fimbriae) promote adherence and virulence, especially for *N. gonorrhoeae.*
  - *N. meningitidis has a polysaccharide capsule which is important for virulence.*

- **Laboratory identification** Neisseria can be identified in the laboratory by the following characteristics:
  - lactose negative, catalase positive, oxidase positive, gram-negative diplococci

Box 2.6

INFECTIONS ASSOCIATED WITH NEISSERIA MENINGITIDIS AND NEISSERIA GONORRHOEAE

N. meningitidis	Meningitis Septicemia Pneumonia Urethritis Arthritis
N. gonorrhoeae	Urethritis Cervicitis Salpingitis Proctitis Septicemia Arthritis Conjunctivitis Pharyngitis Pelvic inflammatory disease

- complex growth requirements; growth on chocolate agar in an atmosphere containing additional CO_2
- isolation on **Thayer Martin medium** (chocolate agar containing vancomycin, colistin, and nystatin) for *N. gonorrhoeae;* this medium is used for specimens obtained from nonsterile areas, such as the cervix and urethra
- fermentation of sugars
  - *N. meningitidis:* glucose positive, maltose positive
  - *N. gonorrhoeae:* glucose positive

Neisseria meningitidis The antigenic determinants of *N. meningitidis* have been classified according to serogroups based on the polysaccharide capsule, serotypes based on the outer membrane protein, and on immunotypes based on lipopolysaccharides. Serogroups A, B, C, Y, and W135 are the most common.

Pathogenesis The organism enters the respiratory tract and mucous membranes and then spreads via the bloodstream.

The virulence factors include the following:

- the **capsule,** which is antiphagocytic
- release of **endotoxin,** which induces fever and increases vascular permeability (potential for shock and petechiae [capillary leakage in skin])
- an IgA protease

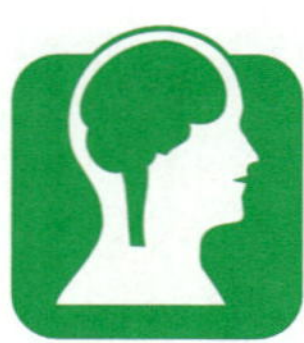

Diseases

1. Meningitis
2. Meningococcemia
   - Acute meningococcemia: occurs with or without meningitis and has a mortality of at least 25%; can be rapidly fatal and should be treated promptly; characterized by fever, shock, and generalized hemorrhage ranging from petechiae to purpura
   - *Waterhouse-Friderichsen syndrome:* a complication of meningococcemia that is charaterized by bilateral adrenal hemorrhage

- Chronic meningococcemia: a milder disease characterized by persistent (for weeks) bacteremia; patient has a low-grade fever, arthritis, and petechial skin lesions

3. Mild febrile disease with pharyngitis, pneumonia, arthritis, or urethritis

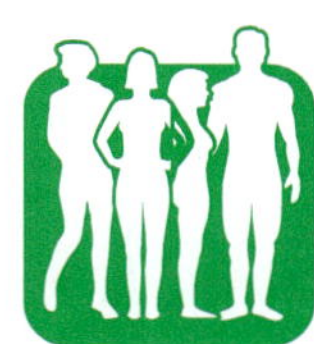

- **Epidemiology**

  Mode of spread: Spread of meningococci occurs by person-to-person transmission from infected persons or from asymptomatic nasopharyngeal carriers via aerosols.

  Populations affected: Individuals at risk include:

  - children under 5 years of age, with the highest risk being for children under 1 year of age
  - patients with deficiency of the terminal components (C5 to C9) of the complement cascade
  - close contacts (in the family, the military, daycare centers)

  Occurrence: The disease occurs worldwide and is more prevalent during the dry months (e.g., winter).

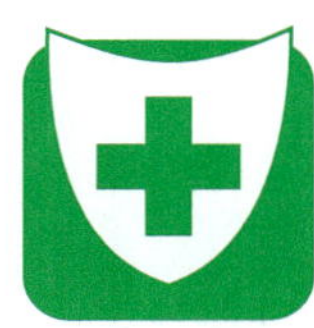

- **Prevention** The incidence of meningitis can be reduced by the following measures:

  - Breast feeding infants for the first 6 months of life
  - Vaccinating children over 2 years of age with a polyvalent conjugate, **anticapsule vaccine** (only for groups A, C, Y, and W135)
  - **Postexposure prophylaxis** with rifampin, quinolones, or sulfonamides (only if the organism is proven susceptible)

- **Treatment** Penicillin is the drug of choice. Other antibiotics that may be used are chloramphenicol, sulfonamides (if susceptible), or cephalosporins (broad spectrum).

Neisseria gonorrhoeae

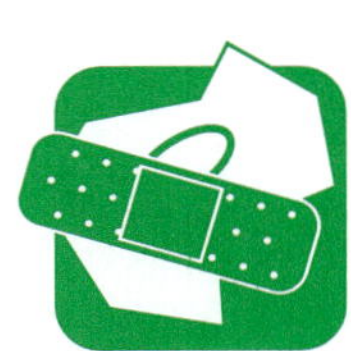

- **Pathogenesis** The organism colonizes epithelium.

  Virulence factors include the following:

  - endotoxin: causes fever, vascular permeability, inflammation, and tissue destruction
  - **pili** (fimbriae): promote adherence to epithelium
  - outer membrane proteins (protein PII): promotes adherence
  - **IgA protease:** breaks down secretory IgA
  - protein I: interferes with neutrophil degranulation

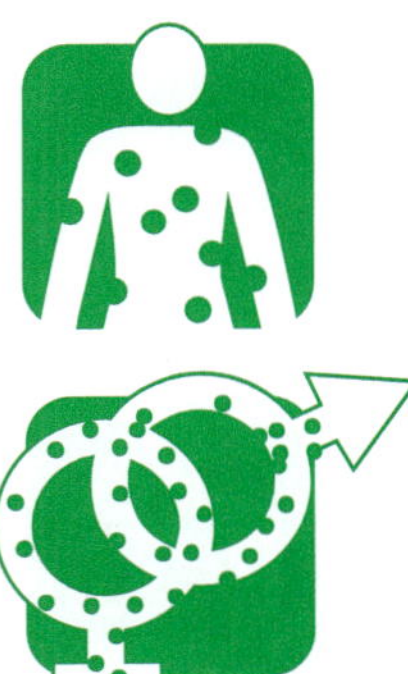

- **Diseases**

  1. Acute gonorrhea

     - In males: Acute gonococcal urethritis is characterized by purulent urethral discharge and dysuria (painful urination).
     - In females: There is vaginal discharge, dysuria, abdominal pain, and fever. Pelvic inflammatory disease (PID) is an ascending infection that involves the pelvis and may result in sterility.

  2. Gonococcal pharyngitis
  3. Anorectal gonorrhea

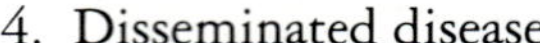

4. Disseminated disease

  - dermatitis-arthritis syndrome
  - bacteremia
  - endocarditis

5. Conjunctivitis in newborns (ophthalmia neonatorum)

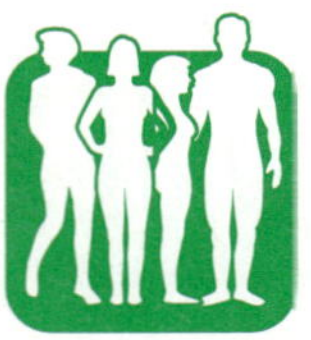

- **Epidemiology**
  Mode of spread: Gonococcal spread is by sexual contact and for newborns, by passage through the birth canal. Asymptomatic disease (especially in males) promotes spread.
  Populations affected: Sexually active individuals with multiple partners are at risk of contracting gonorrhea.
  Patients with terminal complement component deficiencies have a predisposition to disseminated disease.
  Occurrence: The organism is present globally.
- **Prevention** Use of safe sexual practices can reduce the incidence of gonorrhea. Neonatal disease can be prevented by antibacterial eye application at birth.

- **Treatment**
  1. Gonococcal urethritis: Treatment should be directed not only against the gonococcus but also against chlamydial infection, because dual infection is common. Therefore, treatment should include a drug for gonococcus together with a drug for chlamydia.
  Treatment of suspected gonococcal urethritis:

Anti-gonococcal agent	plus	Anti-chlamydial agent
Cefixime (single oral dose)		Tetracycline or doxycycline (multiple doses for at least 7 days)
Ceftriaxone (single intramuscular dose)		Azithromycin (single large dose)
Quinolones: ciprofloxacin or ofloxacin (single oral dose)		

  2. Tuboovarian abscess: Infection is usually caused by a mixture of aerobes and anaerobes, including gonococci and chlamydia. Treatment should include drugs effective against these two agents of sexually transmitted diseases (STDs).
  3. Disseminated or bacteremic illness: Prolonged therapy with penicillin or ceftriaxone is required.

SECTION 2.13 *PSEUDOMONAS*

Pseudomonads are soil bacteria that can live in almost any habitat using exotic carbon sources (e.g., soap). They cause particularly troublesome nosocomial infections in burn patients and cause the respiratory congestion associated with **cystic fibrosis.**

- **General features** The pseudomonads are gram-negative bacilli.

- **Laboratory identification** *Pseudomonas* species are oxidase positive, nonfermenting, gram-negative bacteria. Some species produce diffusible pigments.

Pseudomonas aeruginosa

Pathogenesis

Pathogenesis The mechanisms of pathogenesis include the following:

- pili: promote adherence to respiratory epithelium
- polysaccharide capsule: antiphagocytic and promotes adherence to tracheal epithelium
- exotoxin A and exoenzyme S: inhibitors of protein synthesis
- enzymes—elastase, alkaline protease, phospholipase C: tissue destruction
- leukocidin: inhibition of neutrophil and lymphocyte function
- endotoxin: promotes sepsis, leads to fever, shock, and disseminated intravascular coagulation
- antibiotic resistance: *Pseudomonas* is resistant to many antibiotics

Diseases

1. Skin lesions

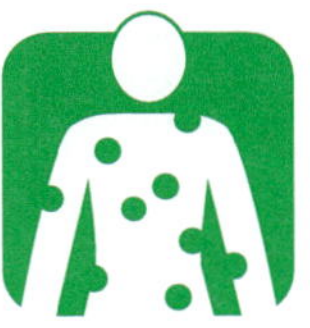

- vesicular and pustular skin lesions; cellulitis, abscesses, and subcutaneous infections
- a more serious form is ecthyma gangrenosum, a focal skin lesion usually seen in patients with neutropenia; characterized by vascular invasion by the bacteria, which results in hemorrhage and focal necrosis

2. Ear infections

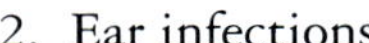

Otitis externa—swimmer's ear

- Malignant external otitis: pain, swelling and discharge from the external auditory canal seen in diabetic patients with poor glycemic control; prognosis is poor, if the infection is not treated promptly with antibiotics or surgical intervention
- Chronic suppurative otitis media

3. Pulmonary infections

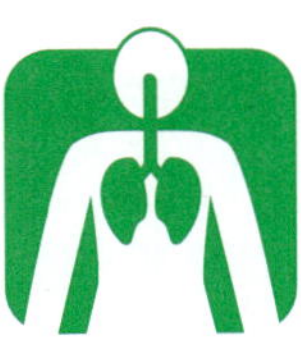

- colonization in patients with cystic fibrosis, other chronic lung diseases, or neutropenia
- pulmonary infection in patients with cystic fibrosis
- pneumonia (diffuse, bilateral bronchopneumonia) is a risk to neutropenic and other immunocompromised individuals

4. Eye infection

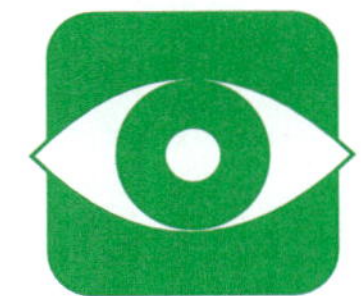

- corneal ulcer and endophthalmitis

5. Gastrointestinal infection: necrotizing enterocolitis in infants
6. Urinary tract infection

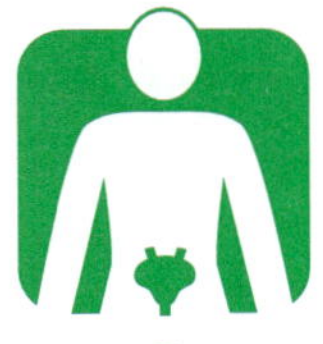

- frequently associated with indwelling catheters and antimicrobial therapy

7. Bacteremia and endocarditis

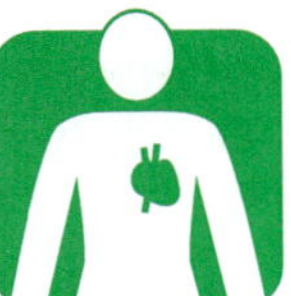

- course is similar to that of other infections caused by gram-

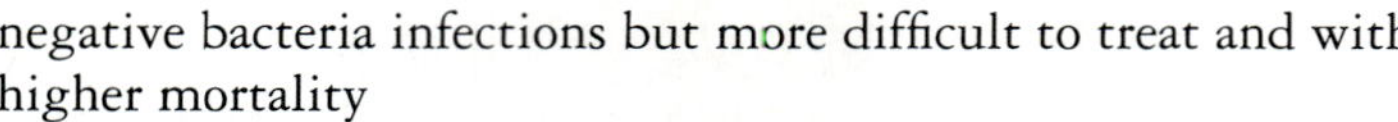

negative bacteria infections but more difficult to treat and with higher mortality

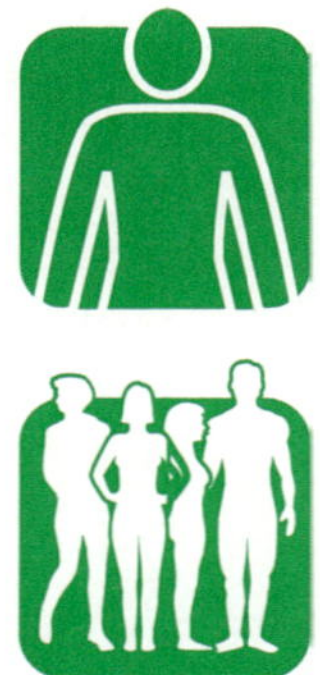

8. Burn infection
   - colonization of burn wounds is followed by vascular damage, tissue necrosis, and bacteremia
   - bacteremia originates from the lower respiratory tract, the urinary tract, or from skin or soft tissue infections in burn patients

- **Epidemiology**

  Mode of action: Pseudomonads are very hardy bacteria capable of growing in almost any environment, because of minimal nutritional needs, tolerance of a wide range of temperatures, and resistance to soaps, many disinfectants, and many antibiotics. They are found in moist environments, such as respiratory therapy equipment, cut flowers, sinks, and bars of soap, in hospitals and other institutions. The bacteria are a common contaminant and are readily acquired from the environment, and from other patients.

  Populations affected: Immunocompromised individuals, such as burn patients, patients with cystic fibrosis or chronic lung disease, and intravenous drug users are at risk of acquiring *Pseudomonas* infection.

  Occurrence: The organisms are ubiquitous.

- **Prevention** Infection control measures must be instituted in hospitals to prevent nosocomial spread.
- **Treatment** A combination of aminoglycoside and beta-lactam antibiotics is used, depending on the susceptibility of the isolate.

Other *Pseudomonas* Infections

- *Pseudomonas cepacia* and *Xanthomonas maltophilia* are frequently associated with hospital acquired infections.
- *Pseudomonas pseudomallei* causes chronic infections. This organism is associated with injuries incurred in Southeast Asia, e.g., in Vietnamese or in veterans of the Vietnam War.

Section 2.14 Vibrionaceae

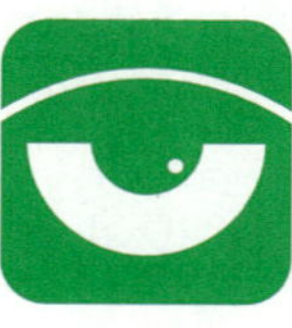

The members of the family Vibrionaceae include the following genera:

- *Vibrio:* Organisms belonging to this genus are curved gram-negative bacteria that are oxidase positive, have polar flagella, and grow in alkaline media. The species pathogenic for humans are summarized in Table 2.22.
- *Aeromonas* causes gastroenteritis
- *Plesiomonas* causes gastroenteritis

Table 2.22 Vibrio *Species Associated With Human Disease*

Vibrio Species	Source of Infection	Clinical Disease
V. cholerae	Water or food	Gastroenteritis
V. parahaemolyticus	Shellfish	Gastroenteritis
V. vulnificus	Shellfish; seawater	Bacteremia; wound infection; cellulitis

Vibrio cholerae

- **Structure** *V. cholerae* is a gram-negative curved (comma-shaped) bacillus.
- **Laboratory identification** *V. cholerae* grows well on most media used for stool culture, including blood agar and MacConkey agar.
- **Pathogenesis** An **exotoxin (of A-B type)** causes the symptoms of cholera (Fig. 2.24). The toxin binds to GM_1 ganglioside on the mucosal cell surface, enters the cell, and activates adenylate cyclase. The increase in cAMP causes secretion of sodium, potassium, and bicarbonate ions and fluid (up to 1 liter per hour), which can lead to severe dehydration and electrolyte imbalance. Resorption is not affected.

  The bacteria adhere to the mucosal epithelium and are thereby prevented from being flushed from the bowel during episodes of diarrhea.

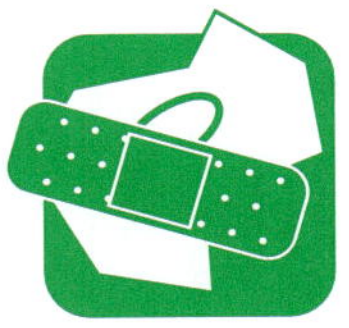

- **Disease** Cholera
  - consists of a **severe diarrhea** leading to dehydration, electrolyte imbalance, and death if not treated
  - results from ingestion of contaminated water or food (fish or shellfish)
  - incubation period is 2 to 3 days
  - symptoms: vomiting and watery diarrhea with mucous flecks (rice-water stools); dehydration; shock, cardiac arrhythmia, renal failure; mortality is 60% unless disease is treated

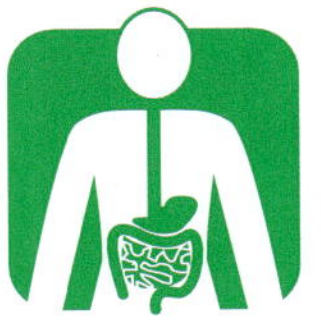

- **Epidemiology**

  Mode of spread: Cholera is spread by the fecal-oral route from contaminated food (fish and shellfish) and water. Large inocula are required to establish infection.

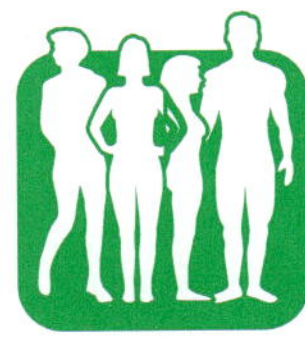

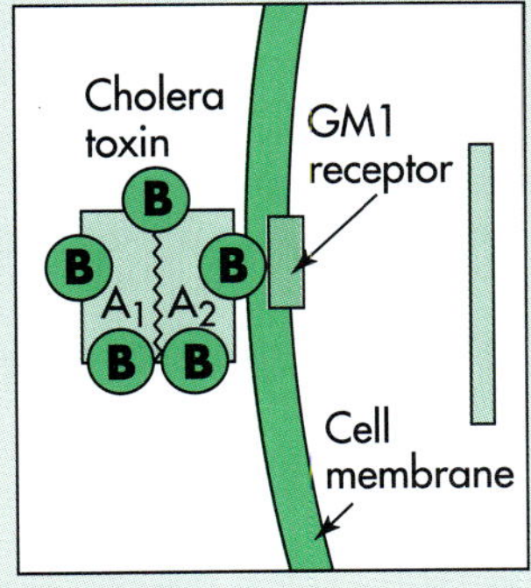

The complete toxin binding to the GM1-ganglioside receptor on the cell membrane via the binding subunits (B).

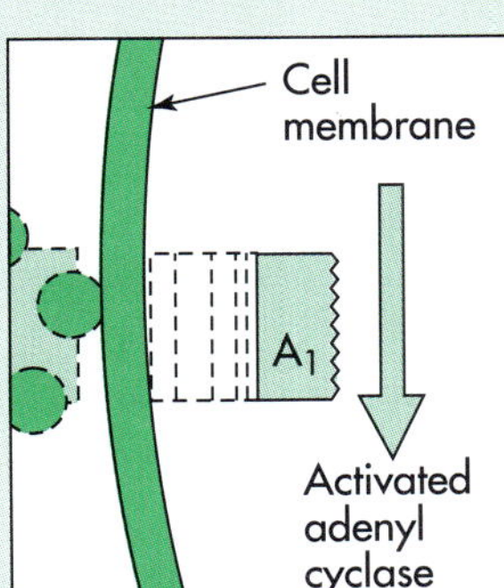

The active portion (A_1) of the A subunit enters the cell and activates adenyl cyclase.

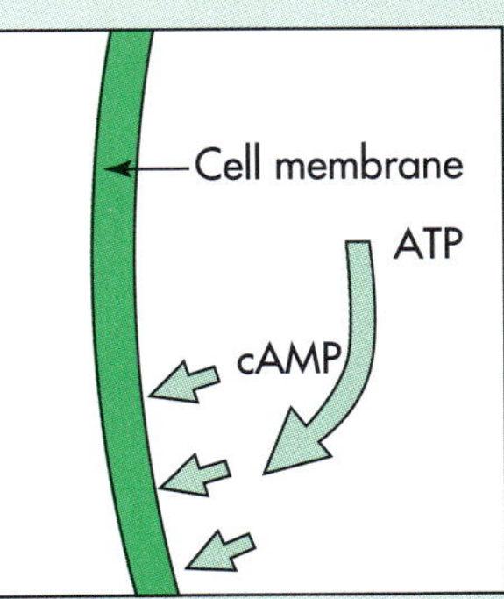

The activity results in accumulation of cyclic adenosine 3′, 5′ mono phosphate (cAMP) along the cell membrane.

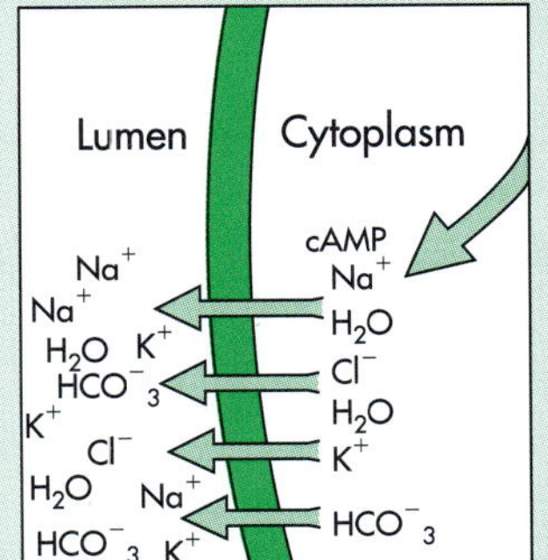

The cAMP causes the active secretion of sodium (Na^+), chloride (Cl^-), potassium (K^+), bicarbonate ($HCO^-{}_3$), and water (H_2O) out of the cell into the intestinal lumen.

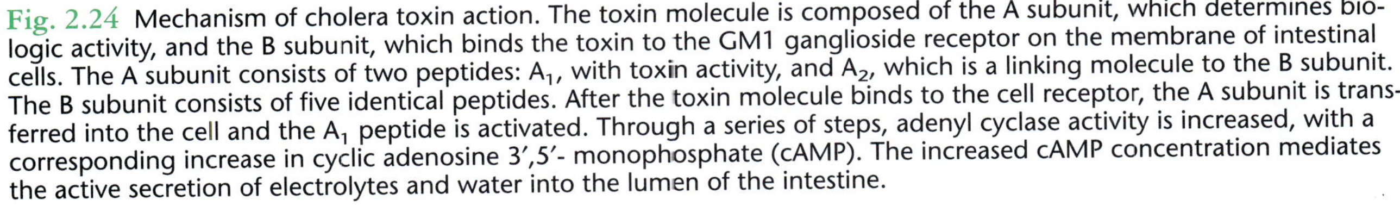

Fig. 2.24 Mechanism of cholera toxin action. The toxin molecule is composed of the A subunit, which determines biologic activity, and the B subunit, which binds the toxin to the GM1 ganglioside receptor on the membrane of intestinal cells. The A subunit consists of two peptides: A_1, with toxin activity, and A_2, which is a linking molecule to the B subunit. The B subunit consists of five identical peptides. After the toxin molecule binds to the cell receptor, the A subunit is transferred into the cell and the A_1 peptide is activated. Through a series of steps, adenyl cyclase activity is increased, with a corresponding increase in cyclic adenosine 3′,5′- monophosphate (cAMP). The increased cAMP concentration mediates the active secretion of electrolytes and water into the lumen of the intestine.

Table 2.23 *Characteristics of* Aeromonas *and* Plesiomonas *Gastroenteritis*

Epidemiologic and Clinical Features	*Aeromonas*	*Plesiomonas*
Natural habitat	Fresh or brackish water	Fresh or brackish water
Source of infection	Contaminated water	Uncooked shellfish
Clinical presentation		
Diarrhea	Present	Present
Vomiting	Present	Present
Abdominal cramps	Present	Present
Fever	Absent	Absent
Blood and PMNs in stool	Absent	Present
Pathogenesis	Enterotoxin (?)	Invasive

Occurrence: The organisms grow in freshwater ponds and brackish water where rivers meet the sea. Outbreaks of cholera occur in areas where there is poor sanitation and sewage processing, mainly in underdeveloped countries.

- **Prevention** Improved sanitation measures can decrease the incidence of disease.
- **Treatment** Supportive care with fluid and electrolyte replacement is the main treatment. Tetracycline may help.

Other Infections by Vibrionaceae (Table 2.23)

- *V. vulnificus* can be found in sea water and can contaminate wound infections resulting in complications. Infection may be initiated by shucking contaminated oysters.
- *V. parahaemolyticus* causes diarrhea that is associated with contaminated seafood. The disease is self-limited, lasting for about 72 hours.
- *Aeromonas: Aeromonas hydrophilia* is acquired from contaminated fresh or brackish water and can contaminate wound infections and cause gastrointestinal disease.
- *Plesiomonas* is acquired from contaminated shellfish (especially uncooked ones) and causes a self-limited gastroenteritis.

Section 2.15 *Campylobacter* and *Helicobacter*

Campylobacter: (Campylobacter jejuni, C. fetus)

Campylobacter organisms are non–spore-forming gram-negative rods.

- ***Campylobacter jejuni***
  - ***Structure*** *C. jejuni* is a gram-negative, motile, non–spore-forming comma-shaped bacillus.
  - ***Laboratory identification*** Organisms are oxidase-positive, catalase-positive bacteria. They require reduced oxygen and an increased carbon dioxide tension and temperature elevated to 42° C for growth. Selective media are needed to isolate *Campylobacter* from stool specimens.

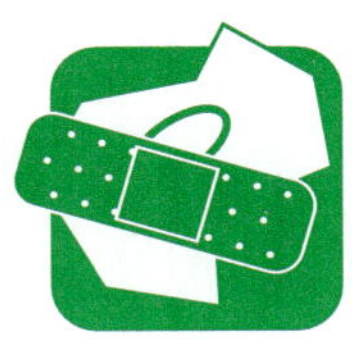

— ***Pathogenesis***

• *C. jejuni* destroys mucosal surfaces of the jejunum, ileum, and colon by unknown means.

• In addition to endotoxin, *C. jejuni* produces enterotoxins and cytotoxins.

— ***Diseases*** Enteritis

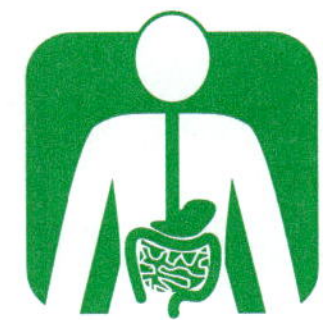

• incubation period is 1 to 7 days after exposure

• *C. jejuni* causes acute enteritis with diarrhea (ten or more bowel movements per day; stools may contain blood), malaise, fever, abdominal pain, and cramps

• difficult to differentiate *C. jejuni* enteritis from *Salmonella* or *Shigella* enteritis on a clinical basis

— ***Epidemiology***

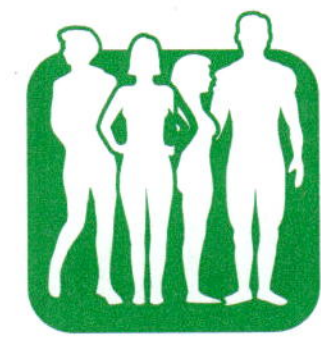

Mode of spread: *C. jejuni* spreads via the fecal-oral route through contaminated food (especially poultry), milk, or water. Asymptomatic carriers promote the spread of bacteria.

Populations affected: Individuals who ingest large numbers of bacteria and who lack gastric acids (which normally inactivate the bacteria) are at risk. People with hypogammaglobulinemia have more severe disease.

Occurrence: Infections occur worldwide, usually during the warm months.

— ***Prevention*** Good sanitation and proper food preparation methods can reduce the incidence of disease.

— ***Treatment*** The disease responds to antibiotic treatment with either erythromycin or quinolones. *C. jejuni* is usually resistant to sulfonamides as well as to trimethoprim-sulfamethoxazole.

● ***Campylobacter fetus*** *C. fetus* is a relatively rare pathogen *except in immunocompromised or elderly individuals.* It spreads from the gastrointestinal tract to the bloodstream and disseminates to several organs.

● ***Helicobacter pylori*** *H. pylori* has been implicated in gastric and duodenal ulcers.

— ***Structure*** *H. pylori* is a small, curved, microaerophilic gram-negative rod.

— ***Pathogenesis*** The following factors contribute to the pathogenesis of *H. pylori:*

- motility: bacteria are able to pass rapidly through a layer of mucus to prevent being eliminated
- adherence: bacteria are anchored at the intracellular junction of enteric cells, below the mucosal layer
- urease production: **urease** can neutralize stomach acid to facilitate growth
- infiltration of inflammatory cells leads to gastrin production and subsequent gastritis and ulceration
- *H. pylori* may cause damage to parietal cells resulting in decreased acid production

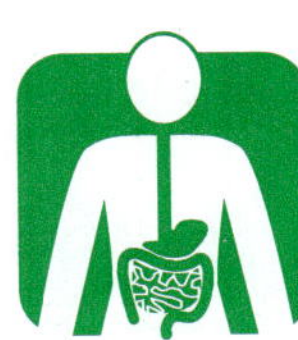

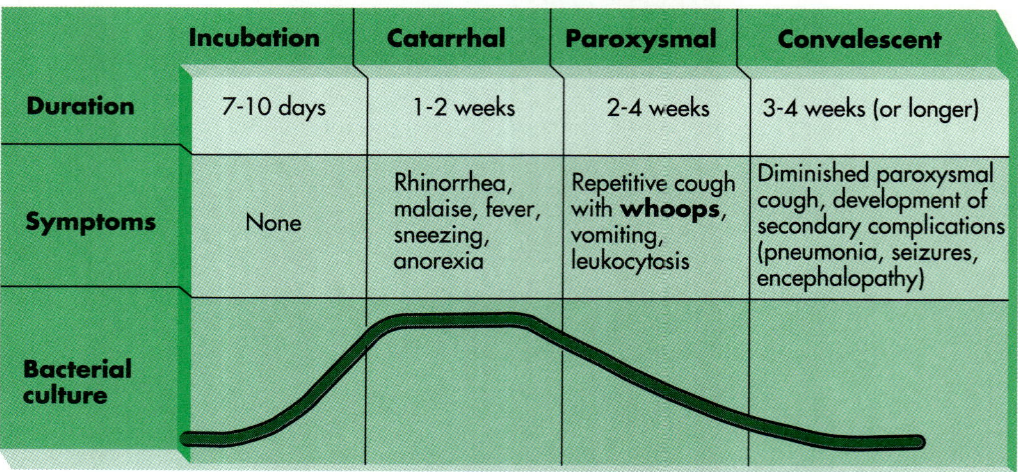

Fig. 2.25 Clinical presentation of *Bordetella pertussis* disease.

- chronic atrophic gastritis and resulting gastric adenocarcinoma

— *Diseases*
1. Gastritis
2. Stomach and duodenal **ulcers**

— ***Epidemiology*** *Helicobacter* is ubiquitous and acquired by ingestion.

— ***Treatment*** *H. pylori* is treated with bismuth salts, metronidazole, amoxicillin, and tetracyclines.

Section 2.16 *Bordetella, Francisella,* and *Brucella*

Bordetella pertussis

- **Structure** *B. pertussis* is a small gram-negative coccobacillus.
- **Pathogenesis** Factors contributing to the pathogenesis of *B. pertussis* are:
  - adherence to ciliated epithelial cells: mediated by a "filamentous hemagglutinin"
  - pertussis toxin: causes ADP ribosylation of G proteins, leading to lymphocytosis and hypoglycemia
  - adenylate cyclase toxin: induces cAMP production, which blocks immune effector function, preventing clearance of the bacteria
  - tracheal cytotoxin: inhibits and damages ciliated tracheal cells
  - endotoxin: causes fever and other pyrogenic responses

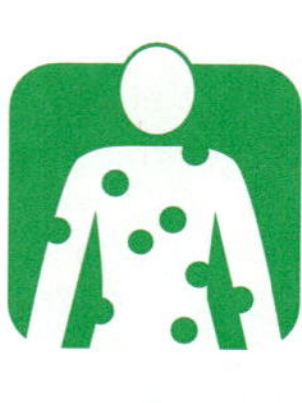

- **Disease** Pertussis or whooping cough (Fig. 2.25)
  - inhalation of bacteria leads to the catarrhal stage in 7 to 10 days: symptoms of a common cold with runny nose, sneezing, malaise, anorexia, and low-grade fever

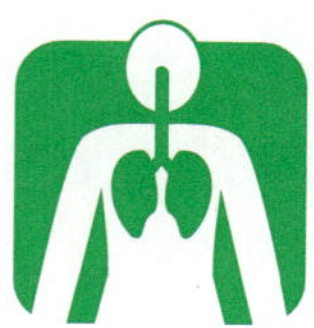

  - in 2 to 4 weeks the paroxysmal stage begins: repeated cough, followed by an inspiratory whoop (whooping cough) occurring 40 to 50 times per day

- impaired clearance of mucus causes airway blockage, leading to coughs
- within 3 to 4 weeks, the convalescent stage begins

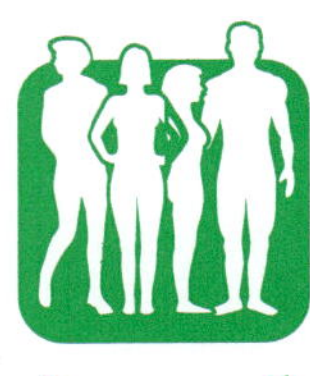

- **Epidemiology**
  Mode of spread: Organisms are transmitted person-to-person, via inhalation before appearance of the characteristic whooping cough.
  Populations affected: Inadequately immunized individuals are at risk.
  Occurrence: Pertussis occurs worldwide.

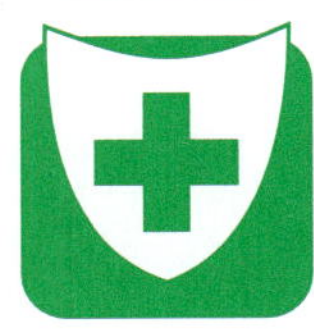

- **Prevention** **A whole-cell, inactivated vaccine** is administered as part of the DPT (diphtheria-pertussis-tetanus) vaccine.
- **Treatment** Treatment of pertussis consists of supportive measures.

Francisella tularensis

- **Structure** *F. tularensis* is a small gram-negative coccobacillus.
- **Pathogenesis**
  - *F. tularensis* is an encapsulated bacterium capable of **growing intracellularly in macrophages.**
  - *F. tularensis* can live in humans, animals, and arthropods (insects).

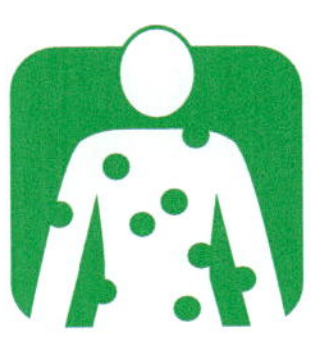

- **Disease** Tularemia
  - 3 to 5 day incubation period
  - abrupt onset of fever, chills, malaise, and fatigue
  - skin ulcers present at the site of infection; lymphadenopathy at the draining lymph node (*glandular fever*)

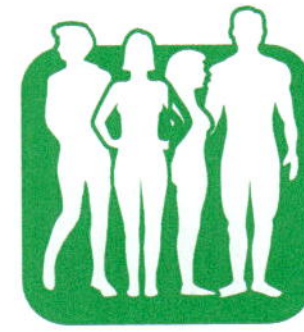

- **Epidemiology**
  Mode of spread: The organisms are spread by bites from **infected ticks** or by **contact with infected animals** (e.g., rabbits). Transmission also occurs by ingestion of contaminated meat or water or by inhalation of infectious aerosols (e.g., while skinning an infected animal).
  Populations affected: Hunters and persons exposed to ticks are most commonly infected.
  Occurrence: The disease occurs worldwide.
- **Prevention** Avoiding tick-infested regions and using gloves while handling furred animals can help protect against infection.
- **Treatment** Streptomycin is the treatment of choice.

Brucella (*Brucella abortus, B. melitensis, B. suis,* and *B. canis*)

- **Structure** *Brucella* are small gram-negative, nonencapsulated coccobacilli.
- **Pathogenesis** *Brucella* are **intracellular parasites growing in macrophages** and evading immune control. The bacteria inhibit neutrophil degranulation.

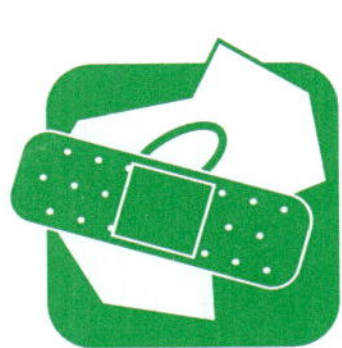

- **Disease** Brucellosis
  - Presentation can be subacute, acute or chronic.
  - Symptoms may include malaise, chills, sweats, fatigue, weight loss, and fever that occurs in waves (intermittent or undulating) (Fig. 2.26).

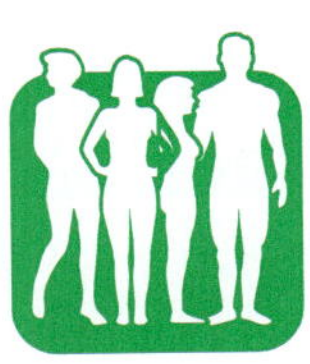

- **Epidemiology**
  Mode of spread: Brucellosis is a **zoonosis,** causing mild or asymptomatic disease in the natural animal hosts: *B. abortus*—**cattle;** *B. melitensis*—

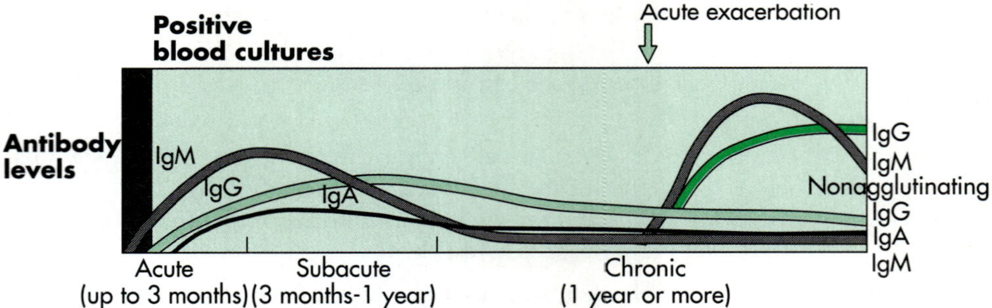

Fig. 2.26 Antibody responses in untreated brucellosis. *(From Mandell GL, Douglas RG Jr, Bennett JE:* Principles and practice of infectious diseases, *ed 2, New York, 1985, Churchill Livingstone.)*

goats and sheep; *B. canis*—dogs. The bacteria are spread by inhalation or by ingestion of contaminated milk.

Populations affected: Brucellosis is an occupational disease of slaughterhouse workers, farmers, and veterinarians who acquire the bacteria through direct contact or by inhalation. Individuals drinking unpasteurized milk are also at increased risk.

Occurrence: Distribution is worldwide. In the United States, the highest incidence is in Texas and California.

- **Prevention** Preventive measures include the control of disease in animals and avoidance of unpasteurized foods.
- **Treatment** A combination of tetracycline and streptomycin or high dose, long-term therapy with trimethoprim-sulfamethoxazole is effective in controlling the disease.

Section 2.17 *Hemophilus* and *Legionella*

Hemophilus

- **General features** All organisms in this group are gram-negative bacilli, with capsules that promote virulence.

- **Laboratory identification**
  - The bacteria can be isolated from cerebrospinal fluid and blood.
  - The organisms require X (hemin) and V (nicotine adenine dinucleotide) factors for growth and hence can grow on **chocolate agar** (heated blood agar; heating releases the X and V factors from blood).
  - Satellite phenomenon: *Staphylococcus aureus* growing on blood agar releases the V factor and allows H. influenza growth of *H. influenzae* as tiny satellite colonies.
  - The capsular antigen is used for serotyping.

Hemophilus influenzae

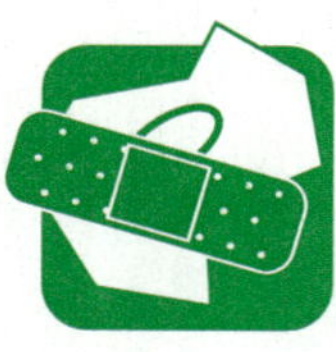

- **Pathogenesis**
  - *H. influenzae* (nonencapsulated) is part of the normal flora of the upper respiratory tract.
  - Encapsulated *H. influenzae* (especially type b) is virulent, invades the mucosa, enters the blood, and causes meningitis.

- The capsule is antiphagocytic.
- Endotoxin induces inflammation and contributes to the symptoms.

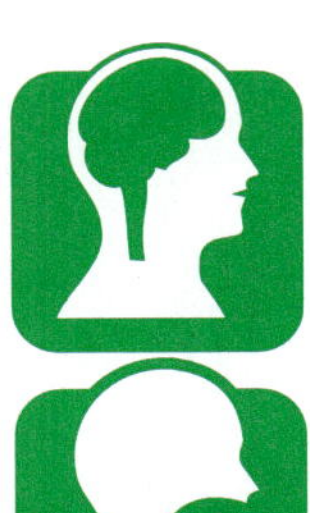

- **Diseases**

    1. Meningitis
        - affects children 3 to 18 months of age
        - 1 to 3 days of mild respiratory disease is followed by bacteremia and then meningitis
    2. Epiglottitis
        - occurs in children 2 to 4 years of age
        - cellulitis and swelling of the supraglottic tissues can block breathing
    3. Cellulitis
        - occurs in the facial region in very young children
    4. Arthritis
        - affects single large joints in children less than 2 years of age
    5. Otitis, sinusitis, and bronchitis
        - caused by nonencapsulated strains of *H. influenzae*

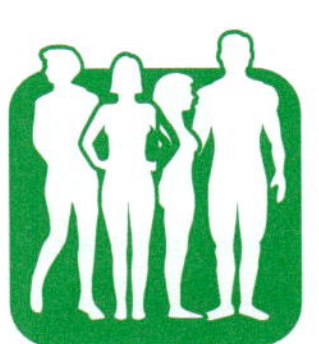

- **Epidemiology**

    Mode of spread: *H. influenzae* are normal flora of the upper respiratory tract. Encapsulated strains are virulent. Bacteria spread within the body by bacteremia.

    Populations affected: Unimmunized children, individuals with a deficiency in complement components, those patients lacking a spleen, and the elderly are at greatest risk for pulmonary disease.

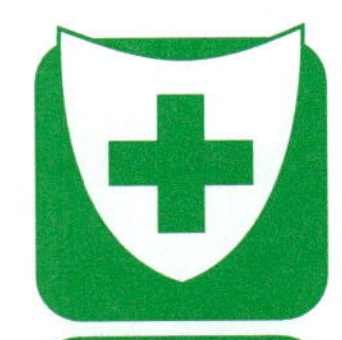

- **Prevention** An effective vaccine consisting of capsular material conjugated to diphtheria toxin protein is administered to infants 2 months and older and has made *H. influenzae* type b infection less prevalent.

- **Treatment** For severe infection, a combination of a beta-lactam antibiotic and a beta-lactamase inhibitor or a beta-lactamase-resistant cephalosporin (such as ceftriaxone), capable of CSF penetration are used. Prompt treatment is essential.

    For mild infection, the same antibiotics as above or the new macrolides (azithromycin, clarithromycin) or tetracycline can be used.

H. ducreyi

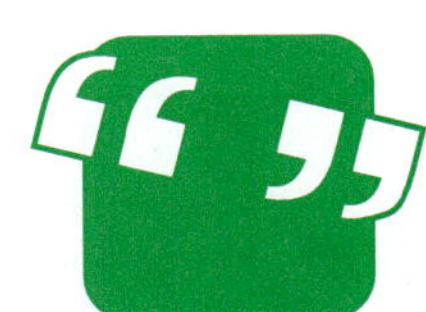

- *H. ducreyi* infection results in **chancroid,** which is a sexually transmitted disease.
- The disease is symptomatic in males but usually asymptomatic in females.
- A painful ulcer on the genitalia or the perianal region, together with inguinal lymphadenopathy develops 5 to 7 days after exposure.
- Diagnosis is by culture of the organisms from clinical samples.
- The disease can be treated with ceftriaxone, azithromycin, or erythromycin.

Legionella pneumophila

- **Structure** *L. pneumophila* is a slender, pleomorphic, gram-negative bacillus.

Table 2.24 ***Comparison of Diseases Caused by* Legionella**

	Legionnaires' Disease	Pontiac Fever
Epidemiology		
Presentation	Epidemic, sporadic	Epidemic
Attack rate	<5%	>90%
Person-to-person spread	No	No
Underlying pulmonary disease	Yes	No
Time of onset	Epidemic disease in late summer or fall; endemic disease throughout the year	Throughout year
Clinical Manifestations		
Incubation period	2-10 days	1-2 days
Pneumonia	Yes	No
Course	Requires antibiotic therapy	Self-limited
Mortality	15% to 20%; higher if diagnosis is delayed	<1%

- **Laboratory identification** *L. pneumophila* requires special media, supplemented with L-cysteine and iron salts (e.g., buffered charcoal yeast extract agar [BYCE]) for growth.

  Detection of antigen in specimens by direct immunofluorescence is an important test for identification.

- **Pathogenesis**
  - Following inhalation, *Legionella* establishes intracellular infection in alveolar macrophages and monocytes.
  - The bacteria coat themselves with C3b (a component of the complement pathway), which promotes uptake into macrophages.
  - Inhibition of phagolysosome fusion prevents contact and intracellular killing by superoxide, hydrogen peroxide, and other toxic metabolites in macrophages.
  - Degradative enzymes can kill cells.
  - Infection is controlled by T cells.

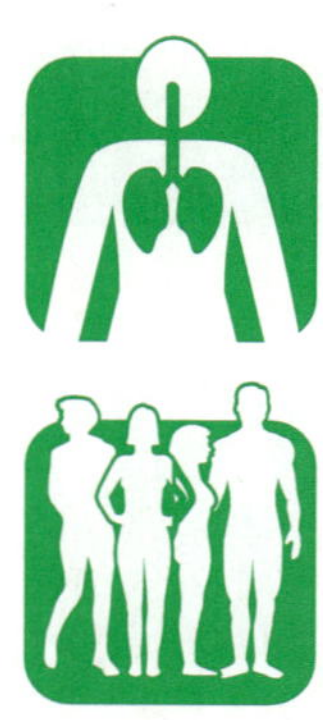

- **Diseases (Table 2.24)**
  1. Legionnaires' disease
  2. Pontiac fever
- **Epidemiology**

  Mode of spread: Inhalation of aerosols from the environment or from interior aquatic habitats, such as air conditioning systems, causes infection.

  Populations affected: Elderly patients with a deficiency in cell-mediated immunity or pulmonary function (including smokers) are at risk of acquiring infection.

  Occurrence: *Legionella* occurs worldwide. The bacteria grow in air conditioning cooling towers, condensers, and water systems, and also in lakes and streams.
- **Prevention** Hyperchlorination of the water supply and heating of water help prevent bacterial growth.

- **Treatment** The drug of choice is erythromycin. Alternative antibiotics are rifampin and fluoroquinolones.

Section 2.18 *Bacteroides*

- **Structure** *Bacteroides* are gram-negative, pleomorphic, encapsulated (polysaccharide capsule) organisms.
- **Pathogenesis**

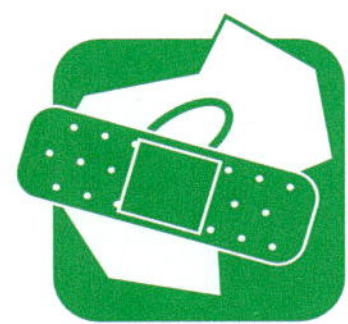

  - *Bacteroides* colonize the bowel and spread endogenously to other body sites via bacteremia and upon surgery.
  - The capsule is antiphagocytic and promotes abscess formation.
  - Bacterial enzymes promote tissue destruction.
  - *Bacteroides* are resistant to many antibiotics.
- **Diseases**

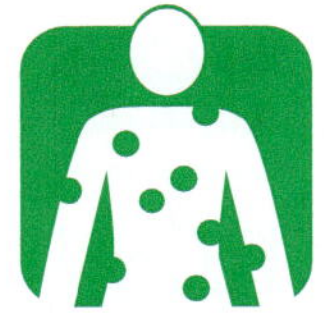

  1. Endogenous infections of normally sterile sites
     - usually found in combination with other organisms (polymicrobic infections)
     - abscess formation is followed by spread to other sites
  2. Intraabdominal infections with abscess formation (100%)
  3. Pleuropulmonary anaerobic infections (15% to 20%)
  4. Suppurative pelvic infections (66%)
  5. Bacteremia
     - more than 75% of all anaerobic gram-negative bacteremias are caused by *B. fragilis*
- **Epidemiology**

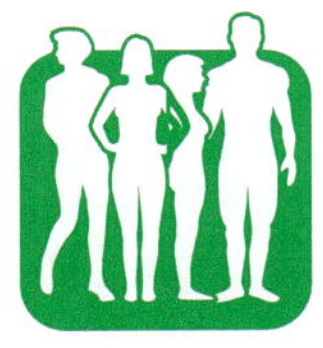

  Mode of spread: *Bacteroides* are part of the normal flora of the colon. Disease occurs after internal spread from the colon.

  Populations affected: Surgical and trauma patients are at risk of developing infection.
- **Prevention** Use of prophylactic antibiotics for planned surgical procedures that disrupt the mucosa can decrease the incidence of disease.
- **Treatment** Treatment consists of surgical intervention together with antibiotic treatment. The antibiotics used are cefoxitin, a beta-lactam antibiotic/beta-lactamase inhibitor combination (e.g., ampicillin/sulbactam, ticarcillin/clavulanate, piperacillin/tazobactam), and imipenem. Because most infections are mixed, antibiotics, such as clindamycin or metronidazole that act on anaerobic organisms, are usually used in combination with an agent such as gentamicin that acts on gram-negative bacteria.

Section 2.19 *Nocardia* and *Actinomyces*

Nocardia

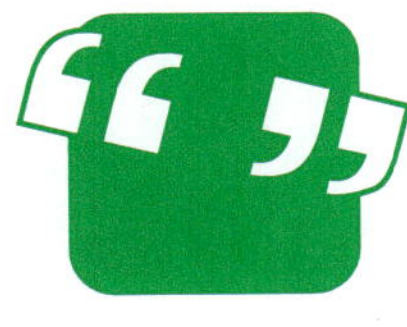

- **General features** *Nocardia* organisms are **soil bacteria** that appear similar to fungi because of their **filamentous** form. They are distinguished from *Actinomyces* that also appear **funguslike** because they are aerobic and produce mycolic acid.

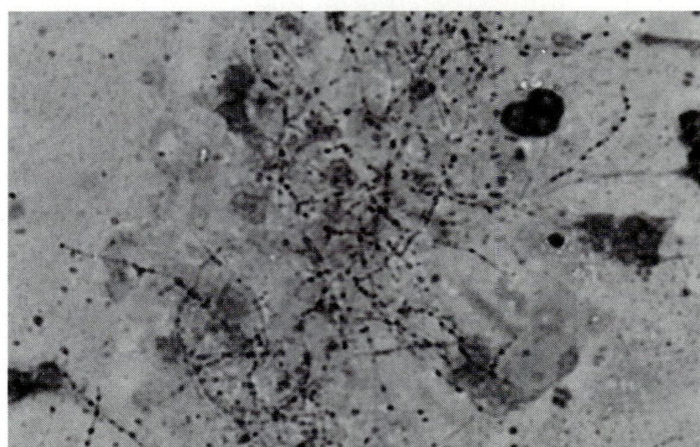

Fig. 2.27 Acid-fast stain of *Nocardia asteroides* in expectorated sputum.

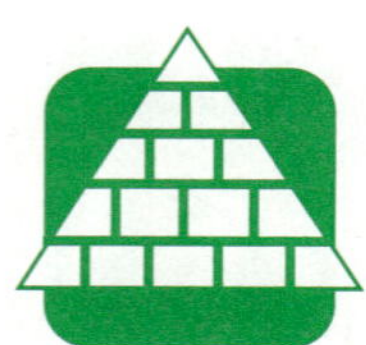

- **Structure** *Nocardia* stains weakly gram-positive. In similarity with the mycobacteria, they contain mycolic acids and are therefore acid-fast.
- **Laboratory identification** *Nocardia* grows very slowly. Sputum, infected tissue, or abscess material are examined for delicate filaments by the acid-fast stain (Fig. 2.27).

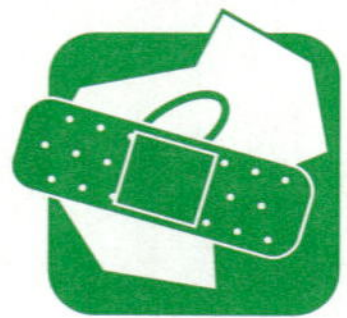

- **Pathogenesis**
  - The bacteria normally grow in soil and are inhaled or injected subcutaneously.
  - The bacteria colonize the oropharynx and are then aspirated into the lower airways.
  - Injection of *Nocardia* into the skin can lead to abscess formation and necrosis.

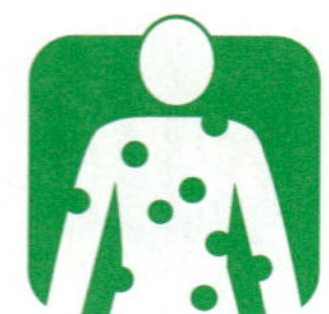

- **Diseases** *Nocardia* is the most common cause of acute or chronic suppurative infections. Nocardioses fall into two categories:
  1. Bronchopulmonary disease
     - cough, dyspnea, and fever with potential pneumonia
     - dissemination to the CNS (forming a brain abscess) or skin may occur
  2. Cutaneous infections, such as cellulitis, pustules, pyoderma, abscesses, and mycetomas

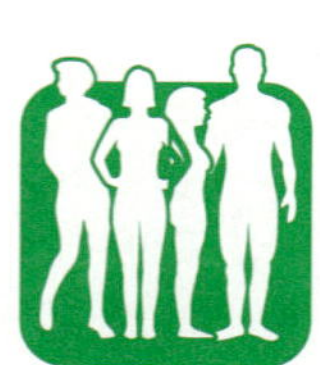

- **Epidemiology**

  Mode of spread: *Nocardia* species are soil bacteria and may be inhaled or enter skin wounds.

  Populations affected: Immunocompromised patients are at highest risk.

  Occurrence: The organisms are ubiquitous.
- **Treatment** Infections are treated by surgical intervention and long-term administration of antibiotics, such as sulfonamides.

Actinomyces

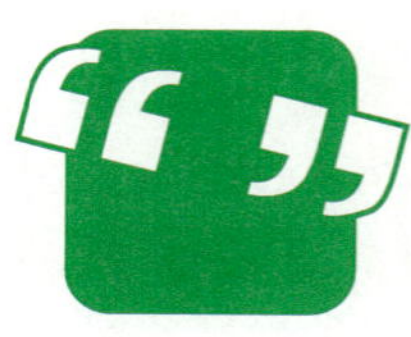

- **General features**
  - *Actinomyces* are **filamentous** bacteria that have the appearance of **fungi.**
  - *Actinomyces* can be distinguished from *Nocardia* (also filamentous) by being **anaerobic** and **non–acid-fast.**

- *Actinomyces* are normal colonizers of the upper respiratory tract, the GI tract, and the female genital tract. *Nocardia* organisms are not normal flora.

- **Pathogenesis**
  - Infection results when *Actinomyces* breaks through a compromised mucosal barrier.
  - The organism causes opportunistic infections that result from internal spread of bacteria.

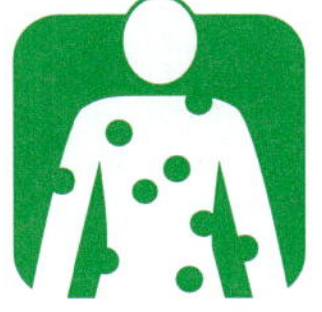

- **Laboratory identification** *Actinomyces* are difficult to identify in the laboratory. In tissue, the organisms appear as *sulfur granules,* which can be stained and examined microscopically for branching, filamentous bacteria. Culture is difficult and requires long-term incubation.

- **Diseases**
  1. Cervicofacial disease
     - tissue swelling, fibrosis, and scarring along sinus tracts along the angle of the jaw and neck
  2. Pelvic, thoracic, abdominal, CNS disease
  3. Chronic granulomatous infections
  4. Mycetomas (swelling with granules)
  5. Salpingitis (occurs with usage of intrauterine devices)

- **Treatment** Actinomycotic disease is treated with surgical debridement, and long-term antibiotic treatment with penicillin.

Section 2.20 *Mycobacterium*

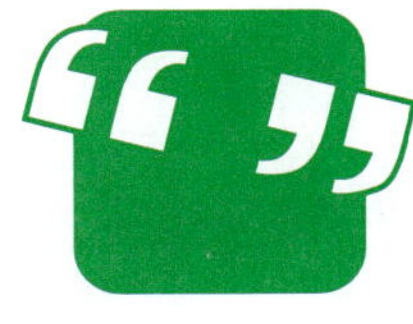

- **General features**
  - Mycobacteria are slow growing, intracellular bacteria that have a unique cell wall structure.
  - Mycobacteria are resistant to disinfection and most antibiotics because of their unique cell wall.
  - Pigment production is used to classify the mycobacteria (Runyon classification).

- **Structure (Fig. 2.28)** The mycobacterial cell wall is surrounded by a hydrophobic surface consisting of proteins and glycolipids and an arabinogalactan layer(s) outside the peptidoglycan. The hydrophobic layer is essential for virulence.

  The cell wall contains (from inside to outside):
  - peptidoglycan
  - arabinogalactan layer: polymer of D-arabinose and D-galactose, with attached mycolic acids
  - **waxes and free lipids**
    - mycolic acid: long-chain fatty acids
    - wax D: immunoadjuvant
    - cord factor: (trehalose dimycolate) correlates with virulence
  - proteins (e.g., purified protein derivative [PPD]): initiate protective immunity and most importantly, delayed type hypersensitivity responses

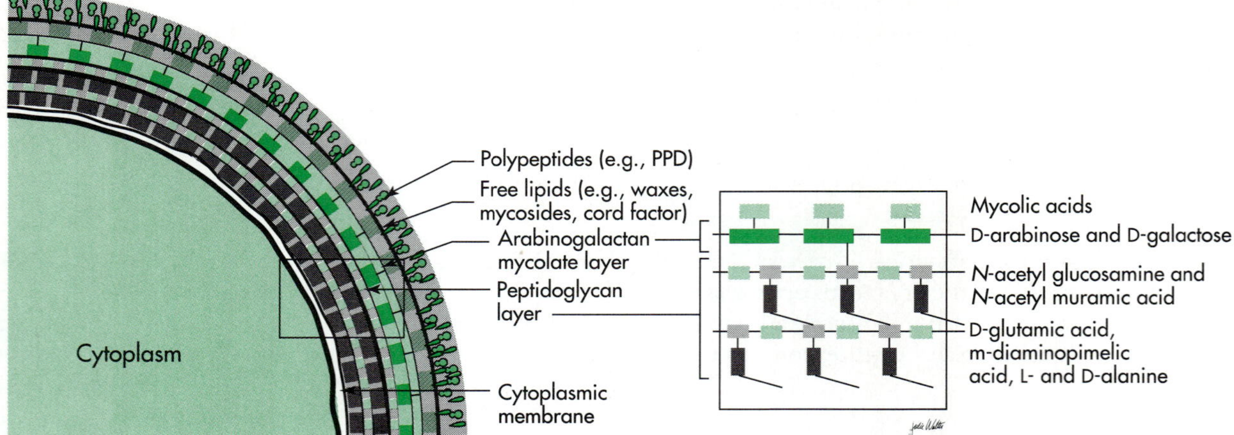

Fig. 2.28 Structural arrangement of mycobacterial cell wall layers. A waxy layer containing PPD antigen surrounds the arabinose-galactose layer which is attached to the peptidoglycan. *(Redrawn from Kubica GP, Wayne LG, editors:* The mycobacteria: a sourcebook, *New York, 1984, Marcel Dekker.)*

Mycobacterium tuberculosis

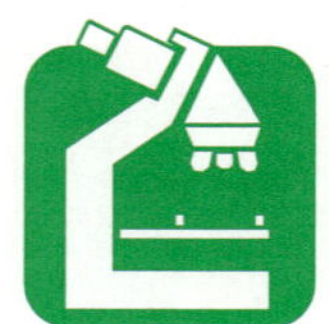

Laboratory identification

- Detection of acid-fast bacilli in sputum or biopsy specimen provides presumptive evidence of disease.
- Isolation *M. tuberculosis* is complicated by its slow growth. The organism grows on egg-based Lowenstein-Jensen media or on other special media.
- Serologic and DNA probes provide a more rapid means of identification.
- The **tuberculin skin test** is a test for delayed type hypersensitivity response to an intradermal injection of PPD and indicates prior exposure.

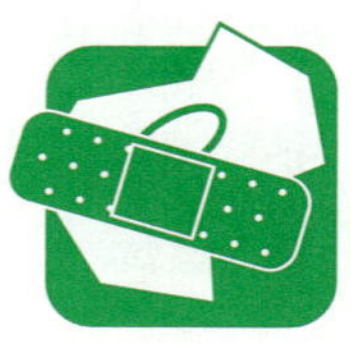

Pathogenesis

- Mycobacteria **grow intracellularly** (especially in macrophages).
- *M. tuberculosis* is inhaled, engulfed by alveolar macrophages, and replicates freely in the phagocytes; other macrophages are attracted to the site, infected cells are killed, and there is spread of the bacteria.
- Tuberculosis may involve any organ but the lungs are the initial and most common site of infection.
- Tissue destruction, fibrosis, and production of granulomas are caused by the host immune response.
- **Granulomas** result from localized collections of macrophages around the initial site of infection.
- Large, caseous granulomas result from large foci of infection. The granuloma gets surrounded by fibrin and the bacteria within remain dormant but viable and can be released later in life.
- The cell wall components prevent bacterial destruction in lysosomes.

Diseases Infection with *M. tuberculosis* can lead to pulmonary or nonpulmonary tuberculosis (TB). TB can remain dormant within the host and be reactivated later in life.

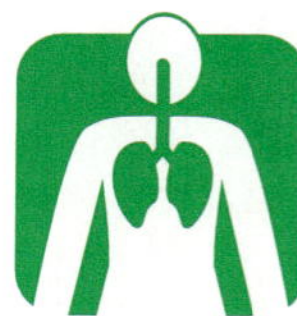

1. Pulmonary tuberculosis
   - A 3 to 6 week incubation period follows the inhalation of myco-

bacteria into the mid to lower lung region. Bacteria replicate and cell-mediated immunity restricts bacterial growth.

- The disease may occur within 2 years of infection (in 5% to 10% of cases) or later in life (in 5% to 10% of cases).
- Symptoms of disease include malaise, weight loss, cough, night sweats, and production of sputum.
- An active disease includes pneumonitis or abscess formation and cavitation in one or both upper lobes of the lungs.
- *The disease may recur, especially if the immune system is weakened.*

2. Extrapulmonary tuberculosis
   - Hematogenous spread of bacteria can lead to tissue destruction at other sites, such as the lymph nodes, the pleura, the genitourinary tract, and the meninges.
3. Tuberculosis in human immunodeficiency virus (HIV)-infected patients
   - The deficiency in $CD4^+$ T cells (the cells responsible for DTH responses) increases the risk of contraction or reactivation of TB and increases the potential for disseminated infection and a rapid progression to death.

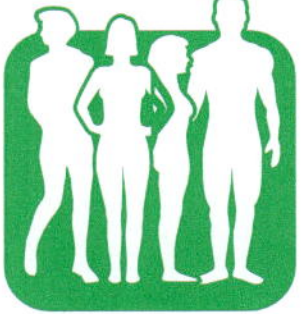

Epidemiology

Mode of spread: Coughing promotes spread of bacteria by aerosols. Bacteria are resistant to disinfection.

Populations affected: Humans are the only natural reservoir of *M. tuberculosis.* Exposure puts an individual at risk. Crowded conditions promote spread of the tubercle bacillus. Immunosuppressed individuals have the highest risk of contracting the disease.

Occurrence: Tuberculosis occurs globally.

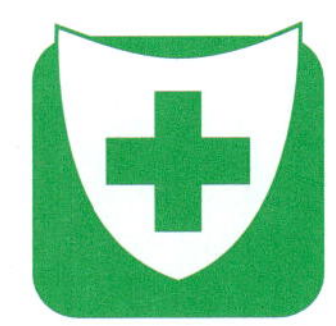

Prevention Surveillance programs using the PPD skin test response identify previously infected individuals. Lung x-ray is the follow-up to a positive PPD response. Vaccination with BCG (bacille Calmette-Guérin) is not used routinely in the United States. Complete treatment of patients prevents further spread.

Treatment Treatment of TB involves long term (6 months) combined therapy with three or four drugs, for example, isoniazid (INH), rifampin, pyrazinamide (2 months only) treatment. Ethambutol or streptomycin may be added. Multi-drug resistant strains are common in developing countries, are prevalent in patients with acquired immunodeficiency syndrome (AIDS), and are becoming more widespread in the United States.

Mycobacterium avium-intracellulare Complex

- This organism is a major mycobacterial pathogen in **AIDS patients,** causing disseminated disease.
- It is asymptomatic in normal adults but can cause pulmonary disease.
- It is resistant to most antibiotics.

Mycobacterium bovis

- *M. bovis* causes tuberculosis in cattle and humans.
- Infections with this organism are rare in the United States. Pasteurization of milk kills the mycobacteria.

Table 2.25 ***Clinical and Immunologic Manifestations of Leprosy***

	Tuberculoid	Lepromatous
Skin lesions	Few erythematous or hypopigmented plaques with flat centers and raised, demarcated borders; peripheral nerve damaged with complete sensory loss; nerves visibly enlarged	Many erythematous macules, papules, or nodules; extensive tissue destruction (e.g., nasal cartilage and bone, ears); diffuse nerve involvement with patchy sensory loss; nerves not enlarged
Histopathology	Infiltration of lymphocytes around center of epithelial cells; Langerhans' cells present; few or no acid-fast bacilli present	Predominantly "foamy" macrophages with few lymphocytes; Langerhans' cells absent; acid-fast bacilli abundant in skin lesions and internal organs
Infectivity	Low	High
Immune response		
Delayed hypersensitivity	Reactivity to lepromin	Nonreactive to lepromin
Immunoglobulin levels	Normal	Polyclonal hypergammaglobulinemia
Erythema nodosum leprosum	Absent	Usually present

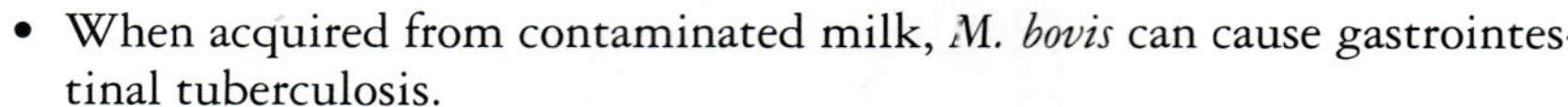

- When acquired from contaminated milk, *M. bovis* can cause gastrointestinal tuberculosis.
- *M. bovis* is the organism used for the BCG vaccine.

■ ***Mycobacterium leprae*** *M. leprae* causes **leprosy (Hansen's disease).** Symptoms include skin lesions, sensory loss, and extensive tissue destruction.

Mode of spread: Infection is spread by person-to-person contact and by inhalation of infected droplets.

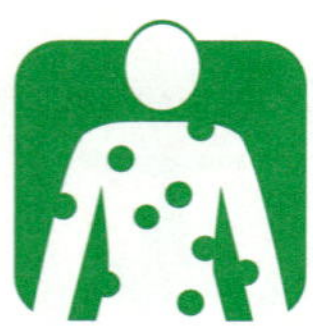

Clinical presentations (Table 2.25):

1. *Lepromatous leprosy* is characterized by a weak immune response and large numbers of *M. leprae* at the site of the lesion.
2. *Tuberculoid leprosy* is characterized by a strong immune response and small numbers of *M. leprae* at the site of the lesion.
3. *Dimorphic leprosy* is characterized by lesions ranging between the tuberculoid and lepromatous forms.

● **Treatment** Leprosy is treatable with dapsone, rifampin, clofazimine, or ethionamide administered for 2 years.

Section 2.21 Spirochetes: *Treponema* and *Borrelia*

● **General features** Spirochetes are thin, helical, gram-negative bacteria. They cause diseases that may have a course lasting from months to years, if not treated. The immune response is responsible for tissue damage.

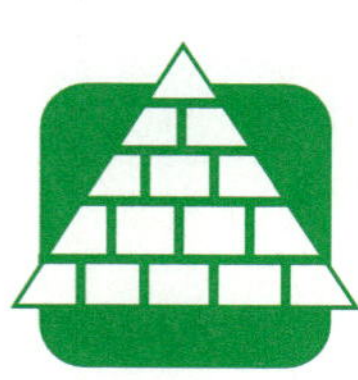

■ **Treponema (*Treponema pallidum, T. pertenue,* and *T. carateum*)**

● **Structure** Treponemes are thin, helical, gram-negative bacteria, visible only by dark-field or fluorescent microscopy. Flagella are present in the periplasmic space (between the peptidoglycan layers and the outer membrane) and run the length of the bacteria.

● **Laboratory identification** Treponemes are slow-growing anaerobes that cannot be cultured in the laboratory. The organisms can be visualized by

Box 2.7

MEDICAL CONDITIONS ASSOCIATED WITH FALSE-POSITIVE TREPONEMAL AND NONTREPONEMAL SEROLOGY TESTS

Nontreponemal Tests
Viral infection
Collagen-vascular disease
Acute or chronic illness
Pregnancy
Recent immunization
Heroin addiction
Leprosy
Malaria

Treponemal Tests
Pyoderma
Skin neoplasm
Acne vulgaris
Mycoses
Crural ulceration
Rheumatoid arthritis
Psoriasis
Systemic lupus erythematosus
Pregnancy
Drug addiction
Herpes genitalis

dark-field microscopy or by direct fluorescent antibody staining of exudate from the lesion.

Serologic tests

1. Nontreponemal tests, such as the **Venereal Disease Research Laboratories (VDRL)** test and the **rapid plasma reagin (RPR)** test are based on the detection of reagin antibodies that develop against lipids released from damaged cells. Since these are nonspecific tests, false-positive reactions can occur (Box 2.7).

2. Treponemal tests, such as the fluorescent treponemal antibody absorption **(FTA-ABS)** test and the microhemagglutination test for *T. pallidum* (MHA-TP), are based on the detection of antigens specific to *Treponema.*

Pathogenesis

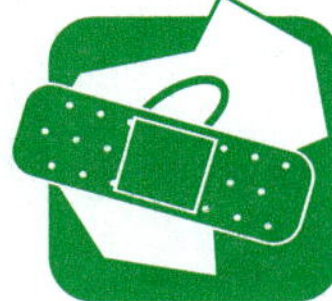

- Bacteria adhere to host cell surfaces and produce hyaluronidase, which promotes invasion.
- Bacteria become coated with host fibronectin to escape phagocytosis and immune recognition.
- Tissue destruction is caused by host immune responses.
- Bacteria enter the blood stream and spread soon after infection.
- The organisms spread to other skin sites. The disease may be controlled by the immune response or there may be spread to other organs, resulting in tissue destruction.
- The bacteria grow slowly and the course of disease may take months to years.
- Syphilis may recur years after the primary infection.

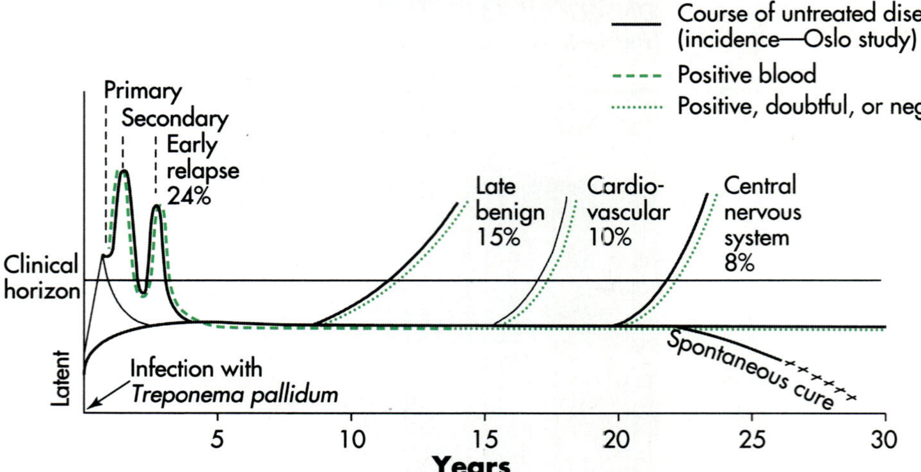

Fig. 2.29 The natural history of untreated syphilis. The incubation period from the time of infection to onset of primary disease varies from 10 to 90 days (average 21 days). Without treatment the chancre will heal in 3 to 6 weeks. Asymptomatic dissemination occurs during this period, and secondary lesions develop from 2 weeks to 6 months (average, 6 weeks) after the initial appearance of the chancre. These lesions will last for 2 to 10 weeks. At the end of the secondary stage of syphilis, patients enter a latent phase during which they can undergo spontaneous cure or relapse into the secondary stage manifestations (observed in 24% of the patients). Tertiary syphilis can occur years later with the development of systemic granulomas (called gummas) in soft tissues (in 15% of the patients), cardiovascular disease (in 10%), or central nervous system lesions (in 8%). *(Modified from* South Med J *26:18, 1933; incidence data from Clark EG, Danbolt N:* J Chron Dis *2:311, 1955.)*

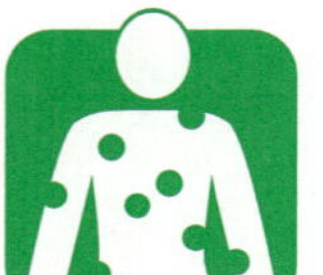

- ***Treponema pallidum***

— ***Diseases (Figs. 2.29 and 2.30)***

1. Syphilis

• The clinical course of syphilis consists of three stages.

a. Primary syphilis: **A chancre** (ulcerated skin lesion) develops at the site of inoculation. **Lymphadenopathy** (swollen lymph glands) develop within 1 to 2 weeks of the chancre indicating the site of bacterial proliferation. Healing of the ulcer *does not* indicate a cure.

b. Secondary syphilis: The disease is **disseminated** and skin lesions that are highly contagious are dispersed over the entire body surface. An influenzalike syndrome, with sore throat, headache, fever, myalgia, anorexia, and generalized lymphadenopathy accompany this stage.

c. Late (tertiary) syphilis: **Gummas** (granulomatous lesions) form in bone, skin, and other tissues. Neurosyphilis and cardiovascular syphilis are life-threatening conditions that may develop.

2. Congenital syphilis

• In utero infection of the fetus in a syphilitic mother causes severe morbidity and mortality in infants.

• Timecourse: Syphilis is a slowly progressing disease that runs its course over a period of months to years.

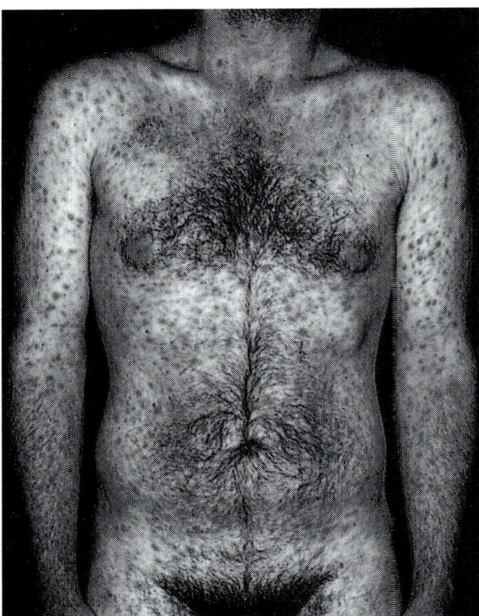

Fig. 2.30 Disseminated rash in secondary syphilis. *(From Habif TP, editor:* Clinical dermatology, *St Louis, 1985, Mosby.)*

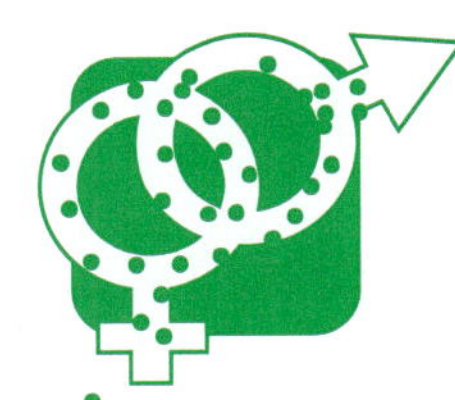

— ***Epidemiology***

Mode of spread: Infection is transmitted by sexual contact or by contact with the rash of secondary syphilis. Congenital syphilis is transmitted in utero to the neonate.

Populations affected: People with multiple sexual partners, newborns of infected mothers, patients with AIDS (neurosyphilis) are at risk.

Occurrence: Syphilis occurs worldwide. It is the third most common STD in the United States.

— ***Prevention*** Use of safe sexual practices can help protect against syphilis.

— ***Treatment*** Penicillin is still the drug of choice.

● ***Treponema pallidum pertenue***

- *T. pallidum pertenue* is the agent of **yaws,** a granulomatous disease with elevated papilloma-like lesions on the skin. Destructive lesions of the skin, lymph nodes, and bones occur later in the disease.
- The organism is spread by direct contact with lesions.
- The disease is found in tropical regions of South America, central Africa, and Southeast Asia.

● ***Treponema carateum*** **Pinta** is caused by *T. carateum.* Skin lesions consist of papules that enlarge into recurrent lesions causing scarring. Disease is limited to the skin. Pinta, also, is spread by contact with lesions.

***Borrelia* (*Borrelia burgdorferi* and *B. recurrentis*)**

● ***Borrelia burgdorferi***

— ***Structure*** The *Borrelia* are larger than treponemes and can be visualized by light microscopy.

— ***Laboratory identification***

• Microscopic examination of blood during the febrile stage (with a Giemsa or a Wright's stain) will show spirochetes.

• The organisms are difficult to culture because of requirements for anaerobic conditions.

• Serologic tests, such as ELISA, can confirm a diagnosis of Lyme disease 2 to 4 weeks after the onset of the rash (erythema chronicum migrans).

• False-positive serologic tests are common and require confirmation by a second test, such as a western blot.

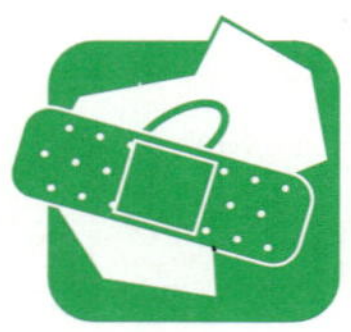

— ***Pathogenesis***

• The organisms are tick borne. The bacteria are deposited in the skin and the blood and then spread to multiple organs.

• *Borrelia* is capable of antigenic variation.

• The immune response to the bacteria in the skin cause the rash.

• Manifestations of late disease are caused by the presence of bacteria in organs, especially the CNS and the heart. A systemic immune response similar to autoimmunity, leads to problems such as arthralgia and arthritis.

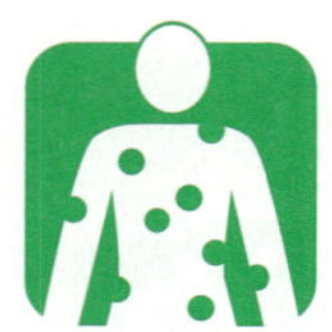

— ***Disease*** Lyme disease

• within 3 to 30 days after a tick bite, the rash starts as a small macule or papule

• approximately 3 weeks later, the rash enlarges, with a red border and a clear center

• initial rash may fade and other rashes may appear

• *early symptoms* (last for 4 weeks)—malaise, severe fatigue, headache, fever, chills, musculoskeletal pains, myalgias, and lymphadenopathy

• *late symptoms* (may occur up to 2 years later)

—Phase 1 consists of neurologic symptoms, such as aseptic meningitis, encephalitis, and peripheral nerve neuropathy (loss of feeling or tingling) including Bell's palsy or cardiac dysfunction, including heart block, myopericarditis, and congestive heart failure

—Phase 2 consists of arthralgias or arthritis (the spirochetes are rarely visualized in affected tissue)

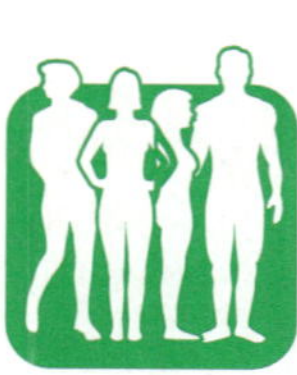

— ***Epidemiology***

Mode of spread: The organisms are borne by the ticks *Ixodes dammini* (in the northeastern United States) and *I. pacificus* (on the West Coast). The natural reservoirs for the ticks are the white footed-mouse and the white-tailed deer; ticks will also infest pets. The adult and nymph stages of the ticks can spread disease.

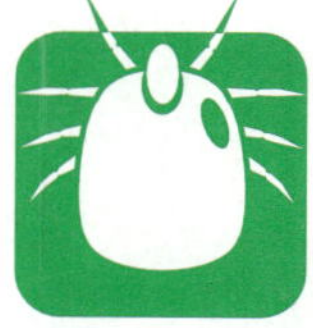

Occurrence: Cases of infection occur in late spring, summer, and early fall, during tick seasons. The disease occurs worldwide. In the United States the three principle foci are in the Northeast (from Massachusetts to Maryland), in the upper Midwest (in Minnesota, Wisconsin, and Michigan), and in the Pacific Northwest (in California, Oregon, and Washington).

Table 2.26 ***Properties of*** **Mycoplasma *and* Ureaplasma**

Properties	Characteristics
Size	0.2 to 0.8 μm
Cell wall	Absent
Growth requirements	Sterols
Atmosphere requirements	Facultatively anaerobic*
Replication	Binary fission
Generation time	1 to 6 hours
Antibiotic susceptibility	
Penicillins	Resistant
Cephalosporins	Resistant
Tetracycline	Susceptible
Erythromycin	Susceptible†

**M. pneumoniae* is an obligate aerobe.
†*M. hominis* is resistant.

— ***Prevention*** Avoidance of tick-infested areas, wearing of protective clothes, and use of insect repellants can help protect against infection.

— ***Treatment*** Doxycycline (tetracycline), amoxicillin, and erythromycin are the antibiotics of choice in treating *B. burgdorferi* infection.

- ***Borrelia recurrentis*** *B. recurrentis* causes louse-borne relapsing fever.

Section 2.22 *Mycoplasma* and *Ureaplasma*

- **General features (Table 2.26)**

  - Mycoplasmas other than *Mycoplasma pneumoniae* form colonies that have a "fried egg" appearance.
  - The organisms require sterols for growth.

- **Structure**

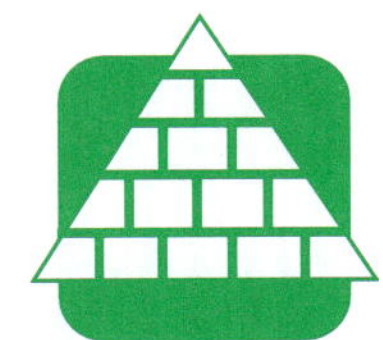

  - *Mycoplasma* and *Ureaplasma* are the smallest, free-living bacteria, capable of passing through a 0.45 μm filter (used normally to remove other bacteria).
  - The organisms lack a cell wall. Because they lack peptidoglycan, these bacteria are resistant to beta-lactam antibiotics.

Mycoplasma pneumoniae

- **Laboratory identification**

  - *M. pneumoniae* is a slow-growing, obligate aerobe forming granular colonies.
  - Serologic tests (measuring antigen specific IgM antibodies) and DNA probe analysis of sputum specimens are used for identification.

- **Pathogenesis** *M. pneumoniae* adheres to respiratory epithelium using bacterial P1 **adherence protein.** The organism disrupts and kills ciliated epithelium, thus facilitating its spread to the lungs.

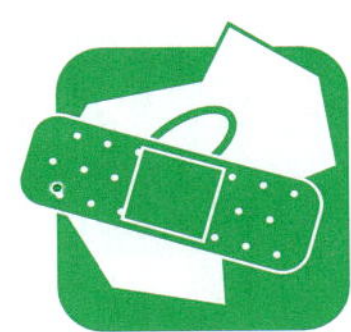

Table 2.27 *Diseases Caused by* **Mycoplasma** *and* **Ureaplasma**

ORGANISM	DISEASES
Mycoplasma pneumoniae	Pneumonia, tracheobronchitis, pharyngitis
Mycoplasma hominis	Pyelonephritis, pelvic inflammatory disease, postabortal fever, postpartum fever
Ureaplasma urealyticum	Nongonococcal urethritis

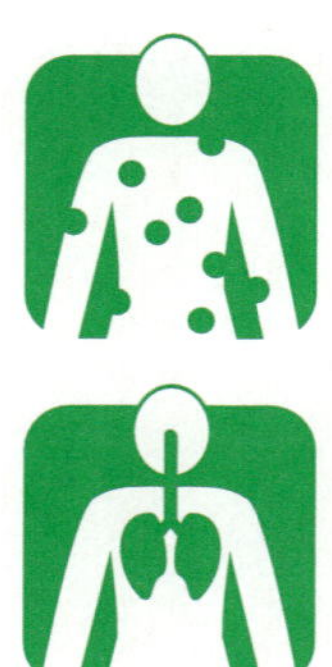

- **Diseases (Table 2.27)**
  1. Primary atypical pneumonia (**walking pneumonia**)
     - comparatively mild, protracted disease with a long incubation period
     - initial symptoms are malaise, low-grade fever, and headache; after 2 to 4 days, nonproductive cough, rales, and rhonchi are present; myalgia and possibly maculopapular rash occur
     - complications include otitis media, erythema multiforme, hemolytic anemia, myocarditis, pericarditis, and neurologic problems
     - resolution is slow
     - infection in adults is more severe than that in children
  2. Tracheobronchitis
     - a common form of the disease, with symptoms similar to pneumonia
     - disease is due to inflammation of the bronchi
     - symptoms include nonproductive **cough,** fever, headache, sore throat, pharyngeal exudates, and cervical lymphadenopathy
  3. Pharyngitis
     - may be the initial or a milder presentation of infection and resembles a group A streptococcal or viral pharyngitis

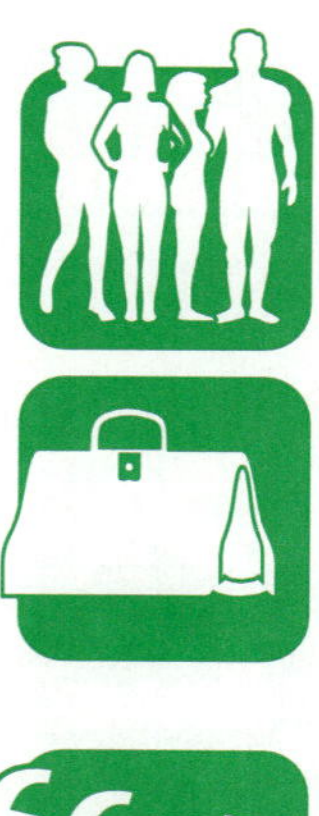

- **Epidemiology**

  Mode of spread: *Mycoplasma* is spread via aerosols. Asymptomatic carriers can also spread the organisms.

  Populations affected: School-aged children and young adults are affected.

  Occurrence: *Mycoplasma* occurs worldwide. Epidemics occur every 4 to 8 years.

- **Treatment** Erythromycin or tetracycline are used. The bacteria are resistant to beta-lactam antibiotics because of the lack of a cell wall.

Mycoplasma hominis

- *M. hominis* is a sexually transmitted pathogen causing genitourinary disease (see Table 2.27).
- The disease is treated with tetracycline or erythromycin, as for chlamydiae infection.

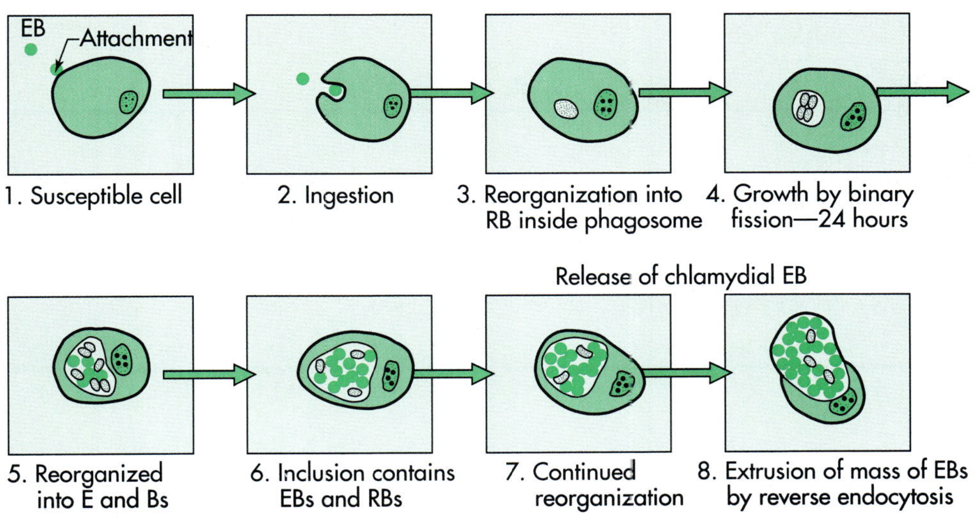

Fig. 2.31 Schematic depiction of the growth cycle of *Chlamydia trachomatis.* *(Redrawn from Batteiger BE, Jones RB:* Infect Dis Clin North Am *1:55-81, 1987.)*

Ureaplasma urealyticum

- *U. urealyticum* is a sexually transmitted organism.
- It requires urea for growth, but media must be buffered in order to decrease the alkalinity.
- Colonies of *U. urealyticum* are tiny.
- The organism causes **nongonococcal urethritis.**
- Infection is treated with tetracycline or erythromycin, as for chlamydiae infection.

Section 2.23 *Chlamydiae* and *Rickettsiae*

Chlamydia

Structure

- *Chlamydiae* are very small, gram-negative bacteria that lack a peptidoglycan. They are, therefore, insensitive to beta-lactam antibiotics.
- *Chlamydiae* exist in two forms:
  - **Elementary body (EB):** a small, infectious form with a rigid outer membrane
  - **Reticulate body (RB):** larger intracellular form, metabolically active, replicating form that is osmotically fragile

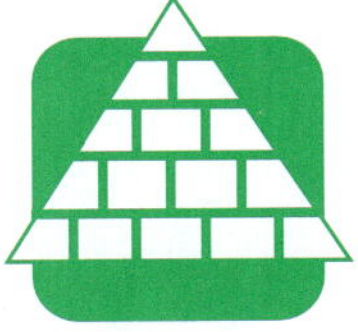

General features

- *Chlamydiae* cannot make ATP and must grow within cells. The reticulate body is capable of replication. Intracellular replication occurs in a cytoplasmic phagosome that becomes an inclusion as it fills with bacteria. Elementary and reticulate bodies are made.
- The growth cycle of *Chlamydia trachomatis* is shown in Figure 2.31.
- The species of *Chlamydiae* are contrasted in Table 2.28.

Table 2.28 *Differentiation of* Chlamydia *Species*

Property	C. trachomatis	C. psittaci	C. pneumoniae
Host range	Primarily human pathogen	Primarily animal pathogen; humans occasionally infected	Human pathogen
Human diseases	Lymphogranuloma venereum (LGV), trachoma, inclusion conjunctivitis, neonatal conjunctivitis, neonatal pneumonitis, urethritis, cervicitis, salpingitis, proctitis, epididymitis, asymptomatic infections	Psittacosis	Pharyngitis, bronchitis, pneumonia, sinusitis

Chlamydia trachomatis

- **Laboratory identification** Laboratory procedures for identification of *C. trachomatis* include the following:
  - cytologic examination for inclusions; *C. trachomatis* inclusions stain with iodine
  - isolation in cell culture
  - antigen or nucleic acid detection in clinical specimens
  - serologic tests

- **Pathogenesis**
  - *C. trachomatis* is spread by contact, the RB binding only to receptor-bearing, nonciliated epithelial cells of mucous membranes.
  - Target cells are found in the urethra, vagina, fallopian tubes, anorectal tract, respiratory tract, and conjunctiva.
  - Strains causing lymphogranuloma venereum infect reticuloendothelial cells, cause systemic infection, and lead to swelling (inflammation) and formation of lesions in the draining lymph node.
  - Symptoms result from destruction of target cells from bacterial replication and severe host inflammatory reactions.

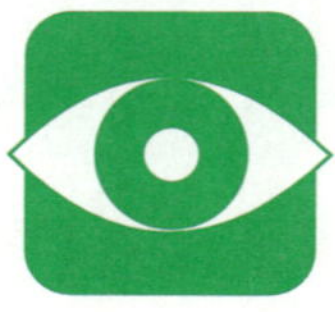

- **Diseases**

  — ***Non–sexually transmitted diseases***

  1. Trachoma
     - chronic keratoconjunctivitis, a leading cause of preventable blindness affecting 500 million individuals
     - initial follicular conjunctivitis with diffuse inflammation of the conjunctiva proceeds to scarring; produces inturned eyelids that cause corneal abrasion, ulceration, scarring, and blindness
     - recurrence is common
     - spread by tears, contaminated clothing, and hands, and promoted by poor hygiene
  2. Adult inclusion conjunctivitis
     - caused by strains associated with genital infections

Table 2.29 *Clinical Urogenital Infections Caused by* **C. trachomatis**

Site of Infection	Clinical Syndrome
Men	
Urethra	Nongonococcal urethritis, postgonococcal urethritis
Epididymis	Epididymitis
Rectum	Proctitis
Conjunctiva	Conjunctivitis
Systemic	Reiter's syndrome
Women	
Urethra	Acute urethral syndrome
Bartholin's gland	Bartholinitis
Cervix	Cervicitis, cervical dysplasia (?)
Fallopian tube	Salpingitis
Conjunctiva	Conjunctivitis
Liver capsule	Perihepatitis
Systemic	Arthritis, dermatitis

From Holmes KK, Mardh PA, Sparling PF, Wiesner PJ: *Sexually transmitted diseases,* New York, 1984, McGraw-Hill.

- characterized by mucopurulent discharge, keratitis, inflammation, and potential scarring
- autoinoculation or oral-genital contact spread the infection

3. Neonatal conjunctivitis
   - acquired upon passage through an infected birth canal
   - occurs in 2% to 6% of neonates
   - symptoms occur 2 to 30 days after birth and may run a course as long as 12 months
   - symptoms consist of swelling of eyelids, extensive purulent discharge with potential conjunctival scarring, and corneal vascularization
   - topical treatment with erythromycin is a routine procedure in most hospitals
4. Infant pneumonia
   - exposure at birth, without treatment may lead to diffuse interstitial pneumonia
   - onset is 2 to 3 weeks after birth, with rhinitis and a distinctive staccato cough; no fever

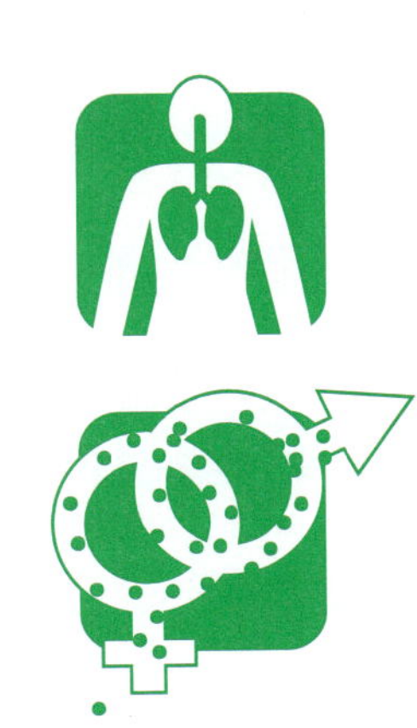

— ***Sexually transmitted diseases (STDs)*** *C. trachomatis* is the most frequent cause of STD in the United States. Most infections are asymptomatic (Table 2.29).

Symptomatic infections produce mucopurulent discharge, with dysuria or pyruria.

1. Reiter's syndrome
   - urethritis non-gonoccal (NGU), conjunctivitis, polyarthritis, and mucocutaneous lesions associated with *C. trachomatis*

2. Lymphogranuloma venereum (LGV)
    - observed more in men than in women
    - after a 1 to 4 wk incubation period, a small, painless, inconspicuous lesion appears at the site of infection, with possible accompanying fever, headache, and myalgia
    - second stage is marked by painful inflammation and swelling of draining lymph nodes (usually inguinal nodes); nodes gradually enlarge and may rupture, forming draining fistulas; systemic responses such as fever, chills, anorexia, headache, myalgias, and arthralgias may occur

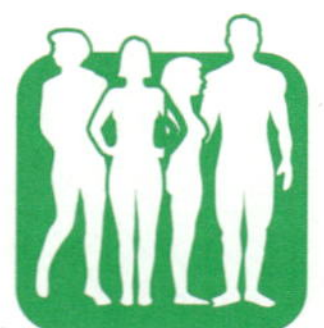

- **Epidemiology**

  Mode of spread: *Chlamydiae* are transmitted by sexual contact or by contact with infected fluids through small breaks in the skin or membranes.

  Populations affected: Sexually active individuals and homosexual males are more at risk for LGV. Neonatal infection is acquired from an infected mother during birth.

- **Prevention** Neonatal conjunctivitis can be prevented by topical erythromycin. Improved personal hygeine and safe sex practices can also reduce the rate of infection.

- **Treatment** Erythromycin and tetracycline are the antibiotics used.

Chlamydiae psittaci

- *C. psittaci* causes **psittacosis** or parrot fever.
- Inhalation of **dried bird excrement** initiates infection. Bird handlers, poultry workers, and similar occupational groups are at risk.
- Symptoms include fever, chills, headache, cough, and pneumonitis, with the potential for serious interstitial pneumonitis, cyanosis, jaundice, and death from lung edema, hemorrhage, and blockage of bronchioles with mucus plugs.

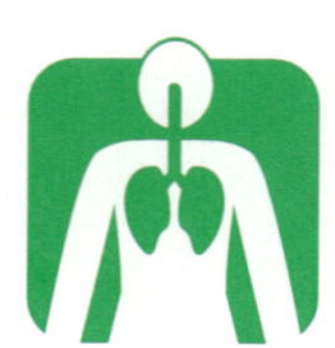

Chlamydia pneumoniae

- Infection with *C. pneumoniae* can cause the symptoms of pharyngitis, sinusitis, bronchitis, or pneumonia, with a persistent cough and malaise.
- The organism is spread by aerosols.
- Infection is treated with tetracycline or erythromycin.

Rickettsiae

- **General features**
    - Rickettsiae are transmitted by arthropods (except for *Coxiella burnetii* and *Rickettsia henselae*).
    - They are tiny gram-negative bacilli.
    - They are obligate intracellular parasites.
    - Their geographic distribution is determined by the distribution of the insect vector.

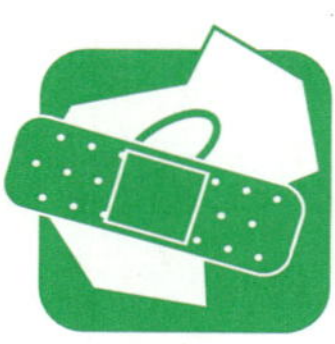

- **Pathogenesis**
    - The rickettsiae are phagocytosed, enter the cytoplasm, and replicate slowly.

Table 2.30 ***Epidemiology of Common Rickettsiaceae Infections***

Disease	Organism	Vector	Reservoir
Rocky Mountain spotted fever	*R. rickettsii*	Tick-borne	Ticks, wild rodents
Ehrlichiosis	*E. chaffeensis*		Ticks
Rickettsialpox	*R. akori*	Mite-borne	Mites, wild rodents
Scrub typhus	*R. tsutsugamushi*		Mites (chiggers), wild rodents
Epidemic typhus	*R. prowazekii*	Louse-borne	Humans, squirrel fleas, flying squirrels
Trench fever	*R. quintena*		Humans
Murine typhus	*R. typhi*	Flea-borne	Wild rodents
Q fever	*C. burnetii*	None*	Cattle, sheep, goats, cats

*Tick vectors may be responsible for animal-to-animal transmission.

- Organisms are continuously shed from the cell and also released by cell lysis.
- Disease is caused by destruction of cells and by the systemic responses to cell damage.
- *R. rickettsii* (agent of Rocky Mountain spotted fever) replicates in endothelial cells and damages blood vessels, causing loss of plasma, shock, and organ failure.

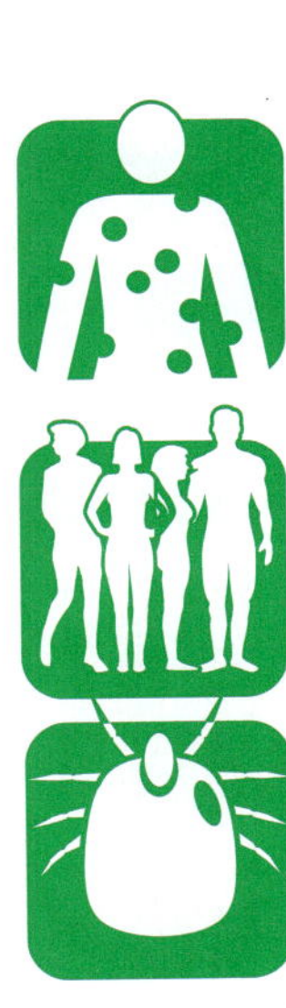

Diseases Tables 2.30 and 2.31 list the features of the various rickettsial diseases.

- Fever, chills, headache, myalgia, and rash are associated with most rickettsial disease.
- The onset of disease is abrupt except for endemic or murine typhus (caused by *R. typhi*), which has a gradual onset.
- Q fever does not produce a rash.

Epidemiology

Mode of spread:

- Rickettsiae are transmitted by insect vectors. Animals are reservoirs of infection and humans are usually accidental hosts.

Table 2.31 *Clinical Course of Common Rickettsial Diseases*

Disease	Average Incubation Period (Days)	Clinical Presentation	Rash	Eschar	Mortality
Rocky Mountain spotted fever	7	Abrupt onset; fever, chills, headache, myalgia	>90%, macular; **centripetal** spread	No	20%*
Rickettsialpox	9 to 14	Abrupt onset; fever, headache, chills, myalgia, photophobia	100%; papulovesicular; generalized	Yes	<1%
Epidemic typhus	8	Abrupt onset; fever, headache, chills, myalgia, arthralgia	40% to 80%; macular; **centrifugal** spread	No	Variable
Endemic typhus	7 to 14	Gradual onset; fever, headache, myalgia, cough	>55%; maculopapular rash on trunk	No	1 to 2%
Scrub typhus	10 to 12	Abrupt onset; fever, headache, myalgia	<50%; maculopapular rash; **centrifugal**	No	7%*
Ehrlichiosis	12	Abrupt onset; fever, headache, myalgia, malaise, leukopenic, thrombocytopenia	20%; nonspecific	No	5%
Q fever (acute)	20	Abrupt onset; fever, headache, chills, myalgia; granulomatous hepatitis	No	No	1%
Q fever (chronic)	Months to years	Chronic disease with subacute onset; endocarditis; hepatic dysfunction	No	No	High

*Mortality in untreated patients.

- Q fever (caused by *C. burnetii*) is the exception, being spread by aerosols or through contaminated milk.

Populations affected: Persons in contact with the vectors are at risk. Poor hygiene (presence of lice) and crowded conditions are associated with epidemic typhus (caused by *R. prowazekii*).

Occurrence:

- Rocky Mountain spotted fever (caused by *R. rickettsii*) usually occurs in the southeastern Atlantic states and south-central states in the United States, *not* in the Rocky Mountains.
- Endemic or murine typhus (causative organism, *R. typhi*) occurs in the southeastern states and near the Gulf of Mexico (especially Texas).

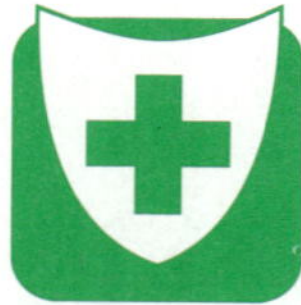

- **Prevention** Avoiding infested areas, wearing protective clothing, and using insect repellant can help to control the disease.

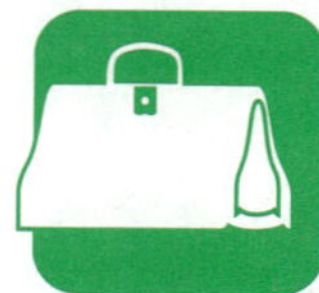

- **Treatment** The standard chemotherapy for rickettscial disease is tetracycline or chloramphenicol.

A summary of bacterias is provided in Tables 2.32 through 2.34.

Table 2.32 ***Gram-positive Bacteria***

Organism	Disease	Identification	Virulence	Epidemiology	Other
Staphylococcus aureus	Food poisoning: diarrhea, vomiting Infections: wounds, bacteremia, endocarditis, impetigo, osteomyelitis, septic arthritis Toxin-mediated: scalded skin syndrome, toxic shock syndrome	Gram (+) cocci in clusters; growth in 7.5% salt; coagulase (+); catalase (+)	Exfoliative toxin; TSST-1; enterotoxins A-E; cytolytic toxin and enzymes; leukocidin; coagulase; protein A	Normal skin flora; growth in lunch meats, creamy foods produce toxin	TSST = superantigen; pus; abscess; methicillin, MRSA-vancomycin
S. epidermidis	Bacteremia; adherence to catheters and prosthetic devices	Gram (+) cocci in clusters; coagulase (–)		Colonizes prosthetic devices	Wound infections Vancomycin
S. saprophyticus	Bacteremia; adherence to catheters, prosthetic devices; urinary tract infection (UTI)	Gram (+) cocci in clusters; coagulase (–)		Colonizes prosthetic devices	
S. pyogenes (Group A streptococcus)	Pharyngitis Scarlet fever, skin infections, necrotizing fascitis Sequelae: glomerulonephritis, rheumatic fever	Gram (+) cocci in chains; catalase (–); β-hemolytic; bacitracin-sensitive (A disk)	M protein Hyaluronic acid capsule Streptolysins S and O Erythrogenic toxins	Transmitted by aerosol droplets	C carbohydrate Dick test Treatment to prevent sequelae; Jones criteria
S. pneumoniae	Pneumonia Sinusitis Otitis media	Gram (+) cocci in chains; α-hemolytic; optochin sensitive (P disk); lysed by bile	Antiphagocytic capsule Pneumolysin	Normal flora of throat, nasopharynx; transmitted by person to person contact and by aerosol droplets	Anti-capsular vaccine
S. agalactiae (Group B streptococcus)	Post partum sepsis Newborn: meningitis	Gram (+) cocci in chains		Gastrointestinal and vaginal flora	
Enterococcus faecalis	UTI	Gram (+) cocci; growth in bile-esculin; salt tolerant			Flora of upper respiratory tract, small intestine; large numbers found in feces
Bacillus anthracis	Anthrax Cutaneous Inhalation Gastrointestinal	Spore forming gram (+) rods easily grown in culture; grow as chains in culture	Anthrax exotoxin: protective factor, edema factor, lethal factor	Contracted from contaminated animals; spores common in soil	Spores can survive in soil for many years

Continued.

Table 2.32 *Gram-positive Bacteria—cont'd*

Organism	Disease	Identification	Virulence	Epidemiology	Other
B. cereus	Gastroenteritis, traumatic eye disease	Spore forming gram (+) rods easily grown in culture; grow as chains in culture	Enterotoxin	Common in soil; present in rice, meats	
Corynebacterium diphtheriae	Diphtheria: pseudomembrane on back of throat, sore throat, meningitis	Gram (+) bacilli with "Chinese character" morphology	Toxgene (encoded by phage); A/B toxin: ADP ribosylation	Asymptomatic carriage; transmission by aerosol droplets	Vaccine: toxoid (DPT)
Propionibacterium acnes	Acne	Gram (+) bacilli with "Chinese character" morphology		Opportunistic skin infections; adherence to synthetic devices, e.g., catheters, prosthetics	
Listeria monocytogenes	Neonatal meningitis	Gram (+) rod; motile; nonspore	Intracellular growth in phagocytes		Baby
Clostridium tetani	Tetanus; spastic paralysis "lockjaw"	Small gram (+) bacilli with terminal spores	Tetanospasmin	Ubiquitous	Vaccine: toxoid (DPT)
C. botulinum	Botulism; bilateral descending paralysis; infantile botulism	Heat-resistant spores; gram (+) bacilli; toxin neutralization tests	Toxin: blocks acetylcholine in cholinergic nerves	Food contamination; raw honey ubiquitous	Avoid food from bulging cans
C. difficile	Antibiotic-associated pseudomembranous colitis	Gram (+) bacilli; spores are rare	Enterotoxin; cytotoxin	Opportunistic intestinal flora	Proliferates in absence of competition in intestine
C. perfringens	Myonecrosis, gas gangrene; food poisoning	Large, boxcar-shaped, gram (+) bacilli; spores are rare; double zone of hemolysis	Phospholipase; hemolysin; collagenase; hyaluronidase; protease	Grows in anaerobic conditions; ubiquitous	40% fatality for wound infections

Table 2.33 ***Gram-negative Bacteria***

Organism	Disease	Identification	Virulence	Epidemiology	Other
Enterobacteriaceae					
Escherichia coli	Urinary tract infections; gastroenteritis; septicemia; neonatal meningitis	Gram (–) bacilli, oxidase (–), lactose (+)		Gastrointestinal tract; common flora	
Enterotoxigenic *E. coli* (ETEC)	Traveler's diarrhea, watery diarrhea, fever		Enterotoxin	Travel	
Enteroinvasive *E. coli* (EIEC)	Dysentery, fever, watery stools; *blood* in stools		Plasmid transferred from *Shigella* allows invasiveness and tissue destruction		
Enteropathogenic *E. coli* (EPEC)	Watery diarrhea; fever; vomiting		Adherence		
Enterohemorrhagic *E. coli* (EHEC) (strain O157:H7)	Bloody diarrhea; hemolytic uremic syndrome; anemia; renal failure		Shiga-like toxin or verotoxin	Undercooked beef (hamburgers)	
Uropathogenic *E. coli* (UPEC)	Urinary tract infection (UTI); pyelonephritis		Fimbriae: adherence		
Salmonella enteritides	Vomiting; nonbloody diarrhea	Gram (–) rods; oxidase (–); lactose (–); H_2S (+)	Antiphagocytic capsule; exotoxin; intracellular growth	Improperly cooked foods: poultry (chicken and turkey), raw eggs, dairy products	
S. typhi	Bacteremia; typhoid fever	Gram (–) rods; oxidase (–); lactose (–); H_2S (+)	Antiphagocytic capsule; exotoxin; intracellular growth	Improperly cooked foods: poultry (chicken and turkey), raw eggs, dairy products	
S. paratyphi	Bacteremia	Gram (–) rods; oxidase (–); lactose (–); H_2S (+)	Antiphagocytic capsule; exotoxin; intracellular growth	Improperly cooked foods: poultry (chicken and turkey), raw eggs, dairy products	
Shigella sonnei, S. flexneri, S. boydii	Self-limiting watery diarrhea; fever; bloody diarrhea	Gram (–) rods; oxidase (–); lactose (–); H_2S (–)	Enterotoxin Invasion	Fecal-oral transmission; young children; long-term patients	
Yersinia pestis	Bubonic plague; pneumonic plague	Gram (–); intracellular growth; biochemical tests	Capsule; intracellular growth; exotoxin; fibrinolysin; coagulase	Transmitted by fleas and droplets	
Y. enterocolitica	Enterocolitis; diarrhea			Contaminated food products and water	

Continued.

Table 2.33 *Gram-negative Bacteria—cont'd*

Organism	Disease	Identification	Virulence	Epidemiology	Other
Klebsiella pneumoniae	Pneumonia; UTI infections	Gram (–) bacilli; oxidase (–); mucoid appearance in culture	Capsule	Community acquired, transmitted by aerosol droplets	
Proteus mirabilis	UTI; urinary stone formation	Gram (–) bacilli; oxidase (–); lactose (–); H_2S (+); urease (+) swarming growth in culture			Highly motile
Non-Enteric					
Neisseria gonorrhoeae	Gonorrhea Septic arthritis	Gram (–) diplococci oxidase (+); sugar fermentation	Pili	Sexual contact; attaches to mucosal cells, then invades	Chocolate agar; Thayer-Martin agar; CO_2; penicillin
N. meningitidis	Meningitis; widespread petechial rash	Gram (–) diplococci oxidase (+); sugar fermentation	Polysaccharide capsule; LPS	Attaches to mucosal cells, then invades; aerosol droplets Neonates at risk	Chocolate agar; Thayer-Martin agar; CO_2; penicillin
Pseudomonas aeruginosa	Wounds; bacteremia; pulmonary: cystic fibrosis; swimmer's ear; *burns*	Gram (–); oxidase (+); flat colonies	Pili; polysaccharide capsule; exotoxin; protease; leukocidin; phospholipase	Ubiquitous; nosocomial and burn infections	Antibiotic resistant; grows on soap
Vibrio cholerae classical	Watery diarrhea; rice-water stools	Gram (–) comma shaped; oxidase (+); flagella	Exotoxin causes increase in cellular cAMP	Infected water; fecal-oral route; more prevalent in poorer, tropical areas	Vaccine
V. cholerae biotype *Eltor*	Often subclinical infection			Better able to survive in fresh water and sets up carrier state	
Campylobacter jejuni	Diarrhea, possibly bloody	Similar to *Vibrio,* but catalase (+)	Ulceration of mucosal surfaces of jejunum	Contaminated food (poultry) or water	
Helicobacter pylori	Gastritis; ulcers	Similar to *Vibrio;* oxidase (+); urease production	Urease (neutralizes stomach acid); mucinase; motility	Transmission unknown but family transmission common	Mucinase and motility allow invasiveness
Bordetella pertussis	Whooping cough	Gram (–) bacillus; fluorescent antibody test	Exotoxin: ADP ribosylation of G proteins; filamentous hemagglutinin	Person-to-person transmission; aerosols from cough	Vaccine

Table 2.33 *Gram-negative Bacteria—cont'd*

Organism	Disease	Identification	Virulence	Epidemiology	Other
Francisella tularensis	Tularemia; skin ulcers; lymphadenopathy	Gram (−) coccobacillus	Capsule; intracellular growth (macrophages)	Transmitted by arthropod vector of infected animal	Intracellular
Brucella spp.	Brucellosis; fever, fatigue, myalgia; granulomas; local abscess at infection site	Gram (−) coccobacillus	Intracellular growth	Zoonosis; contact with contaminated milk or inhalation	
Hemophilus influenzae	Epiglottitis; meningitis; earaches; sinusitis; pneumonia	Gram (−) bacillus; requires Factor X and Factor V for growth; grows on chocolate agar	Polyribose ribitol phosphate capsule	Common oral flora	Hib vaccine: polysaccharide conjugated to protein
Legionella pneumonia	Pontiac fever; *Legionella* pneumonia	Serology; fastidious; difficult to grow	Taken up by macrophages; prevents phagolysosome fusion	Intracellular pathogen able to live in hot water; water-associated, e.g., hot tubs, air conditioning, etc.	
Bacteroides fragilis	Abscess formation; pelvic inflammation; peritonitis	Gram (−) rods, anaerobic; biochemical tests	Polysaccharide capsule; pili (adherence); cytolytic enzymes	Infect mucosal surfaces; normal flora; opportunistic	Surgical patients at risk
Treponema pallidum	Syphilis	Dark field microscopy; serology (VDRL test, FTA-ABS test)	Hyaluronidase; protective outer membrane	Transmitted sexually or by blood exchange	
Borrelia burgdorferi	Lyme disease: rash, fatigue, immune dysfunction; neurologic or cardiac disorders	Serology; Giemsa or Wright's stain of tissue	Immune dysfunction	Tick bite	

Table 2.34 *Other Bacteria*

Organism	Disease	Identification	Virulence	Epidemiology	Other
Mycobacterium tuberculosis	Tuberculosis	Acid-fast stain; slow growth	Cord factor; sulfatides; intracellular growth	Inhalation of aerosol droplets; immunocompromised patients (e.g., with AIDS) at high risk	Highly antibiotic resistant; cell-mediated immunity required; opportunistic infection
M. leprae	Tuberculoid leprosy; lepromatous leprosy	Skin testing; acid-fast stain	Phenolic glycolipid	Unknown	Obligate intracellular parasite
Mycoplasma hominis	Pneumonia	Small colonies; T-strain; "Fried egg" appearance of colonies; no cell wall	Adherence	Attachment to epithelium of respiratory tract	
Ureaplasma urealyticum	Urethritis; chronic lung disease of newborns	Similar to *Mycoplasma;* makes urease			
Rickettsiae	Headache, fever, chills, petechial rash; typhus, Rocky Mountain spotted fever	Gram (–) intracellular parasite		Transmitted by ticks and lice	Rocky Mountain spotted fever—tick; ehrlichiosis—tick; typhus—lice
Coxiella burnetii	Q fever Atypical pneumonia Endocarditis	Gram (–) intracellular parasite		Transmitted by ticks	Endocarditis may manifest quickly
Chlamydia trachomatis	Lymphogranuloma venereum; trachoma (conjunctivitis)	No cell wall	Obligate intracellular parasite; causes swollen glands; elementary body (transmission); reticulate body (replication)	Transmitted during birth or by sexual contact	Cannot produce its own ATP
C. psittaci	Psittacosis (virus-like pneumonia)			Parrots	
C. pneumoniae	Atypical pneumonia			Aerosols	
Nocardia	Mycetoma	Branching; acid-fast		Present in soil	
Actinomyces	Sinus infections	Branching, anaerobic; sulfur granules			

Multiple Choice Review Questions

1. Plasmids differ from bacterial chromosomes by being
   a. capable of carrying antibiotic resistance genes.
   b. capable of carrying toxin genes.
   c. capable of carrying transposons.
   d. dispensable to the cell.
   e. replicons.

2. Which of the following antibiotics is not matched with its correct target activity?
   a. Inhibition of peptidoglycan-crosslinking: ampicillin
   b. Inhibition of topoisomerase: ciprofloxacin
   c. Inhibition of RNA polymerase: rifampin
   d. Inhibition of protein synthesis—initiation step: erythromycin
   e. Inhibition of protein synthesis—elongation step: chloramphenicol

3. Which of the following conditions is not associated with toxin-mediated staphylococcal disease?
   a. Infective endocarditis
   b. Staphylococcal scalded skin syndrome
   c. Toxic shock syndrome
   d. Gastroenteritis
   e. Bullous impetigo

4-6. Match the site of infection to the disease process.
   a. Streptococcal pharyngitis
   b. Streptococcal pyoderma
   c. Both
   d. None

   4. Acute poststreptococcal glomerulonephritis
   5. Acute rheumatic fever
   6. Reiter's syndrome

7-10. Match the bacteria with the test.
   a. Group A streptococcus *(Streptococcus pyogenes)*
   b. Group B streptococcus *(Streptococcus agalactiae)*
   c. *Streptococcus pneumoniae*
   d. None

   7. Optochin sensitive
   8. Bacitracin sensitive
   9. Hydrolysis of hippurate
   10. Bile solubility (sensitivity)

11. Which of the following is *false?*
   a. *Neisseria* can be differentiated from *Moraxella* by the ability of *Neisseria* to produce acid from glucose.
   b. *Neisseria meningitidis,* but not *N. gonorrhoeae* can ferment maltose.
   c. *Neisseria* is oxidase negative.
   d. Asymptomatic infection with *N. gonorrhoeae* is common.
   e. Meningococcal colonization is mediated by pili.

12-16. A 5-year-old boy was admitted to the hospital for bloody diarrhea and dehydration. Match the bacteria to the statement.
   a. *Escherichia coli* O157:H7
   b. *Shigella*
   c. Both
   d. Neither

   12. ferments lactose
   13. grows in sorbitol medium
   14. fecal leukocytes present in stools
   15. causes bacteremia
   16. causes bloody diarrhea

17. Which of the following organisms will not grow in MacConkey medium?
   a. *Escherichia coli*
   b. *Bacteroides fragilis*
   c. *Klebsiella pneumoniae*
   d. *Proteus mirabilis*
   e. *Acinetobacter* species

18. An 18-year-old man had an abrupt onset of severe watery diarrhea speckled with mucous flecks a day after returning to the United States from Chile following a 10-day vacation. Prior to his trip he had been feeling well. He appeared extremely dehydrated on admission. Which of the following statements regarding the most likely causative agent is *incorrect?*
   a. Fluid replacement should be given parenterally because a toxin blocks fluid absorption.
   b. The toxin causes accumulation of cAMP along the cell membrane.
   c. The disease, if untreated, has a mortality greater than 50%.
   d. The disease is indigenous to certain areas in the United States.
   e. Administration of tetracycline will rapidly reduce the number of organisms in the stool and improve prognosis.

19. A 6-year-old girl with cystic fibrosis was hospitalized because of fever and greenish mucoid sputum. A sputum culture yielded mucoid colonies. These colonies showed gram-negative rods that grew aerobically, were non–lactose fermenters, and were oxidase positive. Which of the following microorganisms is the most likely cause of her problem?

    a. *Staphylococcus aureus*
    b. *Klebsiella pneumoniae*
    c. *Hemophilus influenzae*
    d. *Pseudomonas aeruginosa*
    e. *Bacteroides fragilis*

20. A 47-year-old man had a persistent postoperative fever 5 days after exploratory laparotomy for a ruptured appendiceal abscess. In spite of a combination therapy of clindamycin, ampicillin, and gentamicin, fever persisted. His blood culture yielded a gram-negative rod that grew anaerobically and was resistant to bile. Which is the most likely microorganism?

    a. *Prevotella*
    b. *Escherichia coli*
    c. *Veillonella*
    d. *Bacteroides fragilis*
    e. *Capnocytophaga*

21. A 42-year-old man was seen in the office for a chronically draining wound in the jaw. The patient had had multiple tooth extractions 3 months earlier. On examination, he had multiple nodular lesions that drained serosanguinous fluid with small hard granules. You suspect actinomycosis. Which of the following statements is *false?*

    a. Actinomycetes are anaerobic bacteria.
    b. Actinomycetes appear as gram-positive branching filaments on staining.
    c. "Sulfur granules" can be found in the draining fluid.
    d. Actinomycetes are not susceptible to penicillins.
    e. Actinomycetes normally colonize the upper respiratory tract.

22-24. Match the disease with the bacterial agent.

    a. endocarditis
    b. infected animal bite
    c. epiglottitis
    d. chancroid
    e. none of the above

22. *Pasteurella multocida*
23. *Hemophilus ducreyi*
24. *Hemophilus influenzae*

25. A 75-year-old man was admitted for pneumonia. He had started to have fever and cough 2 days previously. On admission, he was febrile and confused. A chest radiograph showed diffuse pulmonary infiltrates. Since other residents of the nursing home had been diagnosed with *Legionella,* antimicrobial therapy directed against *Legionella* was started. Which of the following agents is least active against *Legionella?*

    a. Ampicillin
    b. Erythromycin (macrolide)
    c. Ciprofloxacin (quinolone)
    d. Doxycycline (tetracycline)
    e. Rifampin

26. Which of the following statements about *Mycobacterium* is *false?*

    a. Mycobacteria are intracellular organisms, therefore tissue cultures must be used for isolation.
    b. The most common mode of transmission of *M. tuberculosis* is inhalation of infectious aerosols.
    c. Humans are the only natural reservoir for *M. tuberculosis.*
    d. More bacteria are found in the lepromatous leprosy lesions than in tuberculoid leprosy lesions.
    e. *M. tuberculosis* can remain dormant for years and reactivate.

27. Syphilis can be transmitted by *all* of the following mechanisms *except*

    a. kissing
    b. transplacentally
    c. transfusion of contaminated blood
    d. passage through the infected birth canal
    e. toilet seats

28. Which of the following procedures is *not* used for diagnosis of syphilis?

    a. VDRL test
    b. Culture
    c. FTA-ABS test
    d. Dark field microscopy
    e. Direct fluorescent antibody staining

29. Which of the following diseases is not transmitted by ticks?
    a. Rocky Mountain spotted fever
    b. Ehrlichiosis
    c. Lyme disease
    d. Murine (endemic) typhus
    e. Babesiosis

Chapter 3

Virology

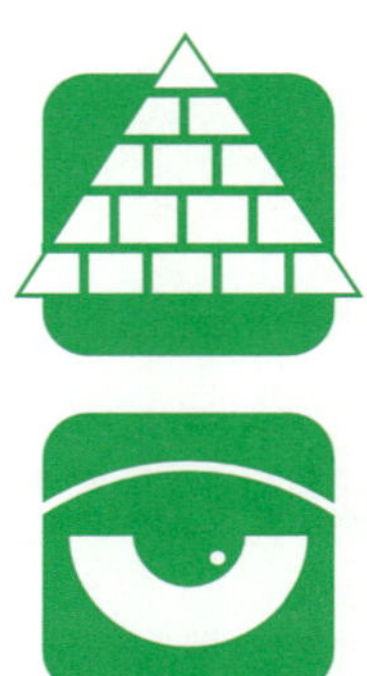

Section 3.1 Viral Morphology

Overview The virion or viral particle consists of a genome packaged in either a naked capsid or a membrane envelope (Fig. 3.1). The structure of the virion will determine many of the properties of the virus. Important generalizations can be made about a virus based on its structure. Learn a prototype virus for each family and generalizations can be made for the other members of the family.

- The classification of viruses into families is based on the physical characteristics of the viruses (such as the size, the genome, and the morphology) and on their mode of replication. Tables 3.1 and 3.2 list the virus families, their members, and their relative sizes.
- The viruses are classified by whether their genome is DNA or RNA. In Tables 3.1 and 3.2 the size of the print for the viral family name corresponds to the relative size of the viruses in that family.
- The size of the virion correlates with the size of the genome, the complexity of the virus, and the number of antigens expressed by the virus. The smallest viruses have DNA or positive sense (+) RNA genomes.

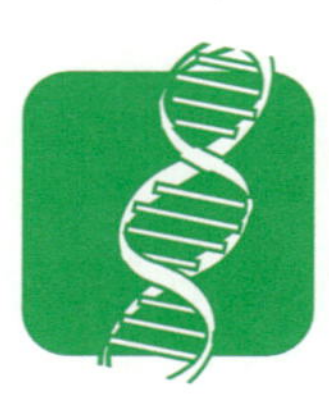

Viral Genome

- Viruses have a genome consisting of either DNA or RNA.

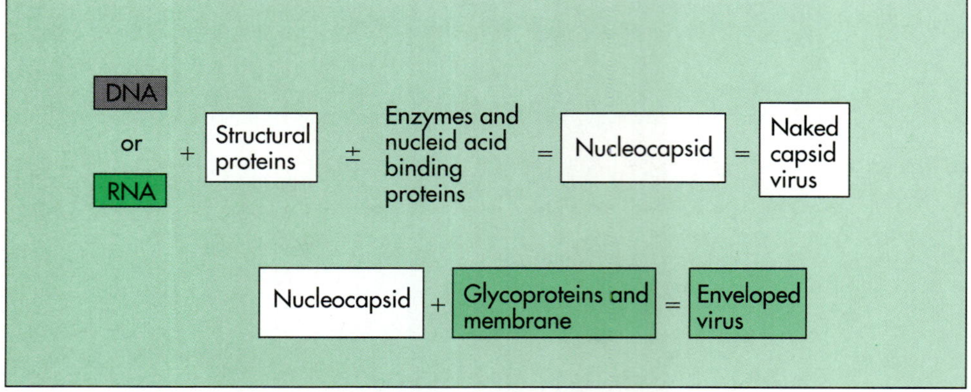

Fig. 3.1 Schematic structure of the basic virion.

• The DNA is usually double stranded, except in the case of parvoviruses, which contain single-stranded DNA (either + or −).

• The genome may be circular, as in the papovaviruses and hepadnaviruses, or linear, as in the parvoviruses, adenoviruses (protein attached to the 5′ end), herpesviruses, and poxviruses.

• RNA genomes can be single stranded or double stranded. Single-stranded RNA can be positive sense (+) (i.e., same as mRNA) or negative sense (−) (i.e., complementary to mRNA, like a photographic negative template) RNA.

Table 3.1 *Families of DNA Viruses and Some Important Members*

Family	Members
Poxviridae*	*Smallpox virus*†, vaccinia virus
Herpesviridae	*Herpes simplex virus* types 1 and 2, varicella-zoster virus, Epstein-Barr virus, cytomegalovirus, human herpesviruses 6 and 7
Adenoviridae	*Adenovirus*
Hepadnaviridae	*Hepatitis B virus*
Papovaviridae	JC virus, BK virus, SV40, *papilloma virus*
Parvoviridae	*Parvovirus B 19,* adeno-associated virus

*The size of the type is indicative of the relative size of the virus.
†The italicized virus is the important or prototype virus for the family.

Table 3.2 *Families of RNA Viruses and Some Important Members*

Family	Members
Paramyxoviridae*	Parainfluenza virus, Sendai virus, *measles virus*†, mumps virus, respiratory syncytial virus
Orthomyxoviridae	*Influenza virus types A*, B, and C
Coronaviridae	*Coronavirus*
Arenaviridae	*Lassa fever virus,* Tacaribe virus complex (Junin and Machupo viruses), lymphocytic choriomeningitis virus
Rhabdoviridae	*Rabies virus,* vesicular stomatitis virus
Filoviridae	*Ebola virus,* Marburg virus
Bunyaviridae	*California encephalitis virus,* LaCrosse virus, Sandfly fever virus, hemorrhagic fever virus, Hanta virus
Retroviridae	Human T cell leukemia virus types I and II, *human immunodeficiency virus,* Animal oncoviruses
Reoviridae	*Rotavirus,* Colorado tick fever virus
Picornaviridae	Rhinoviruses, *poliovirus,* echoviruses, coxsackie virus, encephalomyocarditis virus
Togaviridae	*Rubella virus,* Western, Eastern, and Venezualan equine encephalitis virus, Ross River virus, Sindbis virus, Semliki Forest virus
Flaviviridae	*Yellow fever virus,* dengue virus, St. Louis encephalitis virus
Caliciviridae	Norwalk virus
Delta	Delta agent

*The size of the type is indicative of the relative size of the virus.
†The italicized virus is the important or prototype virus for the family.

• The genomes of (+) RNA viruses (except for retroviruses) and DNA viruses (except for hepadnaviruses and poxviruses) are **infectious by themselves.** Injection of the naked genome into a cell will initiate infection without the need for any other component of the virion.

• The other viruses, (−) RNA viruses, double-stranded RNA viruses (+/−RNA), retroviruses, hepadnaviruses, and poxviruses must **carry a polymerase** in the virion to initiate replication.

Viral Morphology The genome is packaged in either a **capsid** or a membrane **envelope.** These structures are responsible for viral attachment and protection of the genome. Viruses can be characterized further by morphology (Figs. 3.2 and 3.3).

Viral capsid

• Naked capsid, or unenveloped, viruses of humans have an **icosahedral** or an **icosadeltahedral** shape. This shape is an approximation of a sphere with 12 vertices. The icosadeltahedron is an expanded icosahedron.

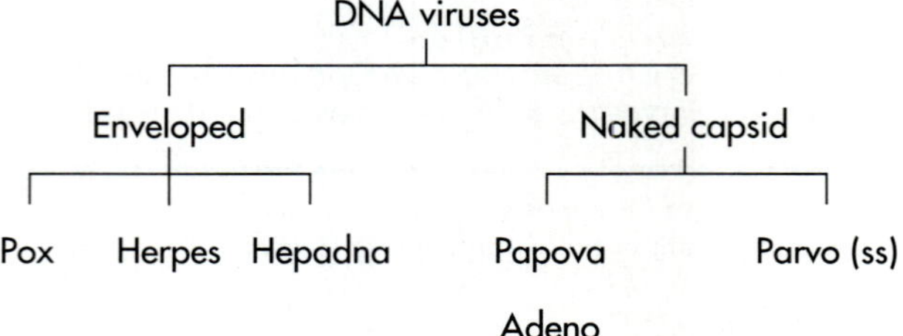

Fig. 3.2 The DNA viruses and their morphology. The viral families are determined by the structure of the genome and the morphology of the virion.

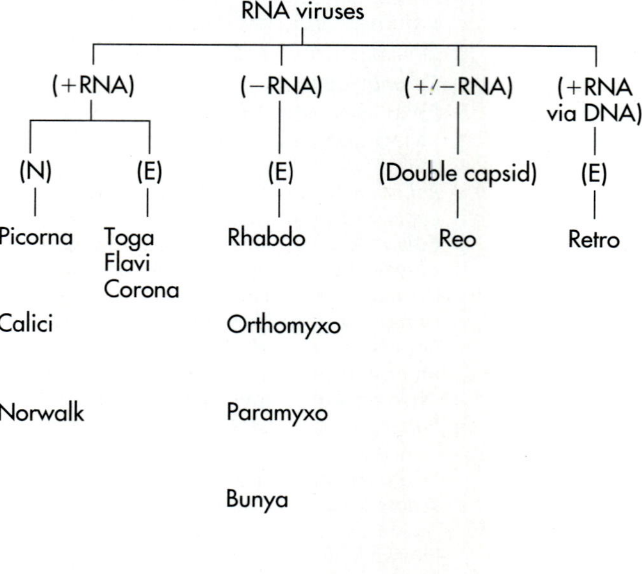

Fig. 3.3 The RNA viruses, their genome structure, and their morphology. The viral families are determined by the structure of the genome and the morphology of the virion.

• The icosahedron is constructed from morphologically distinct **capsomeres** that are made from individual proteins or protein subunits. The capsid structure of poliovirus is presented as the prototype of an unenveloped virus (Fig. 3.4).

• The capsid contains structures that recognize and bind to cell-surface receptors. These structures may take the form of canyons (picornaviruses) or fibers (adenoviruses and reoviruses).

• The protein shell of a naked capsid virus is generally resistant to environmental stresses from agents such as dryness, heat, acid, detergents, and solvents.

Viral envelope

• Enveloped viruses have a characteristic appearance but do not have a defined shape, except for poxviruses (brick shaped) and rhabdoviruses (bullet shaped).

• The envelope is a membrane derived from the host cell and contains lipids, phospholipids, viral proteins, and viral glycoproteins (Fig. 3.5).

• Viral glycoproteins include the **viral attachment protein (VAP).**

• Some viral glycoproteins promote fusion of membranes (e.g., viral F proteins allow fusion of the viral envelope and the plasma membrane of the cell) or have other activities (e.g., neuraminidase [NA]).

• The carbohydrate of the viral glycoproteins is added to the protein in the endoplasmic reticulum and processed in the Golgi apparatus in a manner similar to cellular proteins.

• The viral envelope is a membrane and is therefore disrupted by dryness, detergents, acids, and solvents.

• All (–) RNA viruses are enveloped.

• Enveloped viruses usually initiate an inflammatory response.

• A comparison of naked capsid viruses versus enveloped viruses is presented in Boxes 3.1 and 3.2.

Section 3.2 Viral Replication

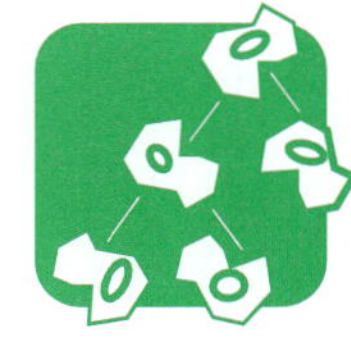

Overview

- Viruses must replicate in order to survive.
- Viruses require an appropriate host cell in which to replicate.

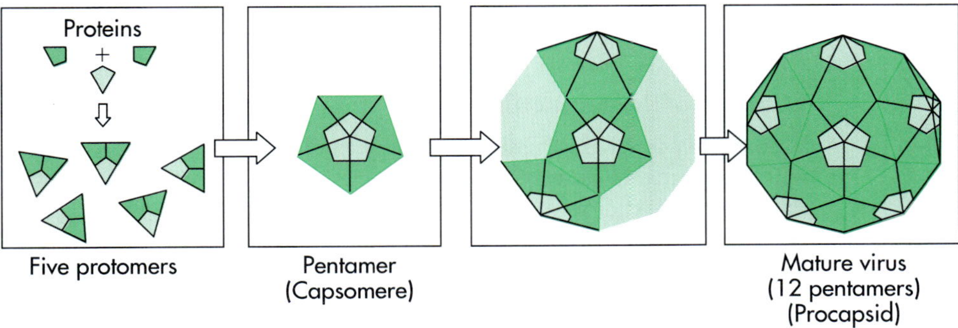

Fig. 3.4 Assembly of the icosahedral capsid of a picornavirus. Individual proteins associate into subunits, which associate into protomers, capsomeres, and an empty procapsid. Inclusion of the (+) RNA genome triggers its conversion to the final capsid form.

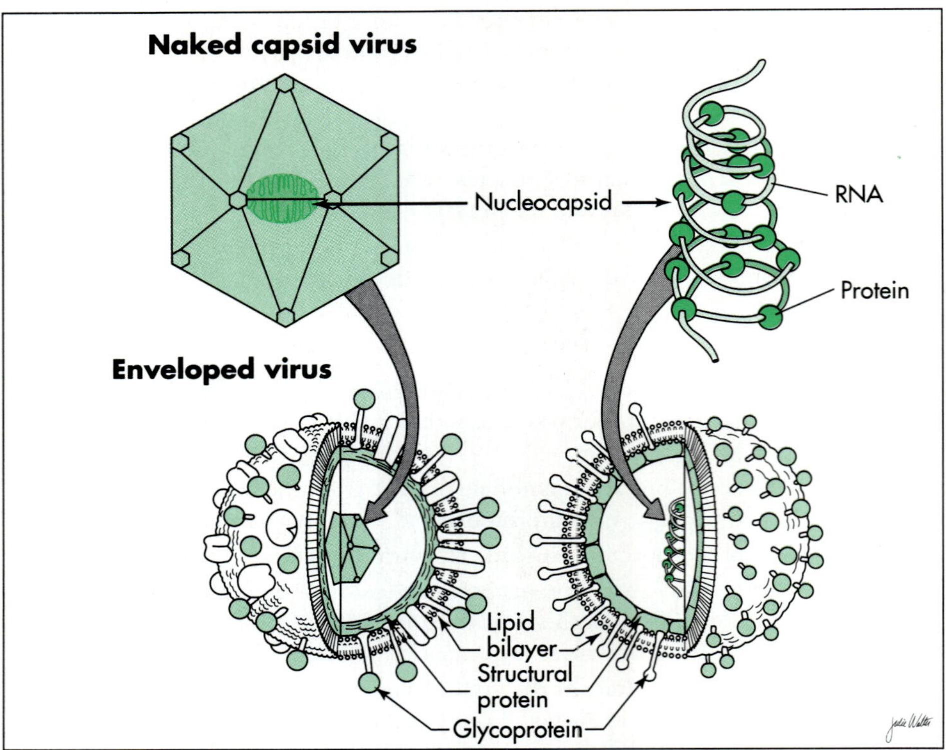

Fig. 3.5 The structures of a naked capsid virus *(top left)* with an icosahedral structure. Enveloped viruses have a membrane that can surround either an icosahedral *(left)* nucleocapsid or a helical *(right)* ribonucleocapsid. The helical ribonucleocapsid is formed by viral proteins (usually components of the RNA-dependent RNA polymerase) with an RNA genome.

- All viruses follow the same steps in replication, but the mechanisms they use depend on the genome structure and on whether the virion has an envelope or a naked capsid.
- Viruses use the biochemical machinery of the cell for replication but must have the gene for any activity that the cell does not provide (e.g., the synthesis of RNA from an RNA template).
- Larger viruses encode nonessential activities that facilitate replication (e.g., the deoxyribonucleotide scavenging enzymes of the herpesviruses).

Basic Steps in Viral Replication Viral replication occurs in several steps (Fig. 3.6 and Box 3.3).

1. Recognition of the target cell
   - Binding of the virus to tissue-specific receptors determines which cell will be infected (*tropism* of the virus) and is a major determinant of the type of disease that will result.
   - Viral binding is mediated by the VAP or any structure that binds a cell-surface receptor for the virus.
   - For naked capsid viruses, a molecular canyon or other structure on the surface interacts with the cellular receptor. The exceptions are the reoviruses and adenoviruses, which have protein fibers that project from the surface of the virion and that contain the VAP.

Box 3.1

VIRUS STRUCTURE: NAKED CAPSID	
Components	**Properties**
Proteins	Environmentally stable to Temperature Acid Proteases Detergents Drying Released from cell by lysis

Consequences

Can be spread easily (on fomites, hand to hand, dust, small droplets)
Can dry out and retain infectivity
Can survive the adverse conditions of the gut
Can be resistant to detergents and poor sewage treatment
Can elicit a protective antibody response

Box 3.2

VIRUS STRUCTURE: ENVELOPED	
Components	**Properties**
Membrane Lipids Proteins Glycoproteins	Environmentally labile: disrupted by Acid Detergent Drying Heat Modify cell membrane during replication Released by budding and cell lysis

Consequences

Must stay wet
Cannot survive the GI tract
Spreads in large droplets, secretions, and organ or blood transplants
Need not kill the cell to spread
Antibody and cell-mediated immune response may be necessary for protection and control
Pathogenesis often due to hypersensitivity and inflammation initiated by CMI

CMI, Cell-mediated immunity; *GI*, gastrointestinal.

- For the enveloped viruses, glycoproteins on the surface of the virion act as the VAPs.
- Cell-surface receptors may be proteins, glycoproteins, or glycolipids (Table 3.3).

2. Attachment: The virus binds to the cell-surface receptor during the attachment step and a tight association is formed.
3. Entry into the cell: The virion can enter the cell by two different mechanisms:

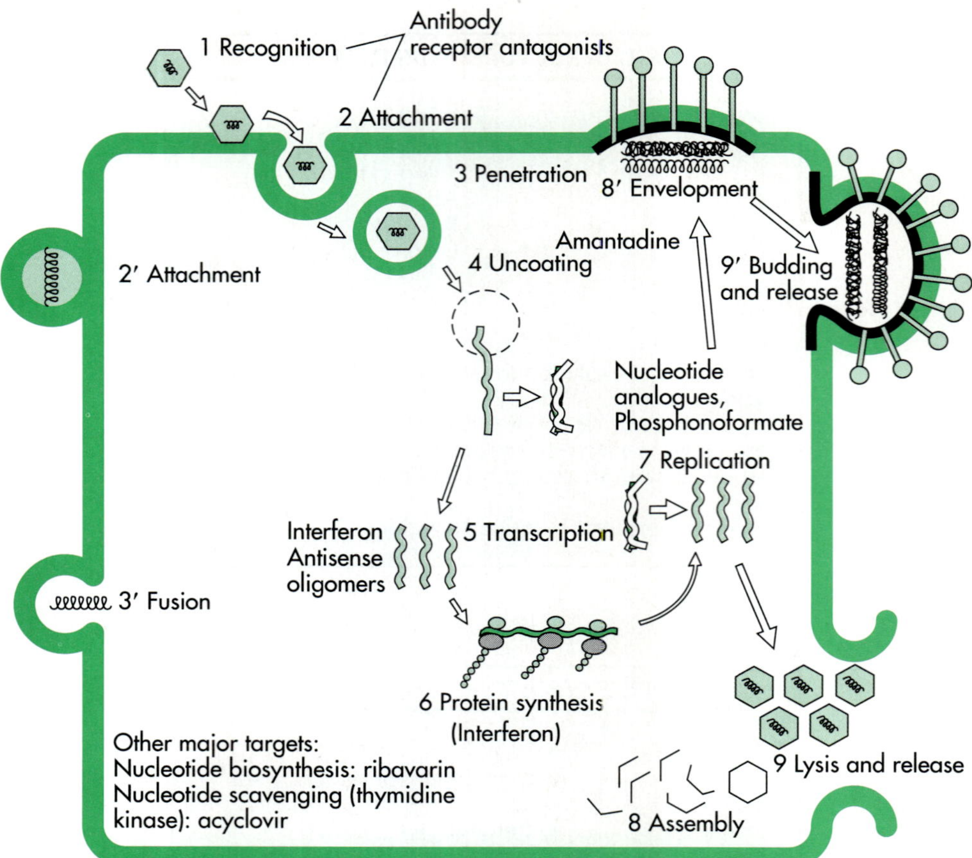

Fig. 3.6 A general scheme of virus replication. Enveloped viruses have alternative means of entry (step 3′), assembly, and exit from the cell (steps 8′ and 9′). The steps in virus replication susceptible to antiviral drugs are listed in color.

Box 3.3

STEPS IN VIRAL REPLICATION

1. Recognition of the target cell
2. Attachment
3. Penetration
4. Uncoating
5. Macromolecular synthesis
   a. Early mRNA and nonstructural protein synthesis: genes for enzymes and nucleic acid-binding proteins
   b. Replication of genome
   c. Late mRNA and structural protein synthesis
   d. Posttranslation modification of proteins
6. Assembly of virus
   a. Budding of enveloped viruses
7. Release of virus

Table 3.3 *Important Virus-Specific Receptors on Human Cells*

Virus	Receptor
Epstein-Barr virus	C3b (complement) receptor (CR2) on B cells and Epithelial cells
HIV and HTLV	CD4 molecule on T cells and macrophages
Rhinovirus	ICAM-1
Poliovirus and other picornaviruses	Protein belonging to the immunoglobulin superfamily
Orthomyxovirus and paramyxovirus	Sialic acid on proteins and lipids

HIV, Human immunodeficiency virus; *HTLV,* human T cell lymphotropic virus.

- receptor-mediated endocytosis (viropexis)
- fusion of the viral envelope with the cell membrane (used by some enveloped viruses, e.g., paramyxoviruses, herpesviruses, and retroviruses)

4. mRNA synthesis
   - The mechanism by which mRNA is synthesized depends on the viral genome (Fig. 3.7).
   - DNA viruses (except for poxviruses) use host machinery for mRNA synthesis.
   - For RNA viruses with a (+) genome, the RNA is the same as mRNA and binds directly to ribosomes for protein synthesis.
   - Viruses with a (–) RNA genome carry RNA-dependent RNA polymerase (transcriptase) in the virion to synthesize a mRNA from the (–) genome template.
   - Viruses with a double-stranded RNA genome carry RNA-dependent RNA polymerase (transcriptase) in the virion to synthesize an mRNA from a (–) genome strand.
   - Retroviruses are RNA viruses that carry a reverse transcriptase (an enzyme that synthesizes a DNA copy [cDNA] of the genome, which gets integrated into the host chromosome and is then transcribed by host enzymes).
   - Many viruses synthesize early and late mRNAs.
     - *Early* mRNA encodes enzymes and controls proteins (e.g., DNA binding proteins).
     - *Late* mRNA encodes structural proteins (e.g., capsid proteins or glycoproteins).

5. Replication of the genome
   - The mechanism of replication depends on the type of genome (see Fig. 3.7).
   - Replication of DNA viruses requires a primer and utilizes host or viral DNA polymerases (Box 3.4).

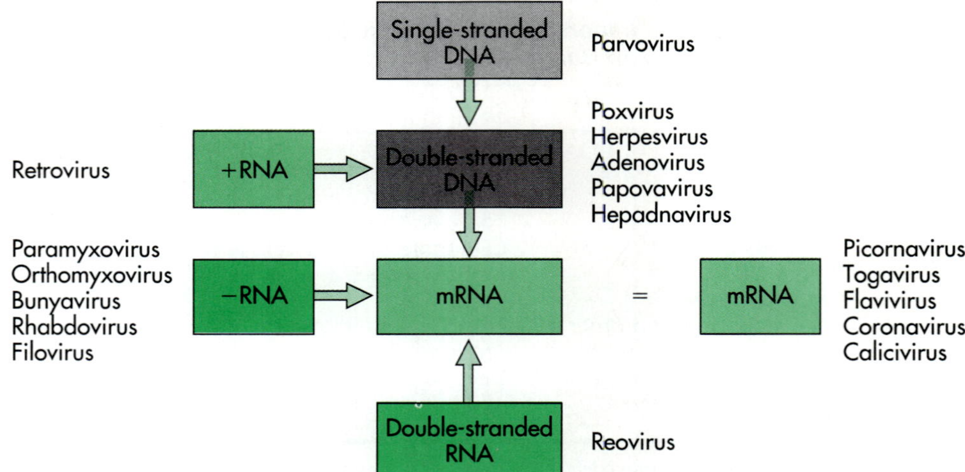

Fig. 3.7 Strategies for production of mRNA. The arrows indicate a synthetic step. *(Based on the Baltimore schema; redrawn from Baltimore D.,* Bacteriol Rev *35:235, 1971.)*

Box 3.4

PROPERTIES OF DNA VIRUSES

1. Viral DNA resembles host DNA for transcription and replication.
   DNA is not transient or labile.
   Viral genomes remain in the infected cell.
   Many DNA viruses establish persistent infections (e.g., latent, immortalizing).
   DNA genomes reside in the nucleus (except for poxvirus).
   Viral genes must interact with host transcriptional machinery (except for poxvirus).
   Viral gene transcription is divided into early and late phases.
   Early genes encode DNA-binding proteins and enzymes.
   Late genes encode structural proteins.
   DNA polymerases require a primer to replicate the viral genome.
2. The larger DNA viruses have more control over the replication of their genome.
   Parvovirus: Replicates in cells undergoing DNA synthesis.
   Papovavirus: Stimulates cell growth and DNA synthesis.
   Hepadnavirus: Stimulates cell growth (?) and encodes its own polymerase.
   Adenovirus: Stimulates cellular DNA synthesis and encodes its own polymerase.
   Herpesvirus: Stimulates cell growth, encodes its own polymerase, encodes enzymes to provide deoxyribonucleotides for DNA synthesis.
   Poxvirus: Encodes its own polymerase, enzymes to provide deoxyribonucleotides for DNA synthesis, replication machinery, and transcription machinery.

- Replication of RNA viruses requires a virally encoded RNA-dependent RNA polymerase (replicase) and an RNA template (Box 3.5).

6. Protein synthesis
   - Viral protein synthesis utilizes ribosomes and other synthetic machinery from the host.
   - Posttranslational modification (e.g., glycosylation, phosphorylation, proteolytic cleavage) is performed by host enzymes, although occasionally viral enzymes may be used.
7. Assembly
   a. Naked capsid viruses

Box 3.5

PROPERTIES OF RNA VIRUSES

RNA is labile and transient.
Most RNA viruses replicate in the cytoplasm.
Cells cannot replicate RNA. RNA viruses must encode an RNA-dependent RNA polymerase.
The genome structure determines the mechanism of transcription (mRNA) and replication.
RNA viruses are prone to mutation.
Picornaviruses, togaviruses, flaviviruses, caliciviruses, and coronaviruses
(+) RNA genome resembles mRNA, is translated into a polyprotein, which is proteolyzed. A (–) RNA template for replication.
Orthomyxoviruses, paramyxoviruses, rhabdoviruses, filoviruses, and bunyaviruses
(–) RNA genome is a template for mRNA, which may also be the (+) RNA template for replication.
Reoviruses
(+/–) segmented RNA genome is a template for mRNA, which may also be encapsulated to generate the (+/–) RNA and more mRNA.
Retroviruses
(+) retrovirus RNA genome is converted into DNA, which is integrated into the host chromatin and transcribed as a cellular gene.

- The capsid proteins self-assemble into distinct subunits called **capsomeres.**
- The capsomeres either assemble into a procapsid (empty shell) and are then filled with the genome or assemble around the genome to form the **nucleocapsid.**

b. Enveloped viruses
- Viral glycoproteins are inserted into host membranes.
- The nucleocapsid associates with the glycoprotein-modified membrane.
- A **matrix** protein may line the glycoprotein-modified membrane (in the case of RNA viruses).
- The membrane forms around the nucleocapsid.
- The virus buds away from the cell membrane.

8. Release
- Virus is released upon cell lysis or by exocytosis.
- Many enveloped viruses are released when they bud from the plasma membrane.

Single Cycle Growth Curve A single round of virus replication, from the addition of the virus to its release, may take different lengths of time and produce different amounts of virus per cell (Fig. 3.8).

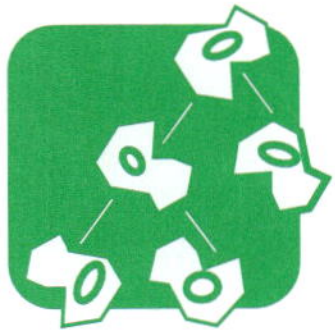

Section 3.3 Mechanisms of Viral Pathogenesis

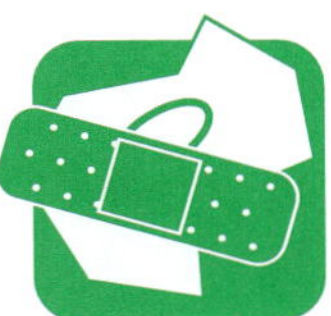

Overview

- Diseases caused by viruses occur either from damage caused by the virus itself or from the immunologic and inflammatory responses to the virus.
- The immunologic or inflammatory reactions may be local or systemic (e.g., the occurrence of influenza-like symptoms).

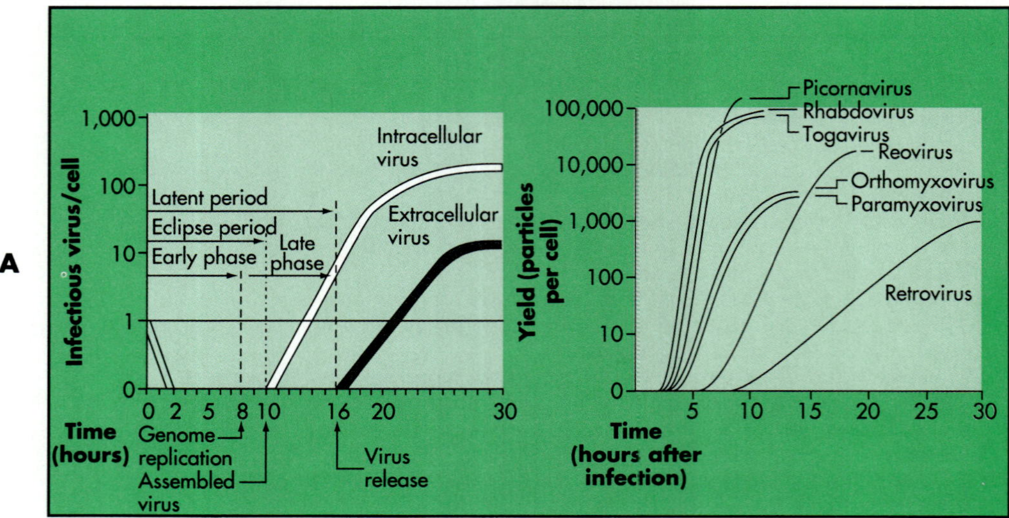

Fig. 3.8 **A,** Single-cycle growth curve of a virus that is released upon cell lysis. The different stages are defined by the absence of visible viral components (eclipse period), absence of infectious virus in the media (latent period), or macromolecular synthesis (early or late phases). **B,** Growth curve and burst size of representative viruses. *(A redrawn from Davis BD, Dulbecco R, Eisen HN, Ginsberg HS:* Microbiology, *ed 4, Philadelphia, 1990, Lippincott;* B *redrawn from White DO, Fenner F:* Medical virology, *ed 3, New York, 1986, Academic Press.)*

- The severity of the disease is determined both by the target organ (e.g., infection of the brain, the central nervous system [CNS], the lungs, the liver, and the heart will have more severe consequences) and by the extent of damage caused.
- The time course of a disease is determined by how long the virus takes to reach the target organ and cause sufficient damage either directly or through inflammatory reactions (Table 3.4). For example, the viruses causing the common cold or influenza cause disease at the site of acquisition (the respiratory tract) and have a short incubation period of 1 day. Measles, mumps, and chicken pox viruses initiate infection in the respiratory tract but must spread through the blood stream (viremia) to other sites before the characteristic disease occurs. The incubation period for these viruses is 9 to 14 days.
- The infection can be asymptomatic or symptomatic.
- The infection may be acute or chronic, depending on whether the immune response can resolve the infection (i.e., eliminate the virus) (Fig. 3.9).

Viral Acquisition, Tropism, and Replication

Acquisition

- Most viral infections are acquired by the oral or the respiratory routes, with infection remaining localized in the nasopharynx, the oropharynx, or the lungs.
- Viruses can also enter the body through breaks in the skin and through the conjunctiva and the urogenital tract. Direct injection of the virus, either by needle or by insect-bite, can also occur.
- Initial replication of the virus usually occurs at the site of infection.
- Many viruses can initiate infection and disease at the site of entry.

Table 3.4 *Incubation Periods of Common Viral Infections*

Disease	Incubation Period* (Days)
Influenza	1-2
Common cold	1-3
Bronchiolitis, croup	3-5
Acute respiratory disease (adenoviruses)	5-7
Dengue	5-8
Herpes simplex virus infections	5-8
Enterovirus infections	6-12
Poliomyelitis	5-20
Measles	9-12
Smallpox	12-14
Chickenpox	13-17
Mumps	16-20
Rubella	17-20
Mononucleosis	30-50
Hepatitis A	15-40
Hepatitis B	50-150
Rabies	30-100
Warts	50-150
AIDS	1-10 years

Modified from White DO, Fenner F: *Medical virology*, ed 3, New York, 1986, Academic Press.

*Until first appearance of prodromal symptoms. Diagnostic signs (e.g., rash, paralysis) may not appear until 2 to 4 days later.

Tropism

- Viral attachment proteins (capsid proteins or the glycoproteins of enveloped viruses) must bind to cell-surface receptors on the target cells.
- The target tissue must express receptors for the virus and possess the machinery for viral replication.
- The virus may spread (usually through the blood stream) from its point of entry to the target tissue. For example, **varicella-zoster virus (VZV)** is acquired by the respiratory route, initiates infection of the lungs, enters the blood stream, spreads to the liver and other organs, initiates a secondary viremia, and then reaches the skin to cause the classic **chicken pox.**
- A virus strain that cannot reach or infect its normal target organ is not virulent (**attenuated strain**). For example, the live polio vaccine (Sabin vaccine) infects the oropharynx and enters the blood stream but cannot reach or infect the brain and therefore does not cause major disease.
- Virus-specific antibodies can block viremic spread to target tissue.

Replication

- The virus must replicate in order to spread and cause disease.
- Not all cells will support the replication of a virus.

1. **Permissive** cells yield productive infections (i.e., virus is produced).
2. **Nonpermissive** cells do not support replication.
3. **Semipermissive** cells may allow some viral functions to occur or may support low levels of virus replication.

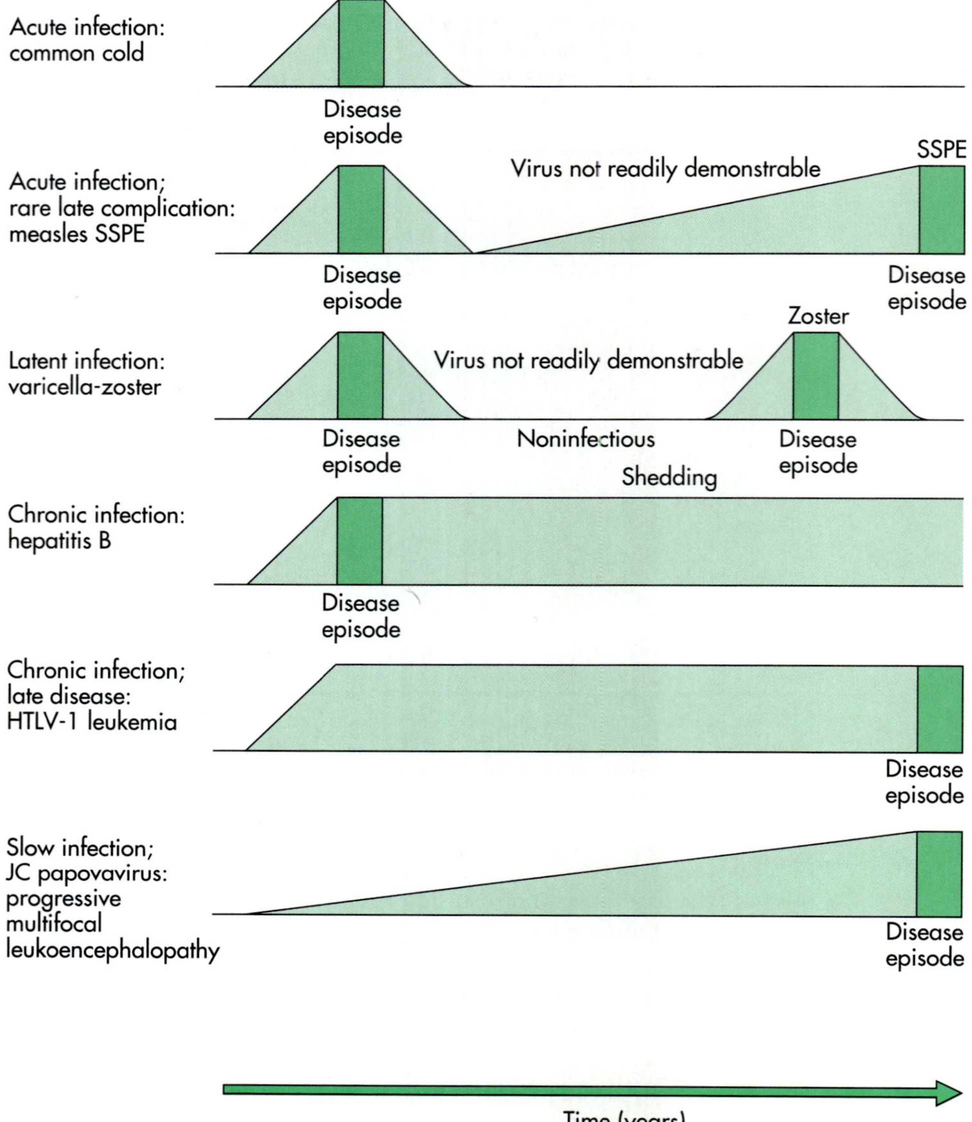

Fig. 3.9 Diagram depicting acute infection and various types of persistent infection, as illustrated by the diseases indicated in the column at the left. Vertical box (green) illustrates disease episode. *SSPE,* Subacute sclerosing panencephalitis. *(Redrawn from White DO, Fenner F:* Medical virology, *ed 3, New York, 1986, Academic Press.)*

- Infection of a cell with a virus may have different effects on the cell.
  1. Virus is produced with death of the cell (**cytolytic infection**).
  2. Virus is produced with little change in the cell (**persistent infection**).
  3. No virus is produced. The virus does not replicate in the cell. Such infections may result in one of the following:
     (a) **latency:** the viral genome is present but no viral protein synthesis occurs or
     (b) **immortalization:** there is restricted viral protein synthesis, which enhances cell growth

Table 3.5 *Mechanisms of Viral Cytopathogenesis*

Mechanism	Representative Viruses
Inhibition of cellular protein synthesis	Polioviruses, herpes simplex virus, togaviruses, poxviruses
Inhibition and degradation of cellular DNA	Herpesviruses
Alteration of cell membrane structure	
Glycoprotein insertion	All enveloped viruses
Syncytia formation	Herpes simplex virus, varicella-zoster virus, paramyxoviruses, human immunodeficiency virus
Disruption of cytoskeleton	Nonenveloped viruses (accumulation), herpes simplex virus
Permeability changes	Togaviruses, herpesviruses
Inclusion bodies	
Negri bodies (intracytoplasmic)	Rabies
Owl's eye (intranuclear)	Cytomegalovirus
Cowdry's type A (intranuclear)	Herpes simplex virus
Intranuclear basophilic	Adenoviruses
Intracytoplasmic acidophilic	Poxviruses
Perinuclear cytoplasmic acidophilic	Reoviruses
Toxicity of virion components	Adenovirus fibers

■ **Cytopathogenesis** In cytolytic infections, viral replication often kills or modifies the target cell. Several mechanisms can lead to cell death (Table 3.5).

1. Inhibition of host DNA synthesis and degradation of host DNA. For example, herpesviruses inhibit host DNA synthesis, degrade the DNA, and use the nucleotides for replication.
2. Inhibition of cellular protein synthesis.
   - Many viruses overpower the cell by production of large quantities of viral mRNA that compete for the ribosomal protein synthesis machinery.
   - Some viruses inhibit host protein synthesis. Poliovirus inactivates elongation factor 1 (EF1) of the ribosome preventing binding of cellular 5′ capped mRNA. Herpes simplex virus (HSV) inhibits transcription of host cell mRNA.
3. Disruption of cellular structures.
   - Inhibition of cellular protein synthesis prevents rebuilding of cell structures and leads to their breakdown.
   - Build up of viral components or virions in the cell disrupts cellular organization. These viral aggregates can be visualized as **inclusion bodies.**
   - Alteration of cell membranes can lead, for example, to cell fusion and the formation of **syncytia** (paramyxoviruses, HSV, human immunodeficiency virus [HIV], and [VZV]).
4. Toxicity of virion components. For example, the fibers on the surface of adenoviruses are cytolytic.

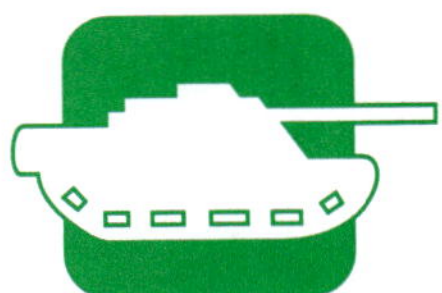

■ **Immune Response**

- Immune resolution of infection is essential for controlling viral disease.
- The virus as well as virus-infected cells must be eliminated. If infected cells are not killed by the virus, then the immune response needs to destroy the cell.

● **Immunogens and antigens** The external structures of the virus, especially the viral attachment proteins (e.g., glycoproteins and capsid proteins) elicit protective **antibody** responses.

Table 3.6 *Interferons*

Type	Number of Subtypes	Stability to Acid	Induction	Principal Source
α	Several	Acid stable	Viruses, etc.†	Most cells, especially leukocytes and epithelial cells
β	One	Acid stable	Viruses, etc.	Mainly fibroblasts
γ*	Three	Acid labile	Mitogens	NK cells and T cells

*Interferon-γ activity resembles that of lymphokines. It activates macrophages. The response of viral infection is a later event. *NK,* Natural killer.
†There are other stimuli for interferon α and β.

Box 3.6

INTERFERONS

Induction

Interferon production is stimulated by viral infection.
1. Double-stranded RNA (e.g., RNA virus intermediate).
2. Viral inhibition of cellular protein synthesis.

Mechanism of Action

1. Release from an initial infected cell.
2. Bind to a specific cell-surface receptor on another cell.
3. Induce the "antiviral state:" protein kinase, 2-5A synthetase, and RNase L.
4. Virus infection of the cell activates these enzymes.
5. Inhibition of viral and cellular protein synthesis.

The internal and external components of the virus must be presented by MHC class I molecules to elicit recognition by **cytolytic** T cells ($CD8^+$ cells).

- **Components of the antiviral immune response**
  - ***Antigen nonspecific responses:***
    1. **Interferons** (Table 3.6, Boxes 3.6 and 3.7)
       - Interferon production is the earliest antiviral response elicited by the infected target cell. The interferon initiates an antiviral state in other cells, preventing viral replication and stimulating other components of the immune response.
       - There are three major types of interferons: α, β, and γ.
    2. **Natural killer (NK) cells** NK cells are large granular lymphocytes that can be activated by interferons and can kill virus-infected cells (Box 3.8).
    3. **Monocytes and macrophages**
       - Monocytes and macrophages phagocytize fragments of lysed infected cells and virions and present viral antigens to T cells.
       - These cells are activated by interferon γ to kill infected cells.
  - ***Antigen specific responses***
    1. **T cell responses** (Box 3.9) T cell responses are mediated by two types of T cells.

Box 3.7

ACTIVITIES OF INTERFERONS

Antiviral Actions

Interferons initiate an antiviral state in cells.
Interferons block viral protein synthesis.
Interferons inhibit cell growth.

Immunomodulatory Actions

Interferons α and β activate natural killer (NK) cells.
Interferon γ activates macrophages.
Interferons increase MHC antigen expression.
Interferons regulate the activities of T cells.

Other Actions

Interferons regulate inflammatory processes.
Interferons regulate tumor growth.

MHC, Major histocompatibility complex.

Box 3.8

CELLULAR COMPONENTS OF ANTIVIRAL IMMUNITY

NK Cells

Are large granular lymphocytes
Act as the local militia
Are activated by interferon
Are important for controlling infections caused by enveloped or noncytolytic virus

Mononuclear Phagocyte System

Consists of monocytes, macrophages, Kupffer cells, and alveolar macrophages
Phagocytizes particles
Produces lymphokines (e.g., TNF, IL-1)
Presents antigen
Causes cytolysis of infected cells

NK, Natural killer.

- $CD4^+$ T helper/delayed-type hypersensitivity cells. $CD4^+$ T cells recognize peptide antigens presented by macrophages and B cells in association with **MHC class II antigens.** These cells release lymphokines that activate other responses, such as T and B cells and inflammatory responses. An essential function of $CD4^+$ T cells is to activate other immune defenses.
- $CD8^+$ T cytolytic/suppressor cells. $CD8^+$ T cells recognize peptide antigens on infected target cells presented by **MHC class I antigens** (HLA-A, HLA-B, or HLA-C). These cells bind to target cells and kill them. An essential function of $CD8^+$ T cells is to eliminate noncytolytic viruses, e.g., enveloped viruses and viruses that cause persistent infections.

2. **Antibody production** (Box 3.10 and Table 3.7)

Box 3.9

T CELL IMMUNE RESPONSES

T cell responses are important for controlling enveloped and noncytolytic virus infections

$CD4^+$ T Cells

Respond to antigen-MHC class II protein complex (antigen presenting cells [APC])
Release lymphokines (e.g., Interleukin-2)
Activate other T cells
Activate B cells (cause immunoglobulin class switch)
Initiate delayed-type hypersensitivity responses

$CD8^+$ T Cells

Respond to viral antigen-MHC class I protein complex (infected-cell)
Kill infected cells

MHC, Major histocompatibility complex.

Box 3.10

ANTIVIRAL ANTIBODY RESPONSES

Neutralize extracellular virus
  Block viral attachment proteins
  Destabilize viral structure
Opsonize virus for phagocytosis
Activate the complement cascade
Responsible for antibody directed cellular cytotoxicity (ADCC)
Block viremic spread to target tissue

IgM

Early antibody
Indicator of recent or current infection

IgG

More effective antibody than IgM
Main component of the later response and the secondary response

IgA

Secretory and serum antibody
Transient response

- IgM, IgG, and secretory IgA are responsible for neutralization and opsonization of viral particles.
- **Neutralization** (inactivation) of virions occurs by the binding of an antibody to virion attachment proteins to prevent viral interaction with the target cell. Neutralization of viruses may also be caused by destabilization of the virion structure by the antibody.
- **Opsonization** of virions by the antibody promotes uptake of virions by macrophages.
- Antibodies can cause cytolysis of viruses by initiating

Table 3.7 Summary of Antigen-Specific Immunity

	Antibody	T Cell
Target	Molecules Virions Infected cells	Viral antigen on cells ($CD4^+$ cells: viral antigen + MHC class II antigens) ($CD8^+$ cells: viral antigen + MHC class I antigens)
Mechanism	Neutralization Opsonization ADCC Complement activation	Delayed-type hypersensitivity ($CD4^+$ cells) Cytolysis ($CD8^+$ cells) Suppression ($CD8^+$ cells)
Protective antigen	VAP (glycoproteins, capsid proteins)	Viral peptides (glycoproteins, nucleoproteins, etc.)
Type of infection resolved	Lytic viruses Viremia	Nonlytic or enveloped viruses

complement action and through antibody dependent cellular cytotoxicity (ADCC).

- The essential function of antibodies is to block virus spread by inactivating an extracellular virus. This is especially important for **controlling viremia.** The antibody is sufficient for controlling a cytolytic viral infection because the virus kills the infected cell while the antibody inactivates the free virus.

Escape From Immune Responses Several mechanisms permit viruses to evade the immune response.

1. Viruses can escape detection by the immune response by
   - direct cell-cell spread (by formation of syncytia): HSV, VZV, paramyxoviruses, and retroviruses
   - initiating latent-recurrent infections: HSV, VZV, and retroviruses
   - changing antigenicity: influenza A virus, HIV
2. Viruses can inactivate the immune response by
   - killing or injuring the lymphocytes: HIV kills $CD4^+$ cells
   - preventing interferon action: adenovirus, hepatitis B virus
   - inactivating complement: HSV
3. Viruses can block the immune response by
   - production of competing antigen: HBsAg of hepatitis B virus

Immunopathogenesis Viral-induced immunopathogenesis is responsible for many of the symptoms associated with disease (Table 3.8).

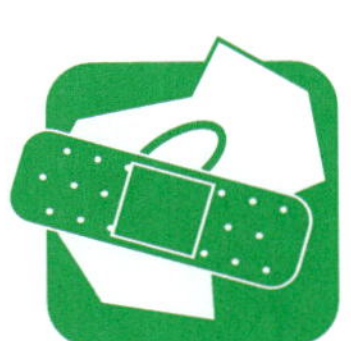

Chronic, Latent, and Immortalizing Infections

- In chronic infections the virus remains in the host without immune resolution. Examples of chronic infections are infections with hepatitis B virus, HIV, and HTLV.
- There is continual production of the virus or viral components.
- There may be an immune complex formation with the antibody, for example, hepatitis B virus.
- The continued presence of the virus leads to immune elimination of the target cell as is seen in measles and postmeasles encephalitis.

Table 3.8 *Viral Immunopathogenesis*

Immunopathogenesis	Immune Mediators	Examples
"Influenza-like symptoms"	Interferon/lymphokines	Respiratory viruses, arboviruses (viremia-inducing viruses)
DTH and inflammation	T cells, PMNs, etc.	Enveloped viruses
Immune-complex disease	Antibody, complement, PMNs	Hepatitis B virus
Hemorrhagic disease	T cells antibody/complement	Dengue virus
Postinfection cytolysis	T cells	Enveloped viruses (e.g., postmeasles encephalitis)
Immunosuppression		HIV, cytomegalovirus, measles virus, influenza virus

DTH, Delayed-type hypersensitivity; *PMNs,* polymorphonuclear leukocytes.

• The presence of the virus alters the immune system, in HIV infection, for example.

- **Latent infections**

In latent infections, the virus remains hidden until reactivated by immune suppression or stress. Such infections are characteristic of the herpesviruses and retroviruses.

- **Immortalizing infections**

In immortalizing infections, the virus stimulates the growth of the cell. This may be a possible initiation step to cancer.

Tumor Viruses (Fig. 3.10)

- **DNA viruses**

• Examples of DNA tumor viruses are papovaviruses, adenoviruses (not in human cells), Epstein-Barr virus, and hepatitis B virus.

• Expression of late genes (which results in virus production) would preclude (prevent) transformation. (The production of the virus would kill the cell.)

• DNA tumor viruses transform cells by the following mechanisms:

  • The virus can prevent the activity of the growth suppressor proteins p53 or RB (papovaviruses and adenoviruses).
  • The virus acts as a mitogen and activates cell growth (Epstein-Barr virus).
  • The virus prevents apoptosis (Epstein-Barr virus).

- **RNA viruses**

• Examples of RNA tumor viruses are the retroviruses (the animal oncoviruses, HTLV-1).

• Viral replication occurs in retrovirus-transformed cells.

• The virus carries an oncogene. Oncogenes are genes that encode proteins that are in the growth stimulatory pathway of hormones, for example, receptors, protein kinases, and DNA binding proteins.

• The virus integrates into a host chromosome and transactivates a host gene, which stimulates cell growth (e.g., HTLV-1).

• The virus makes a transactivating protein that activates the transcription of a growth-stimulating protein, for example, the HTLV-1 tax protein stimulates IL-2 and IL-2 receptor expression, which promotes T cell growth.

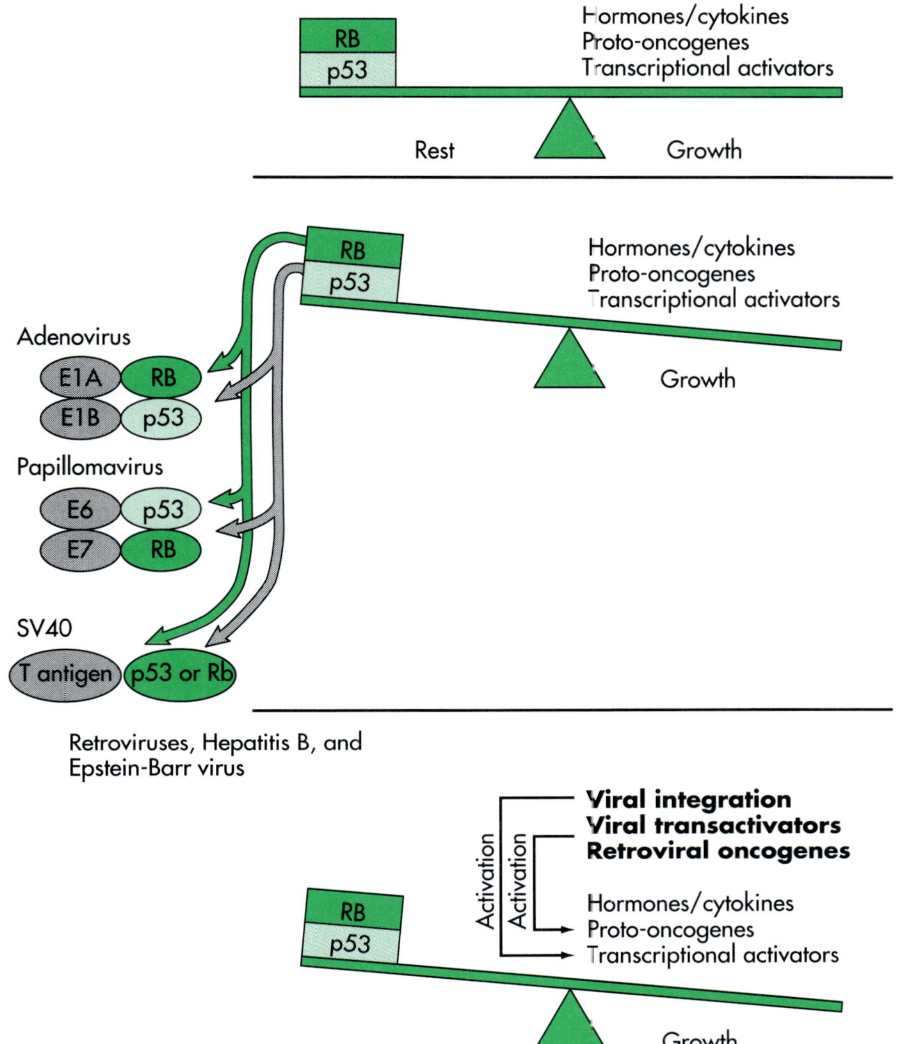

Fig. 3.10 Mechanisms of viral transformation or immortalization. Cell growth is controlled by the balance of external and internal growth activators (accelerators) and growth suppressors (brakes), such as p53 and the retinoblastoma gene product (RB). Oncogenic viruses alter the balance by removing the brakes or enhancing the accelerators.

Section 3.4 Antiviral Drugs and Vaccines

Antiviral Drugs

- **Overview** Antiviral drug targets are viral proteins or activities (Tables 3.9 and 3.10; Figs. 3.11 through 3.13).
  - Most antiviral drugs are nucleotide analogues.
  - Most antiviral drugs are targeted to herpesviruses or HIV.
  - Acyclovir is activated by the HSV- or VZV-encoded thymidine kinase and then inhibited by the viral DNA polymerase (see Fig. 3.12).

- The viruses treatable by antiviral drugs are
  - Herpes simplex virus
  - Varicella-zoster virus
  - Cytomegalovirus
  - HIV
  - Influenza
  - Respiratory syncytial virus

Table 3.9 *Targets for Antiviral Drugs*

Replication Step Targeted	Agent	Virus
Attachment	Receptor	All viruses
	Viral attachment protein peptide analogues	All viruses
	Antibody	All viruses
Penetration and uncoating	Amantadine and rimantadine	Influenza A viruses
		Picornaviruses
DNA replication	Nucleotide analogues	Herpesviruses, HIV
	Phosphonoformate and phosphonacetic acid	Herpesviruses
Nucleotide biosynthesis	Ribavarin	Respiratory syncytial virus
Nucleotide scavenging (thymidine kinase)	Nucleotide analogues	HSV, varicella-zoster virus
Transcription	Interferon α	Hepatitis B virus, hepatitis C virus, papilloma virus
Protein synthesis	Interferon α	Hepatitis B virus, hepatitis C virus, papilloma virus
Glycoprotein processing		HIV
Viral enzymes (protease)	Saquinavir	HIV

HIV, Human immunodeficiency virus; *HSV*, herpes simplex virus.

Table 3.10 *Approved Antiviral Drug Therapies*

Virus	Antiviral Drug	Tradenames
Herpes simplex	Acyclovir	Zovirax
	Valacyclovir	Valtrex
	Famciclovir	Famvir
	Adenosine arabinoside (ara-A, vidarabine)	Vira-A
	Iododeoxyuridine	Stoxil, Idoxuridine
	Trifluorothymidine	Viroptic, Trifluridine
Cytomegalovirus	Ganciclovir	Cytovene
	Phosphonoformate	Foscarnet
Human immunodeficiency virus	Zidovudine (azidothymidine)	Retrovir
	Dideoxycytidine (DDC)	Zalcitabine
	Dideoxyinosine (DDI)	Didanosine
	Saquinavir	
Influenza virus type A	Amantadine	Symmetrel
	Rimantadine	
Hepatitis B virus	Interferon α	
Hepatitis C virus	Interferon α	
Papilloma virus	Interferon α	

Fig. 3.11 Structures of nucleoside analogues that are antiviral drugs. The chemical distinctions between the natural deoxynucleosides and the antiviral drug analogues are in color.

- (Other viruses may also be sensitive to antiviral drugs.) (Table 3.10)

Antiviral Vaccines

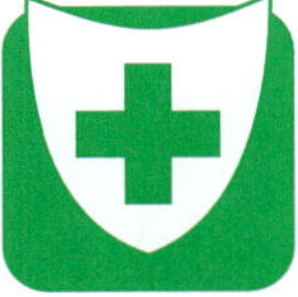

- **Passive immunization** Passive immunity to viruses can be conferred by immunoglobulin administration. For example, varicella-zoster immune globulin protects immunocompromised children, such as those with leukemia. Rabies gamma globulin is administered immediately after infection to block progression of the virus. Hepatitis A virus gamma globulin can be given to block infection after exposure.
- **Active immunization**
  - ***Live vaccines*** Live vaccines are prepared from attenuated strains of the same virus, which cannot cause serious disease. Alternately, the vaccine may be prepared from the virus from another species that elicits a protective response in humans (e.g., the smallpox vaccine is prepared from vaccinia virus).

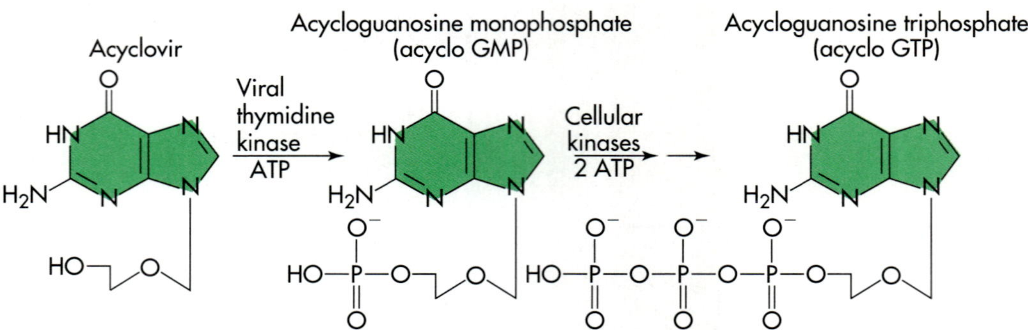

Fig. 3.12 Activation of acyclovir (acycloguanosine) in herpes simplex virus-infected cells. Acyclovir is converted to acycloguanosine monophosphate (acyclo GMP) by the herpes-specific viral thymidine kinase and then to acyclo GTP by cellular kinases.

Amantadine hydrochloride

Rimantadine hydrochloride

Arildone

Phosphonoformic acid (Foscarnet)

Phosphonoacetic acid

Fig. 3.13 Structures of some nonnucleoside antiviral drugs.

— ***Inactivated vaccines*** Inactivated vaccines may contain a whole virus that is chemically inactivated or heat inactivated, or they may be subunit vaccines, which contain viral fragments that are prepared by genetic engineering.

Some commonly used viral vaccines are listed in Table 3.11. Table 3.12 provides a comparison of live and inactivated vaccines. Table 3.13 presents a vaccine schedule for children.

Section 3.5 Laboratory Identification of Viruses

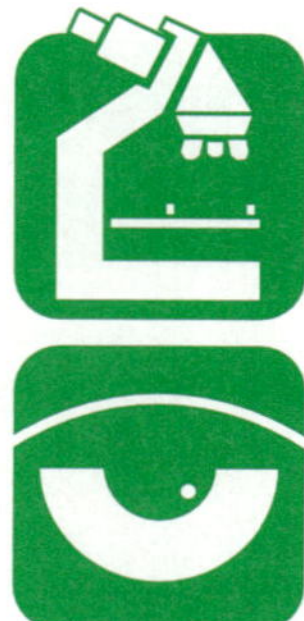

■ **Overview** A bacterial or fungal etiology for an infection must first be excluded.

Laboratory procedures for diagnosis of viral infections include the following (Table 3.14):

- Cytologic examination
- Electron microscopy
- Virus isolation and growth
- Detection of viral proteins (antigens and enzymes)
- Detection of viral genetic material
- Serology

Table 3.11 *Viral Vaccines**

Virus	Vaccine Components	Indications
Polio	Inactivated (IPV; Salk vaccine)	Children
	Attenuated (OPV; Sabin vaccine)	Children
Measles	Attenuated	Children
Mumps	Attenuated	Children
Rubella	Attenuated	Children
Influenza	Inactivated	Adults, especially medical personnel and elderly
Hepatitis B	Subunit	Newborns, health care workers, high-risk groups (promiscuous individuals, IV drug abusers)
Smallpox	Vaccinia	No longer necessary
Varicella-zoster	Attenuated	Children
Hepatitis A	Inactivated	Travelers
Rotavirus	Bovine or rhesus rotavirus (share common antigen)	Experimental

*Listed in order of frequency of use. *IPV,* Poliovirus vaccine inactivated; *OPV,* poliovirus vaccine live oral.

Table 3.12 *Advantages and Disadvantages of Live vs. Inactivated Vaccines*

Property	Live	Inactivated
Route of administration	Natural* or injection	Injection
Dose of virus; cost	Low	High
Number of doses	Single†	Multiple
Need for adjuvant	No	Yes‡
Duration of immunity	Many years	Generally less
Antibody response	IgG, secretory IgA§	IgG; serum IgA
Cell-mediated immune response	Good	Poor
Heat lability in tropics	Yes‖	No
Interference¶	Occasional	No
Side effects	Occasional mild symptoms#	Occasional sore arm
Reversion to virulence	Rarely	No

From White DO, Fenner F, *Medical virology*, ed 3, New York, 1986, Academic Press.
*Oral or respiratory, in certain cases.
†A single booster may be required or desirable after about a decade
‡However, no satisfactory adjuvants are licensed for human use.
§IgA if delivered via oral or respiratory route. OPV can prevent wild poliovirus from multiplying in the gut and thus facilitate near eradication of the virus from the community.
‖$MgCl_2$ and other stabilizers, and maintenance of refrigeration or cold storage assist preservation.
¶Interference from other viruses or diseases.
#Especially rubella and measles.

Cytologic Examination Clinical specimens can be examined for virus-induced histologic changes in cells and tissue.

- Viral cytopathic effect (CPE) includes vacuolization, necrosis, syncytia formation, and other changes in cell morphology.
- Some viruses form characteristic **inclusion bodies**, which can be identified in tissues. Examples of such viruses are the following:
  - Cytomegalovirus: owl's eye nuclear inclusion bodies

Table 3.13 *Recommended Schedule of Vaccinations for All Children*

Birth	2 Months	4 Months	6 Months	15 Months	4-6 Years (before school)
	DPT	DPT	DPT	DPT	DPT
	Polio	Polio		Polio	Polio
	Hib	Hib	Hib	Hib	
				MMR	MMR
HBV	HBV			HBV	
				VZV	

DPT, Diphtheria/Pertussis/Tetanus vaccine; *Polio,* live oral polio vaccine (OPV) or killed (inactivated) polio vaccine (IPV); *MMR,* measles, mumps, rubella live vaccines; *Hib,* haemophilus influenzae type b conjugate vaccine; *HBV,* hepatitis B vaccine; *VZV,* varicella-zoster live virus vaccine. (From Centers for Disease Control)

Table 3.14 *Specimens for Viral Diagnosis*

Common Pathogenic Viruses	Specimens for Culture	Comments
Respiratory		
Adenovirus, influenza, enterovirus (picornavirus)*, rhinovirus, paramyxovirus†, rubella virus, herpes simplex virus	Nasal washing, throat swab, nasal swab, sputum	*Enterovirus is also shed in stool; measles and mumps may also be in urine†
Gastrointestinal		
Reovirus, rotavirus, adenovirus, Norwalk virus, and calicivirus	Stool, rectal swab	Samples are analyzed by electron microscopy and antigen detection; viruses are not cultured
Maculopapular Rash		
Adenovirus, enterovirus (picornavirus) Rubella virus and measles virus	Throat swab and rectal swab	
Vesicular Rash		
Coxsackievirus, echovirus, herpes simplex virus, and varicella-zoster virus	Vesicle fluid, scraping or swab	Initial diagnosis of HSV and VZV can be obtained from vesicle scraping (Tzanck smear)
Central Nervous System (Aseptic Meningitis, Encephalitis)		
Enterovirus (picornavirus)	Stool	
Arboviruses (togaviruses, flaviviruses, bunyaviruses, etc.)	Viruses rarely cultured	Diagnosis by serologic test
Rabies virus	Tissue, saliva, brain biopsy	Diagnosis by immunofluorescence analysis for antigen
Herpes simplex virus, cytomegalovirus, mumps virus, measles virus	Cerebrospinal fluid, brain biopsy	Virus isolation and immunofluorescence analysis for antigen
Urinary		
Adenovirus, cytomegalovirus	Urine	Cytomegalovirus may be shed without apparent disease
Eye		
Adenovirus, herpes simplex virus, enterovirus (picornavirus)	Conjunctival swab or scraping, throat swab	

*Data from Cherneskey MA, Ray CG, Smith TF: *Laboratory diagnosis of viral infections*, Washington, DC, 1982, Cumitech 15.

†American Society of Microbiology; and Hsiung GD: *Diagnostic virology*, New Haven, 1982, Yale University Press.

- Herpes simplex virus: Cowdry's type A nuclear inclusion bodies
- Rabies virus: Negri bodies

• Immunologic reactivity can be used to detect viral antigens. Immunofluorescence and enzyme immunoassay are the most common immunologic techniques used.

• The presence of a viral genome can be detected by in situ hybridization or by the **polymerase chain reaction (PCR).** The reverse transcriptase PCR (RT-PCR) is used for RNA viruses.

Electron Microscopy Visualization of virions in cells or stool can be detected directly or enhanced by antibody (immune electron microscopy).

Viral Isolation and Growth

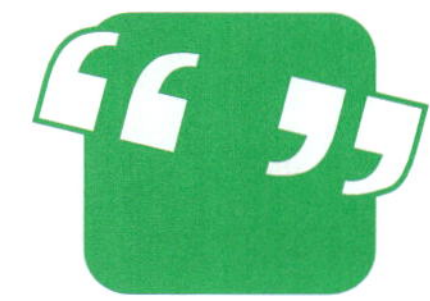

- Special cell culture systems support the growth of specific viruses.
- Types of cell culture systems:
  - Organ culture
  - Embryonated eggs
  - **Primary cells:** dissociated tissue cells grown in culture; these cells can be maintained for only two to three passages
  - **Diploid cell lines:** normal cells that can be maintained for up to 100 doublings. (This represents several passages.)
  - **Transformed cell lines:** immortalized cells
- The characteristic viral CPE can be detected in cell culture (see above).
- Viral antigens and viral nucleic acids can also be detected in cell culture.

Detection of Viral Proteins

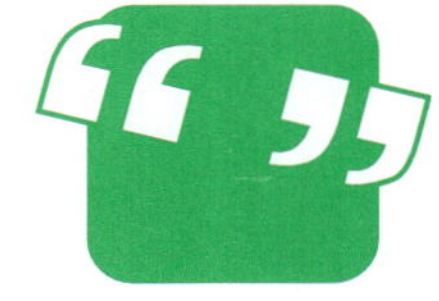

Detection of viral proteins on cells

Hemagglutination: Some viruses produce glycoproteins that bind to erythrocytes of specific species and cause the erythrocytes to clump (e.g., influenza virus).

Hemadsorption: Expression of hemagglutinin proteins on the cell surface allows erythrocytes to adsorb (bind) to the cell surface.

Immunohistochemistry: Immunofluorescence (IF) or enzyme immunoassay (EIA) can detect viral proteins (Fig. 3.14).

In situ hybridization: Viral DNA or RNA can be detected using genetic probes that are either radiolabeled or labeled with a fluorescent marker.

Detection of free virions or proteins

— ***Enzyme linked immunosorbent assay (ELISA) or radioimmunoassay (RIA)*** Specific antibodies are used to detect and quantitate free virus or viral antigens. For ELISA, an antibody is affixed to a plastic plate or to beads and is used to capture the antigen from the sample. A second antibody is then bound to the antigen, followed by a third antibody that is linked to an enzyme. The enzyme converts a substrate to a colored product. (ELISA is similar to EIA.)

For RIA, a previously prepared radioactive antigen is displaced from immune complexes by an antigen from the sample. Immune complexes are separated from the unbound antigen and quantitated by comparison with a standard curve.

— ***Western blot*** Viral proteins are separated by sodium dodecyl sulfate-polyacrylamide gel electrophoresis, the proteins are transferred

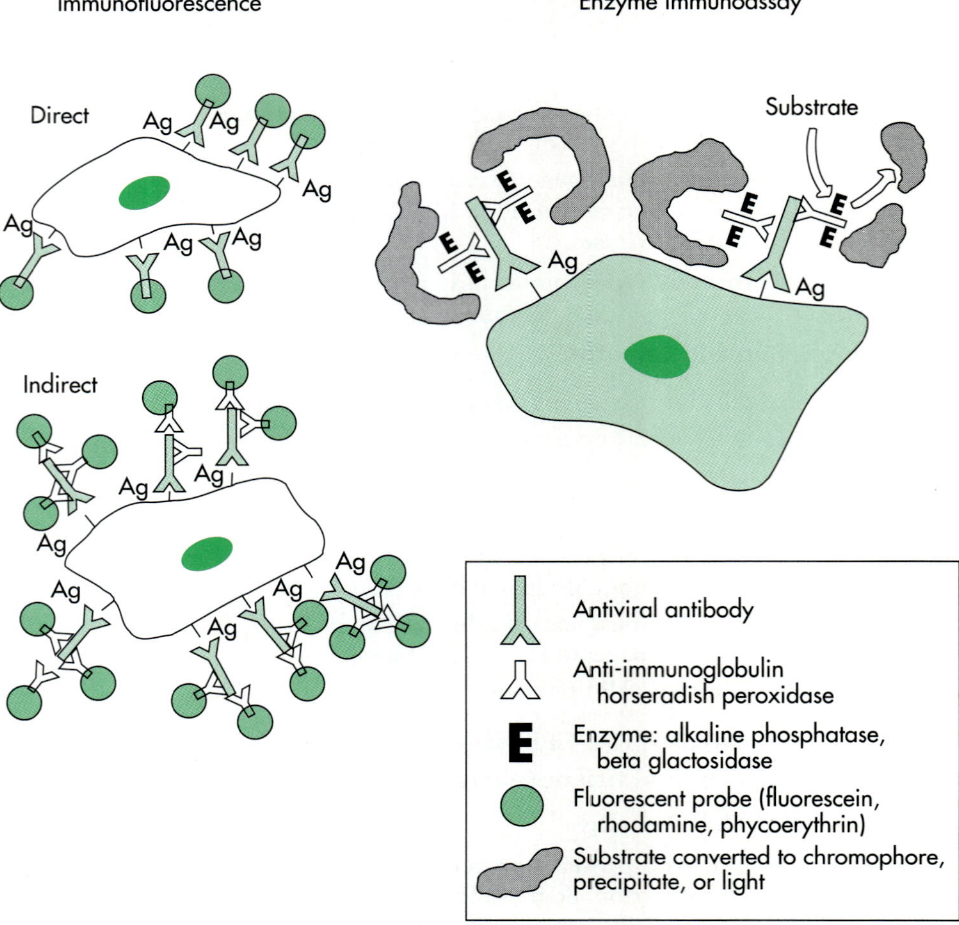

Fig. 3.14 Immunofluorescence (IF) and enzyme immunoassays (EIA) for antigen localization in cells. Antigens can be detected by direct assay with an antiviral antibody modified covalently with a fluorescent or enzyme probe or by indirect assay using antiviral antibody and chemically modified antiimmunoglobulin. The enzyme converts the substrate to a precipitate, a chromophore, or a light emitting compound.

to nitrocellulose paper, and the relevant viral proteins are identified using specific antibodies and enzyme immunoassay techniques.

- **Detection of Viral Genetic Material** Viral nucleic acid can be detected in tissues by Southern blotting, Northern blotting, and PCR.
- **Serology**

  - Serology provides information on the clinical history of an individual.
  - The finding of IgM antibodies indicates current or recent infection.
  - A fourfold increase in antibody titer is required to indicate recent infection.
  - The presence and titers of an antibody to key viral antigens can describe the stage of disease for infection with certain viruses, such as Epstein-Barr virus and hepatitis B virus.

- Serologic assays

  Complement fixation: Immune complexes formed after addition of an antigen to a patient's serum will fix (use up) the complement (that is also

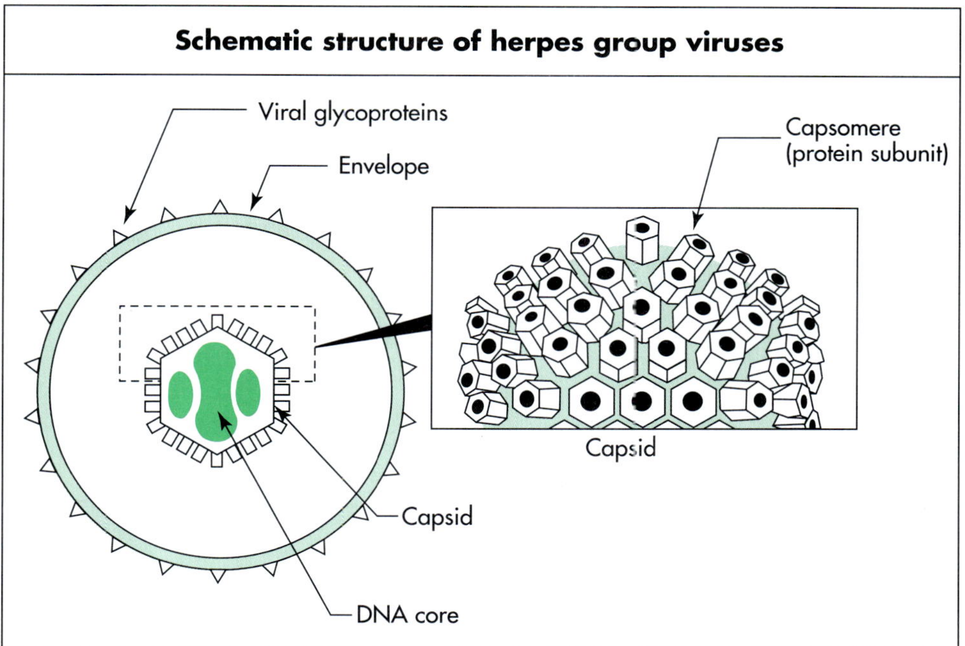

Fig. 3.15 General schematic structure of the herpesviruses. The DNA genome is surrounded by an icosahedral capsid and a membrane envelope. Several viral glycoproteins are inserted into the envelope.

added). The residual complement is measured by its activity on antibody-coated erythrocytes.

Neutralization: An antibody added to the virus will block viral infection. This test is also useful for defining the serotype of the virus.

Hemagglutination inhibition: An antibody is used to block hemagglutination. This test is also useful for defining the serotype of the virus.

Latex agglutination: Latex particles are coated with an antigen. Addition of an antibody causes the particles to clump.

ELISA: An immobilized antigen is used to capture a specific antibody from the patient's serum. A second antibody labeled with an enzyme is added, followed by a substrate. The production of color by enzymatic action is quantitated.

RIA: Immune complexes between antibodies in the patient's serum and radioactive antigen can be quantitated.

Western blot: Antibody specific antigens can be detected as described earlier. (See discussion on detection of viral proteins.)

Section 3.6 Herpesviruses

General Features

- The herpesviruses are important human pathogens.
- The herpesviruses are large DNA viruses. The genome is enclosed in an icosahedral capsid that is surrounded by a membrane envelope (Fig. 3.15).
- All of the herpesviruses establish infections of the **latent-recurrent** type.
- **Cell-mediated immune responses** are required for control of herpesvirus infections.
- The herpesviruses are categorized by target cell tropism (Table 3.15).

Table 3.15 *Properties Distinguishing the Herpesviruses*

Subfamily/Virus	Primary Target Cell	Site of Latency	Means of Spread
Alpha-Herpesvirinae			
Herpes simplex type 1 (HSV-1)	Mucoepithelial	Neuron	Close contact
Herpes simplex type 2 (HSV-2)	Mucoepithelial	Neuron	Close contact
Varicella-zoster virus (VZV)	Mucoepithelial	Neuron	Respiratory and close contact
Gamma-Herpesvirinae			
Epstein-Barr virus (EBV)	B lymphocyte and epithelial cells	B lymphocyte	Close contact (kissing disease)
Beta-Herpesvirinae			
Cytomegalovirus (CMV)	Monocyte, lymphocyte, and epithelial cells	Monocyte, lymphocyte, and ?	Close contact, transfusions, tissue transplant, and congenital
Herpes lymphotropic virus (HHV6)	T lymphocytes and ?	T lymphocytes and ?	Respiratory and close contact?
Human herpesvirus 7 (HHV7)	T lymphocytes and ?	T lymphocytes and ?	?

? indicates that other cells may also be the primary target or site of latency.

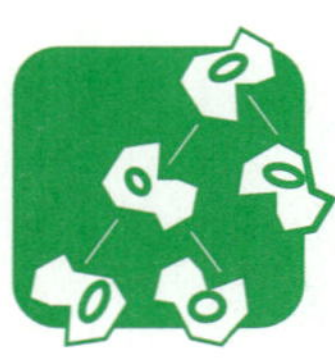

Replication of Herpesviruses (Fig. 3.16)

- Viruses bind to specific receptors and enter a cell by fusion of the viral envelope with the cell membrane.
- Viral DNA reaches the cell nucleus where replication and mRNA synthesis occur.
- mRNA and protein are synthesized in three phases: immediate-early, early (DNA synthesis), and late.
- Capsids are assembled and filled in the nucleus and are enveloped at the nuclear membrane.
- Virus is released by exocytosis and upon cell lysis.
- Latent infection occurs if early mRNA, early protein, or DNA synthesis does not occur.
- The host cell type determines whether latency will occur. For example, herpes simplex virus sets up a latent infection in neurons.

Herpes Simplex Viruses Type 1 and Type 2 Herpes simplex viruses (HSVs) type 1 and type 2 are closely related viruses differing mainly in their means of transmission. Infection with HSV-1 usually involves the mouth or throat, whereas HSV-2 is involved in genital infections.

Laboratory identification

- The sample for diagnosis usually consists of vesicle fluid or a biopsy sample from affected tissue.
- The virus replicates and causes extensive cytopathic effects in most tissue culture cells.
- Many strains of HSV cause **syncytium** formation (formation of multinucleated giant cells).
- **Cowdry's type A nuclear inclusion bodies** can be seen upon staining.
- Distinction of HSV-1 from HSV-2 is done using immunologic tech-

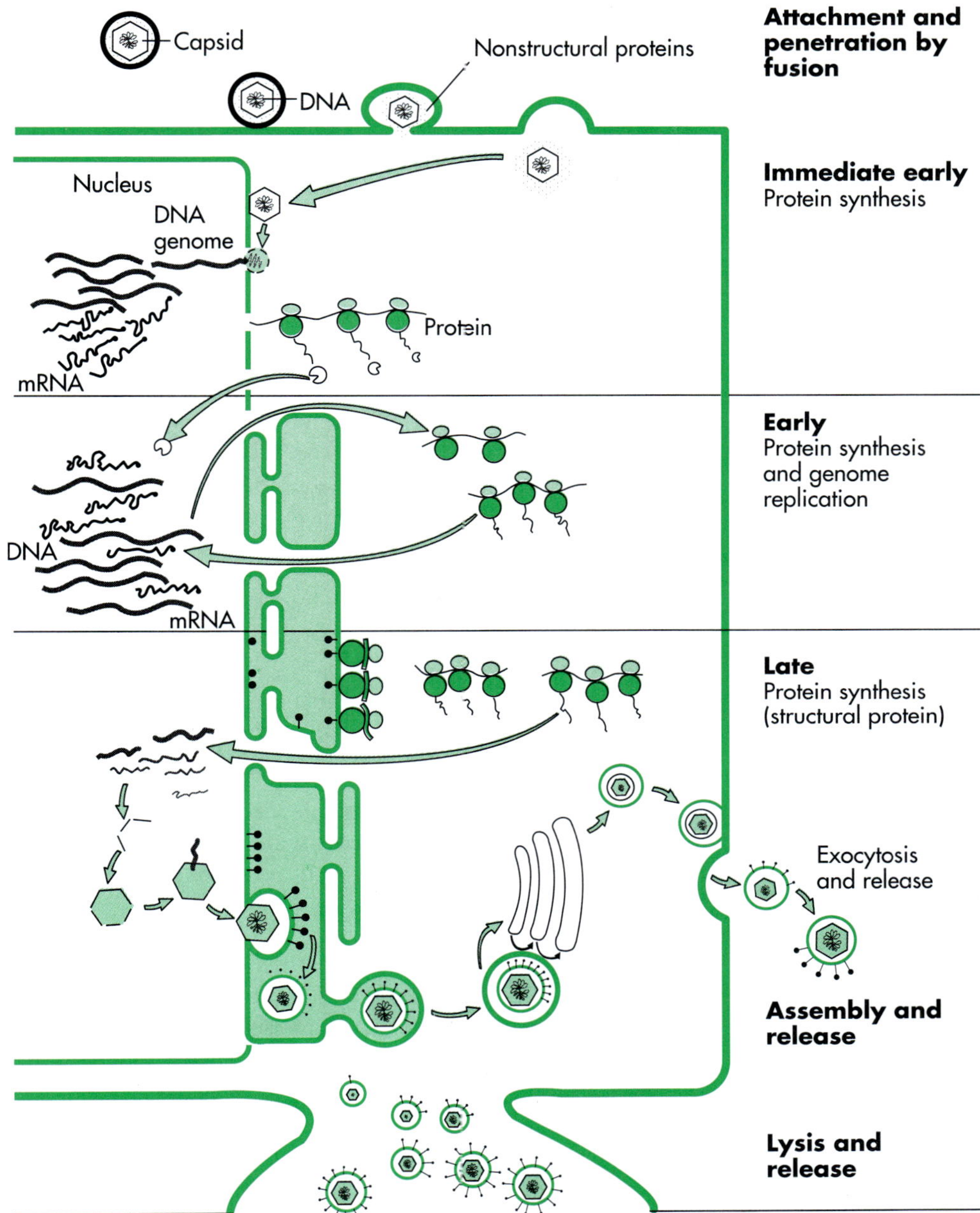

Fig. 3.16 Replication of herpes simplex virus (HSV), a complex enveloped DNA virus. HSV binds to specific receptors and fuses with the plasma membrane. The nucleocapsid then delivers the DNA genome to the nucleus. Transcription and translation occur in three phases: immediate-early, early, and late. Immediate-early proteins promote the takeover of the cell; early proteins consist of enzymes, including the DNA-dependent DNA polymerase; and the last proteins are structural proteins, including the viral capsid and glycoproteins. The genome is replicated before transcription of the late genes. Capsid proteins migrate into the nucleus, assemble into icosadeltahedral capsids, and are filled with the DNA genome. The viral glycoproteins are co-translationally glycosylated in the endoplasmic reticulum and diffuse to the contiguous nuclear envelope. The capsids filled with genomes bud through these modified membranes and are transferred to the Golgi apparatus, the glycoproteins are processed, and the virus is released by exocytosis.

niques (IF or ELISA) or by DNA probe techniques on biopsy tissue or infected cell cultures.

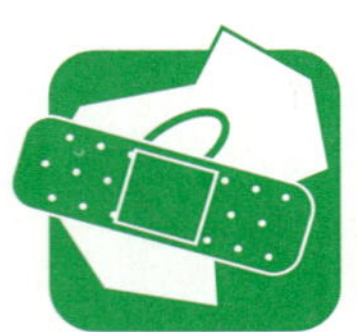

- **Pathogenesis**
  - HSV encodes a **thymidine kinase** and is **neurotropic**.
  - HSV causes a lytic infection in most types of cells and a latent infection in neurons.
  - HSV initially infects mucoepithelial cells and then the innervating neuron.
  - Tissue damage results directly from virus replication and from inflammatory reactions.
  - The virus may remain latent in neurons without expressing any proteins or replicating the genome for the life of the individual.
  - Reactivation can be induced by emotional or physical stress (sunburn, menstruation), certain foods, and immune suppression.
  - The virus spreads directly from cell to cell, escaping antibody control.
  - Life-threatening, disseminated infection may result in neonates and in individuals with compromised cell-mediated immunity.

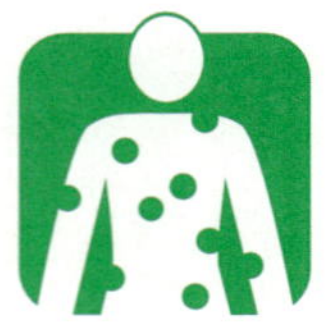

- **Diseases (Fig. 3.17)**
  - HSV disease is determined by the type of tissue infected.
  - Recurrent disease is less severe than the primary infection and may be asymptomatic.
  - Infection or recurrence in the immunocompromised host can cause serious morbidity and mortality, even if treated.
  - HSV-1 infections include the following:

1. Oral infections: These infections are the most common and include gingivostomatitis and herpes labialis.
2. Infections of the eye: Keratoconjunctivitis is a potential cause of blindness.
3. Encephalitis (serious)
4. Whitlow: This is a herpetic infection of the fingers.
5. Genital disease
6. Neonatal disease: This infection can be disseminated and life threatening.

  - HSV-2 also causes all of the above infections, but the three predominant diseases are genital disease, oral disease, and meningitis.
  - Classic HSV lesions are vesicular with an erythematous base (they have the appearance of a dewdrop on a rose petal). The lesions appear approximately 3 days after contact and can last for up to 2 weeks (primary herpes).

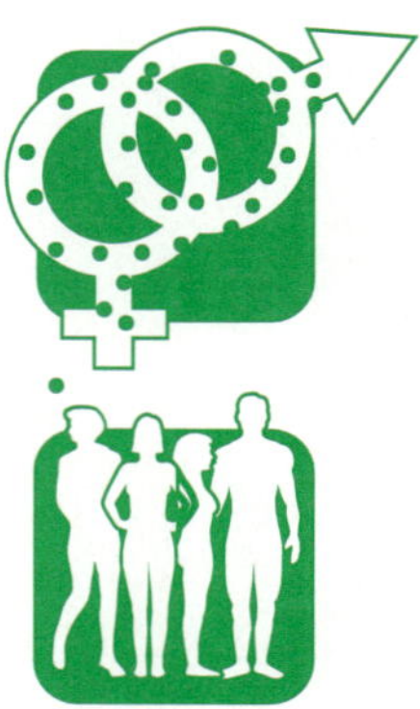

- **Epidemiology**

  Mode of spread: HSV is spread by direct contact with vesicle fluid or virus-containing mucus, for example, by kissing, sharing utensils, sexual transmission, or autoinoculation. Neonates may be infected upon traversing the birth canal if lesions are present in the mother. Recurrences can be asymptomatic, thereby promoting spread of the virus.

  Populations affected:

  - HSV-1 is ubiquitous and more than 90% of the population have been infected.

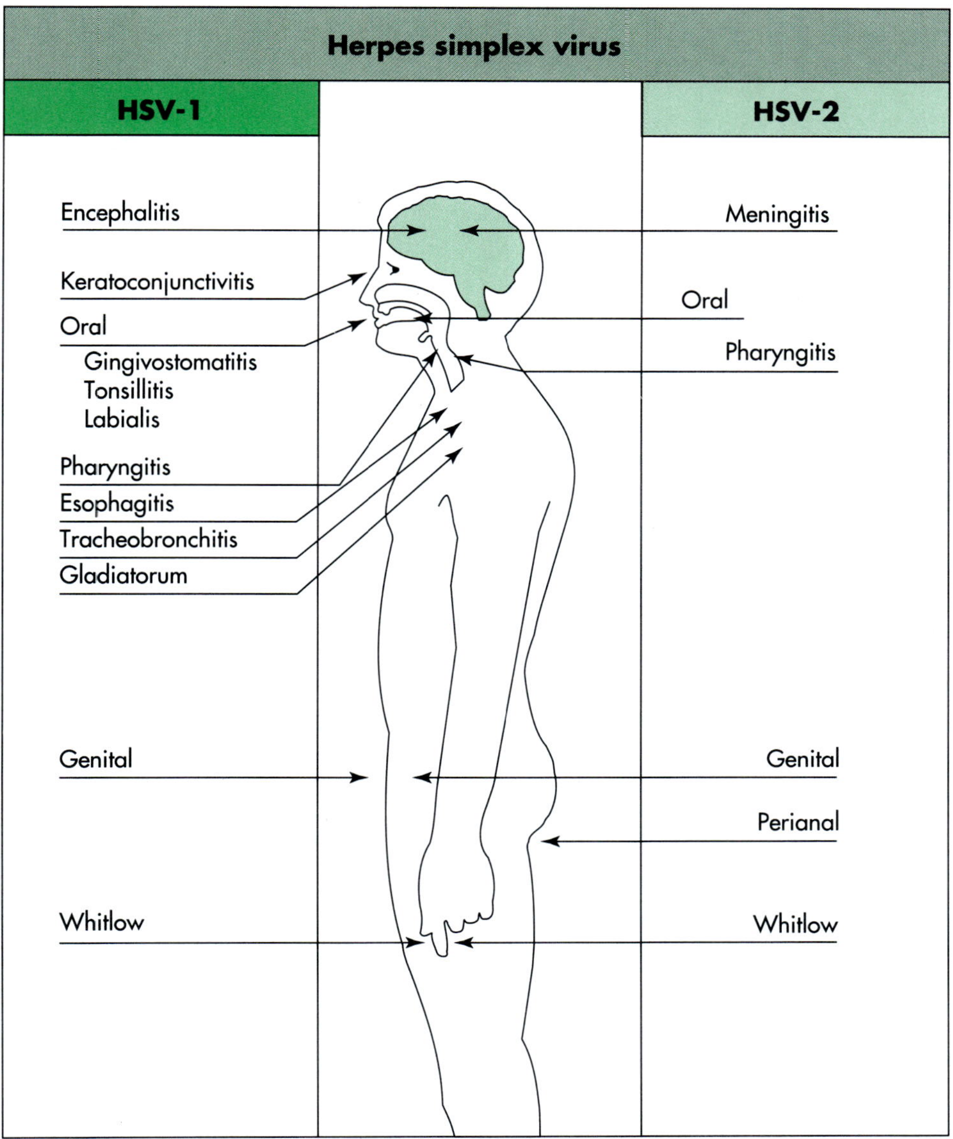

Fig. 3.17 Disease syndromes of herpes simplex viruses. HSV-1 and HSV-2 can infect the same tissues and cause similar diseases but have a predilection for the sites and diseases indicated. Alternatively, the virus may be released upon cell lysis.

- HSV-2 is usually transmitted sexually and acquired later in life by approximately 30% of the population.

Occurence: There is no seasonal or geographic distribution. Unlike arboviral encephalitis, HSV disease can occur year round.

- **Prevention** Good hygiene can help lower the risk of contracting HSV infections.
- **Treatment**

- Acyclovir, famciclovir, and valacyclovir are the drugs of choice and are approved by the Food and Drug Administration (FDA). Other active drugs

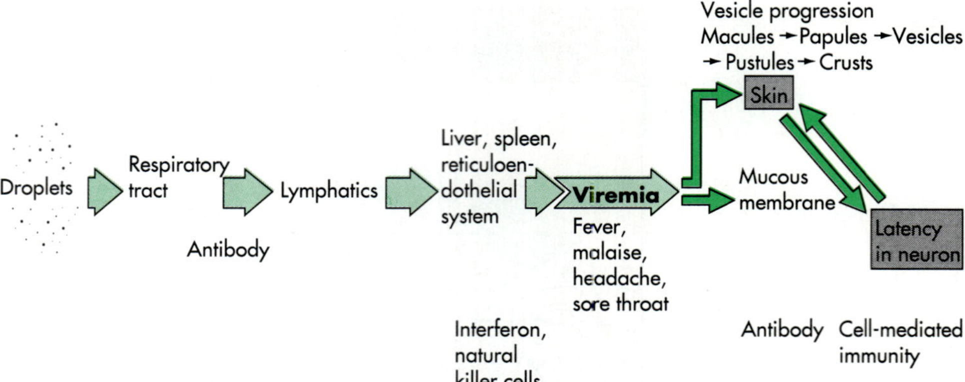

Fig. 3.18 Mechanism of spread of varicella-zoster virus (VZV) within the body. VZV initially infects the respiratory tract and is spread by the reticuloendothelial system and by viremia to other parts of the body. The spread can be blocked by the immune response at the stages indicated below the progression.

are ganciclovir, phosphonoformate, adenosine arabinoside, iododeoxyuridine, and trifluorothymidine.

- Acyclovir, famciclovir, valacyclovir, and ganciclovir are activated by the virally encoded **thymidine kinase** and inhibit the **viral DNA polymerase.**
- Resistance develops (through mutations in target enzyme genes) in AIDS patients who are on prophylactic treatment.
- No vaccine is available for herpes simplex viruses.

Varicella-Zoster Virus (VZV)

Laboratory identification

- VZV can be identified in vesicle fluid or biopsy specimens.
- Identification of the infection is usually made on the basis of the clinical symptoms.
- VZV can be isolated in cell culture.
- The diagnosis can be confirmed by antibody staining and DNA probe techniques.

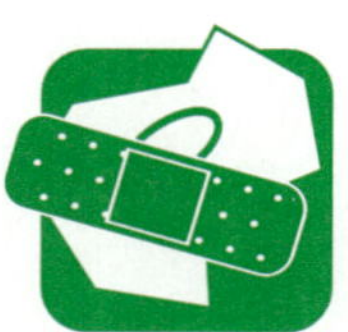

Pathogenesis (Fig. 3.18)

- VZV is very similar to HSV. It encodes **a thymidine kinase** and is **neurotropic.**
- VZV initiates infection in the lungs and then spreads by **viremia** to the organs and skin.
- Lesions at different stages of development can be observed on the skin.
- Cell-mediated immunity is important for control of VZV infection.
- Latency is established in neurons.
- Varicella infection can recur as herpes zoster later in life, with lesions occurring along a single dermatome.

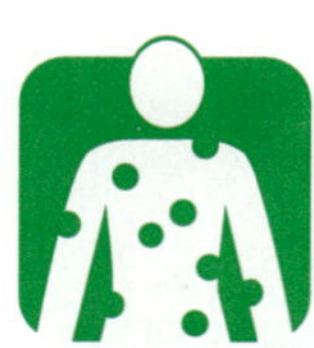

Diseases

1. Primary disease: chicken pox
   - Approximately 10 to 14 days after exposure (maximum, 90 days), lesions appear first on the trunk and then on the peripheral regions of the body.

- Lesions progress in the following order: macule—papule—vesicle—ulcer—scab.
- Lesions in different phases can be present at the same time (unlike smallpox).
- The disease is more severe in adults, with significant potential for pneumonia to develop.
- The disease can be life threatening in immunocompromised children, e.g., those with leukemia.

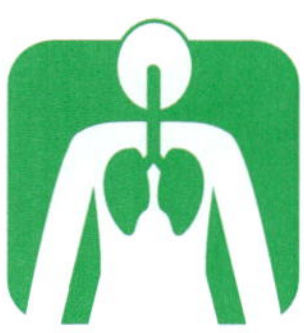

2. Recurrent disease: zoster (shingles)

- Lesions and severe pain occur along a single dermatome, e.g., a beltlike presentation along a thoracic dermatome.

Epidemiology

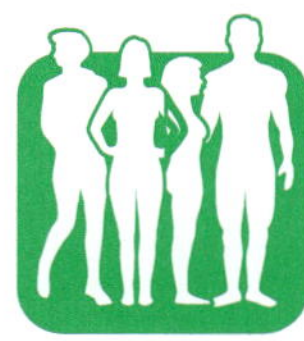

Mode of spread: The virus is spread by aerosols before the onset of symptoms. It can be spread by contact with lesions. The disease is very contagious.

Populations affected: Infection in children is usually relatively benign. Primary infection of adults is often severe. Infection of immunocompromised individuals (leukemics) and neonates can be life threatening.

Occurrence: VZV is ubiquitous.

Prevention

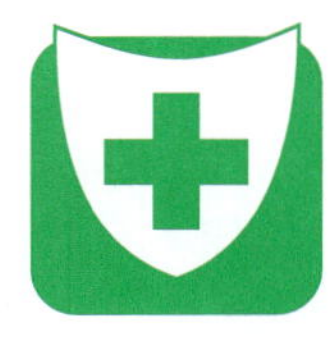

- Careful isolation procedures should be used for immune deficient individuals at risk of getting infected.
- Varicella-zoster immune globulin (VZIG) can be used for prophylactic treatment of immunosuppressed individuals.
- A live attenuated varicella vaccine was approved in 1995.

Treatment

- VZV infections can be treated with acyclovir, famciclovir, or valcyclovir but they are less effective than with HSV, requiring much higher doses.
- Treatment is mainly for individuals at high risk of morbidity.

Epstein-Barr Virus (EBV)

Laboratory identification

- EBV cannot be cultured.
- The diagnosis of EBV infection is based on the clinical features, presence of **atypical lymphocytes** (Downey cells), and the presence of a heterophile antibody and a specific antibody to viral antigens.
- Monospot tests are used to detect a **heterophile antibody**, which is an early IgM response directed to the Paul Bunnell antigen on sheep or bovine erythrocytes.
- Antibody titers to viral antigens defines the course of the disease.
- ELISA tests are available to detect a heterophile antibody, as well as a specific viral antigen and antibodies.

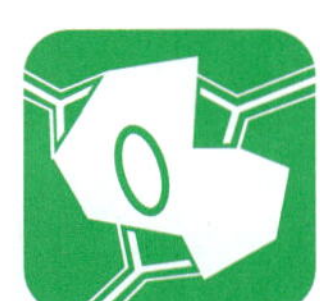

— *Viral antigens and antibodies*

- Several EBV antigens have been identified in infected cells.
- Epstein-Barr nuclear antigen (EBNA) is present in all infected cells.
- Viral capsid antigen (VCA) is present only in virus-producing cells.

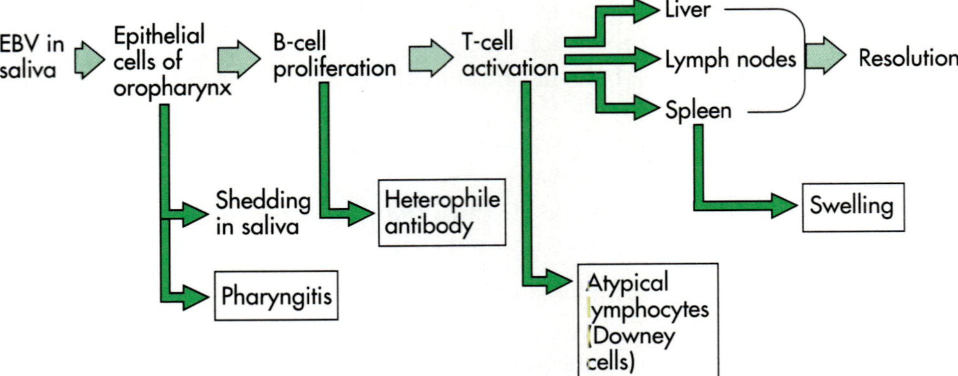

Fig. 3.19 Pathogenesis of EBV. EBV is acquired from saliva and infects epithelial cells and B lymphocytes. The resolution of the EBV infection and many of the symptoms of infectious mononucleosis result from activation of T lymphocytes in response to the infection.

- Early antigen (EA) is present only in virus-producing cells.
- Membrane antigen (MA) (envelope) is present only in virus-producing cells.
- Antibodies to EA and VCA occur during active infection.
- The presence of antibodies to EBNA signifies resolution of infection.

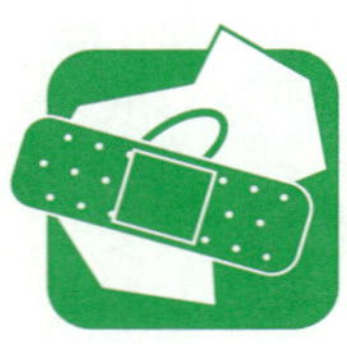

- **Pathogenesis (Fig. 3.19)**
  - The virus is spread via saliva.
  - EBV binds only to B lymphocytes and epithelial cells.
  - EBV establishes a lytic infection of epithelial cells, which produce a virus.
  - EBV infection of B cells is blocked and only the EBNA, latent period (LP), and latent membrane proteins (LMP) are produced.
  - EBV induces the proliferation of B cells and can immortalize the cells.
  - In the absence of T cell-mediated immunity, EBV-induced proliferation of B cells causes a leukemia-like disease.
- **Diseases**
  1. Infectious mononucleosis **(heterophile antibody positive)** (Fig. 3.20)
     - It has an incubation period of up to 2 months.
     - Symptoms include sore throat, swollen glands, hepatosplenomegaly (enlarged liver and spleen), and severe malaise and fatigue.
     - Blood tests show an abundance of atypical lymphocytes (Downey cells) that are T cells.
     - Resolution may take weeks or months.
     - Symptoms in younger children are milder.

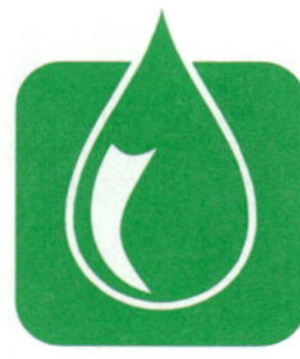

  2. Hairy oral leukoplakia
     - It is observed only in immunosuppressed patients (e.g., AIDS patients).
     - There are white lesions in the mouth, especially on the tongue.
  3. African Burkitt's lymphoma

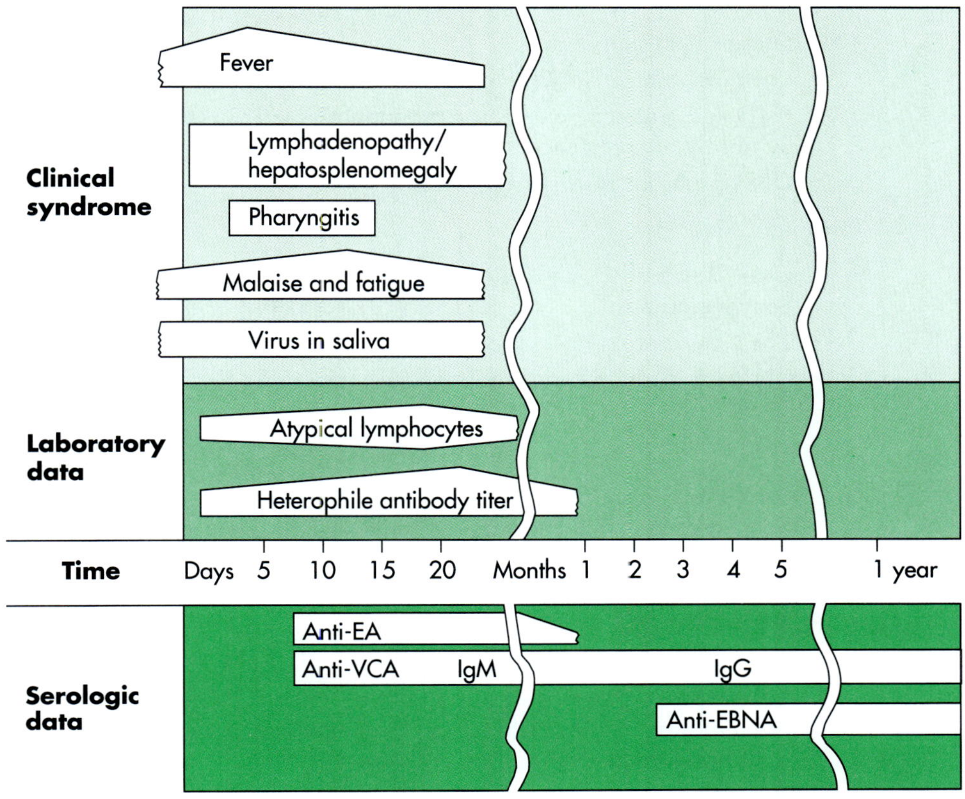

Fig. 3.20 Clinical course and laboratory findings of infectious mononucleosis. EBV infection may be asymptomatic or produce the symptoms of mononucleosis. The incubation period can be as long as 2 months.

- EBV and malaria are associated with this neoplasm.
- All tumor cells contain EBV.

4. Nasopharyngeal carcinoma
   - It is common in China.
   - EBV is associated with this neoplasm.

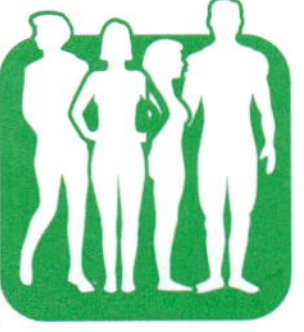

- **Epidemiology**

  Mode of spread: EBV is spread in saliva and potentially by blood transfusions. Asymptomatic infection with virus production is common.

  Populations affected: The virus is ubiquitous and most members of the population are seropositive. Children generally have milder symptoms. Teens and adults have more classic symptoms of mononucleosis.

  Occurrence: The virus is ubiquitous and present worldwide.

- **Prevention** No preventive measures can be taken to reduce infection.
- **Treatment** Treatment consists of supportive care.

■ **Cytomegalovirus (CMV)** CMV is the most common viral cause of congenital disease.

- **Laboratory identification**
  - CMV can be grown from secretions, saliva, semen, urine, and blood.

- Infected cells are swollen (cytomegalic) and have a large owl's eye nuclear inclusion body.
- The virus can be isolated on human lung fibroblast cells.
- Early antigens can be detected in biopsy tissue or infected cell culture by immunofluorescence.
- DNA probe analysis speeds detection.

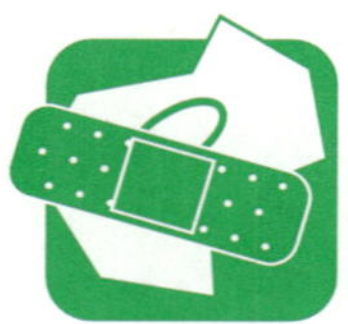

- **Pathogenesis**
  - CMV is spread through saliva, blood, organ transplants, and most body secretions.
  - The virus infects most types of cells but is not greatly cytolytic.
  - CMV establishes latency in monocytes, macrophages, and lymphocytes.
  - Immunosuppression allows reactivation of the virus.

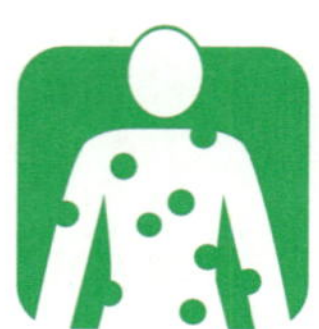

- **Diseases** Infection with CMV is usually asymptomatic.
  1. Mononucleosis syndrome (heterophile antigen negative)
     - usually follows a blood transfusion
  2. Congenital CMV
     - acquired in utero after a primary infection of the mother
     - causes severe morbidity and mortality in the neonate
     - symptoms include rash, cerebral calcification, hepatosplenomegaly, deafness, microcephaly (small head), and mental retardation
  3. Opportunistic disease
     - occurs in AIDS patients, immunosuppressed individuals, or transplant patients
     - manifested as chorioretinitis, pneumonia, esophagitis, colitis, hepatitis, or encephalitis

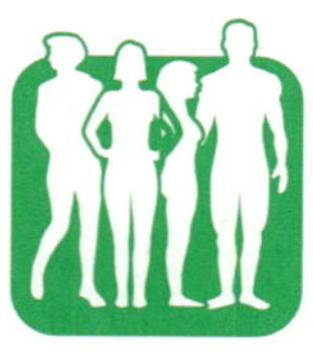

- **Epidemiology**

  Mode of spread: CMV is spread through saliva, blood transfusion, organ transplants, urine, semen, cervical secretions, and breast milk.

  Populations affected: Babies are at risk of developing CMV infection. Babies from mothers who seroconvert during term are at high risk for congenital defects. Infection also occurs in sexually active individuals, blood and organ recipients, and burn patients. Immunosuppressed individuals can have serious disease.

  Occurrence: CMV occurs worldwide.

- **Prevention** Screening of blood and organ donors can help prevent infection.
- **Treatment** Ganciclovir and foscarnet are antiviral drugs that can be used to treat CMV disease.

Human Herpesvirus 6 (HHV6)

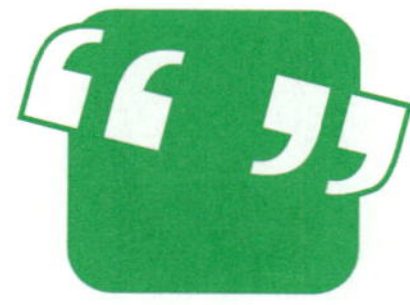

- **Roseola** is a common benign disease of children.
- The rapid onset of high fever for 3 days is followed by a whole body rash for 1 to 2 days.
- The virus is ubiquitous and almost all people are seropositive.

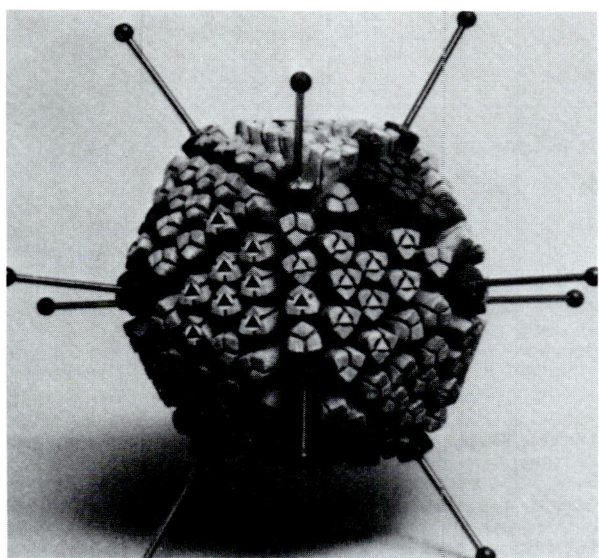

Fig. 3.21 Model of an adenovirus virion with fibers. *(From Ginsberg HS:* The adenoviruses, *New York 1984, Plenum Publishers.)*

Section 3.7 Adenoviruses

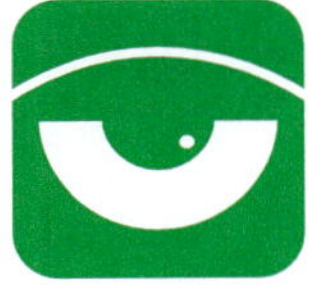

- **General Features** Adenoviruses cause relatively benign infections of the eye, the oropharynx, and the gastrointestinal tract. Adenoviruses have transforming potential in animals.

- **Structure (Fig. 3.21)**
  - Adenoviruses are mid-sized DNA viruses in a **naked** icosadeltahedral capsid.
  - **Fibers** extend from the vertices of the penton and are the viral attachment structures.
  - The genome is linear double-stranded DNA with a protein covalently attached to each 5′ end.

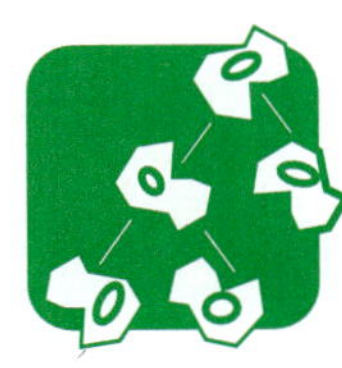

- **Replication**
  - Adenovirus binds to specific receptors on epithelial cells.
  - Both strands of the genome are transcribed into proteins.
  - Genes are encoded on both strands of the DNA and differential splicing of the RNA transcript produces several different mRNAs.
  - Early proteins include a DNA polymerase and host shut-off proteins.
  - The early proteins E1A and E1B bind to cellular growth suppressor genes and promote cell growth.
  - The late mRNA codes for structural proteins.
  - The virus is assembled in the nucleus.
  - The virus is released by cell lysis.

- **Laboratory identification**
  - Identification is made by observing for CPE in appropriate tissue culture cells.
  - Intranuclear inclusion bodies are diagnostic of adenoviruses.

Table 3.16 *Illnesses Associated With Adenoviruses*

Illness Category	Most Common Serotypes
Endemic respiratory disease	1, 2, 5
Acute respiratory disease of military recruits	3, 4, 7, 14, 21
Adenoviral pneumonias	3, 4, 7b, 14, 21
Epidemic keratoconjunctivitis	8, 19
Pharyngoconjunctival fever	3, 7
Less common syndromes	
Pertussis syndrome	1, 2, 3, 5
Acute hemorrhagic cystitis	1, 4, 7, 11, 21
Hepatic disorders	3, 7
Gastroenteritis	9, 12, 13, 18, 25, 26, 27, 28, 40, 41, 42
Intussusception	1, 2, 5
Musculoskeletal disorders	7
Genital infections	19
Skin infections	2, 4, 7, 21
Infections in immunocompromised hosts	32, 34, 35, 36

From Liu C: Adenoviruses. In Belshe RB, editor: *Textbook of human virology*, ed 2, St Louis, 1991, Mosby.

- Identification of adenovirus types is accomplished by immunoassay or DNA probe analysis.
- Immunoelectronmicroscopy can be used to concentrate and identify adenovirus types 40, 41, and 42 from stool specimens.

- **Pathogenesis**
  - The viral fiber proteins determine the target cell specificity and serotype.
  - The virus infects epithelial cells of the mucous membranes in the respiratory tract, the gastrointestinal tract, conjunctiva, and cornea.
  - Adenovirus infection is lytic in epithelial cells and causes inflammation.
  - Viremia may occur.
  - Adenovirus persists in lymphoid tissue (e.g., tonsils, adenoids, and Peyer's patches).
  - Adenoviruses can transform rodent cells and are oncogenic in rodents but are not involved in human cancer.

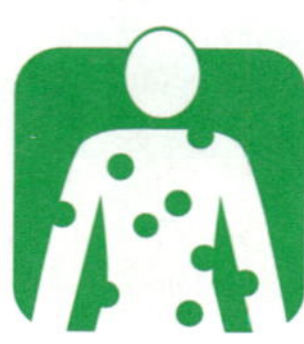

- **Diseases (Table 3.16)**
  1. Pharyngitis (with fever) occurs in young children (less than 3 years of age).
  2. Pharyngoconjunctival fever occurs in older children.
  3. Acute respiratory disease: Fever, cough, pharyngitis, and cervical adenitis are seen in outbreaks (e.g., in military recruits).
  4. Other respiratory diseases: Laryngitis, croup, bronchiolitis, and pneumonia can occur in children and adults.
  5. Conjunctivitis and epidemic keratoconjunctivitis (inflamed, "pebbled or nodular" conjunctiva [pink eye]) may occur in outbreaks from a common source (e.g., swimming pools).
  6. Gastroenteritis and diarrhea are common.

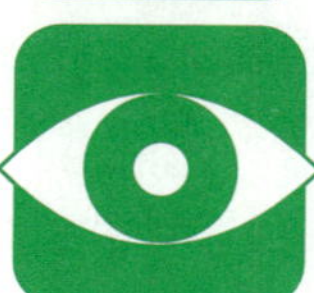

The incubation period for adenovirus infections can be 4 to 9 days. The virus may be released for long periods, even after the resolution of symptoms.

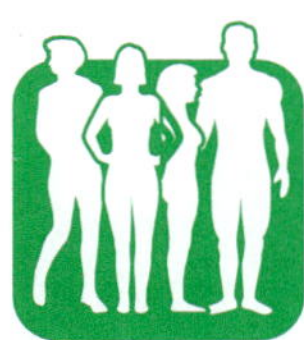

- **Epidemiology**
  Mode of spread:
  - As naked capsid viruses, adenoviruses are resistant to drying and detergents. They are very contagious.
  - The virus is spread in aerosols, from objects (e.g., towels), by close contact, and in inadequately chlorinated swimming pools.

  Populations affected: Seronegative children and individuals who live in close quarters (e.g., military camps and daycare centers) are at risk.
  Occurrence: The adenoviruses have a worldwide distribution.
- **Prevention** A live oral vaccine has been developed for military recruits against adenovirus types 4 and 7.
- **Treatment** Supportive care is used to treat adenoviral infections.

Section 3.8 Papovaviruses

General Features

- Papovaviruses are viruses with a small, **naked** (nonenveloped) icosahedral capsid.
- The genome consists of double-stranded, **circular DNA.**

Human Papillomaviruses (HPV)

- **Replication**

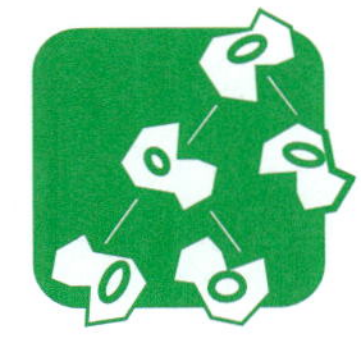

  - The plus strand of the DNA encodes the viral proteins.
  - The early proteins, E1 to E8, are involved in replication and transcription.
  - The late proteins, L1 and L2, are structural proteins.
  - The early proteins, E6 and E7 of HPV-16, are transforming proteins. These proteins inactivate cellular growth suppressor proteins: E6 inactivates the p53 suppressor protein; E7 inactivates the RB protein.
  - The viral DNA is usually in a circular form, but may integrate into the host cell chromosome.
- **Laboratory identification**

  - Warts can be identified histologically by hyperplasia of the prickle cells, by hyperkeratosis, and by the presence of vacuolated squamous epithelial cells (koilocytosis).
  - HPV can be identified histologically on peroxidase-antiperoxidose (PAP) smears.
  - Immunofluorescence and immunoperoxidase are used to identify viral antigens in tissue.
  - Southern blot hybridization with DNA probes can be used to detect viral nucleic acid in cervical tissue and swabs.
  - No method is available for culture of the virus.
- **Pathogenesis**

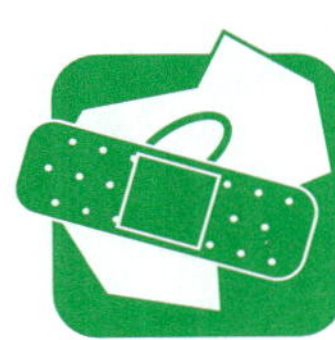

  - Papillomaviruses infect and replicate in epithelial tissues, both cutaneous and mucosal, where they induce cellular proliferation leading to the formation of benign tumors or warts.

- HPV-16 and HPV-18 are associated with cervical cancer.

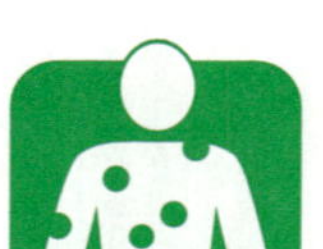

- **Diseases**
  1. Skin warts
  2. Benign head and neck tumors
  3. Laryngeal papillomas
     - HPV-11 is involved
     - tumors are benign but can be life threatening in children because of airway obstruction

  4. Anogenital warts *(condyloma acuminata)*
     - warts of the squamous epithelium of the external genitalia and the perianal region
     - caused by HPV-11 and HPV-6
     - the benign growths may become malignant

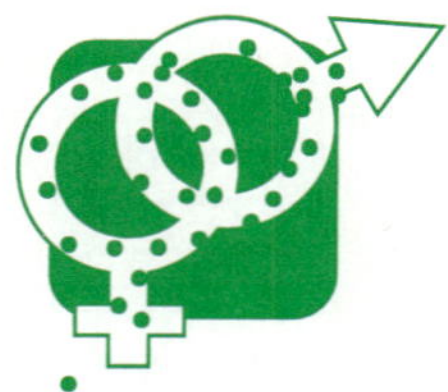

  5. Cervical dysplasia and neoplasm
     - HPV-16 and HPV-18 are involved in human cervical carcinoma
     - presence of koilocytotic cells (cells with enlarged nuclei and cytoplasmic vacuoles) in Papanicolaou-stained cervical smears
     - dysplasia may regress spontaneously in 40% to 70% of the cases
     - dysplasia may progress to cancer

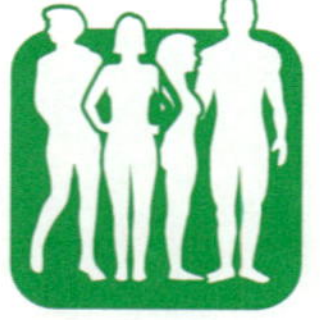

- **Epidemiology**

  Mode of spread: Transmission of the virus occurs by direct contact with warts, venereally, or during birth.

  Populations affected: Plantar, common, and flat warts are prevalent in children and young adults. Genital warts occur in sexually active individuals; 20% of women may be infected. Laryngeal papillomas occur in children and middle-aged adults.

  Occurrence: Human papillomaviruses occur throughout the world.

- **Prevention** Avoiding close contact with infected individuals can prevent infection with HPV.

- **Treatment** Warts can be removed by cryotherapy, electrocautery, or with chemicals (salicylic acid or podophyllin); recurrences, however, are common. Surgery has been used for laryngeal papillomas. Interferons may be used for treatment.

Polyomaviruses (Human Viruses: BK and JC Viruses; Prototype Tumor Virus: SV40)

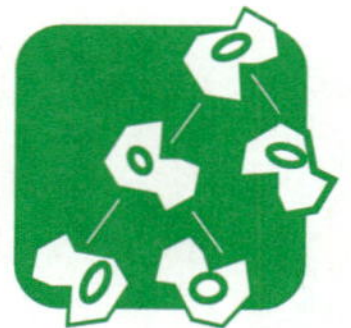

- **Replication** The polyomavirus genome codes for early proteins (transformation or T proteins) and late proteins (capsid proteins VP1, VP2, and VP3) (Fig. 3.22).

- **Laboratory identification**
  - In progressive multifocal leukoencephalopathy, which is caused by a polyoma virus, brain tissue histology shows abnormal oligodendrocytes near areas of demyelination.
  - Nucleic acid hybridization can be used to identify polyomaviruses.

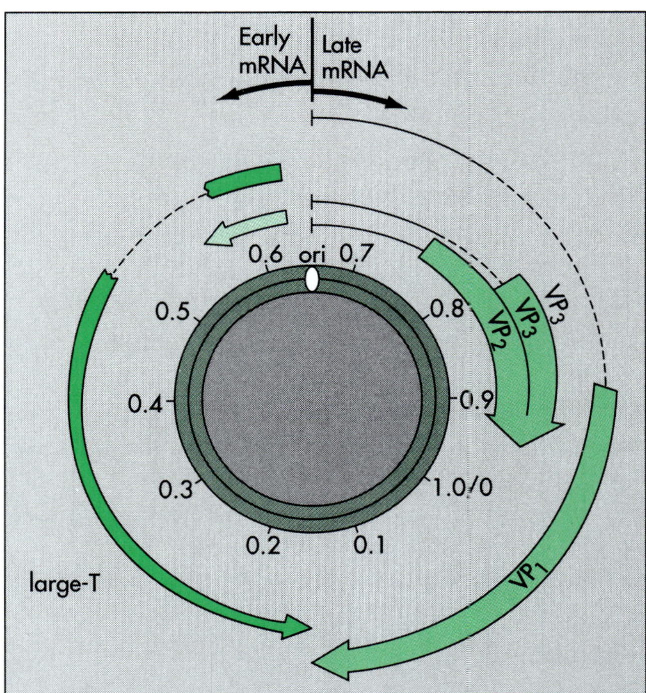

Fig. 3.22 Genome of SV-40 virus. The SV-40 genome is a prototype of other polyoma viruses and contains early, late, and noncoding regions. The noncoding region contains the start sequences for both the early and the late genes and for DNA replication *(ori)*. The individual early mRNAs and late mRNAs are processed from larger nested transcripts. *(Redrawn from Butel JS, Jarvis DL:* Biochem Biophys Acta *865:171, 1986.)*

Pathogenesis

- The polyomavirus displays host and target-tissue specificity.
- It establishes a latent infection.
- Reactivation of the virus may occur from suppressed T cell function.
- Polyomaviruses can cause tumors in hamsters, but there is no evidence that they are oncogenic in humans.

Diseases

1. Primary infection is generally asymptomatic and becomes latent.
2. In immunodeficient individuals, the JC virus causes progressive multifocal leukoencephalopathy (PML), a disease characterized by impairment of speech, sight, coordination, and mental abilities, paralysis, and death.

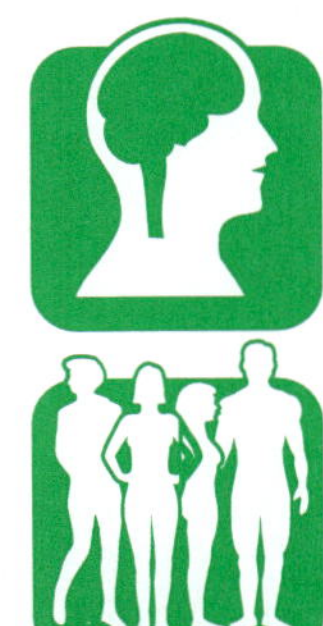

Epidemiology

Mode of spread: The viruses are spread by the respiratory route.

Populations affected: Most humans are infected by 15 years of age. Reactivation of latent infection occurs in immunocompromised individuals (AIDS patients, transplant patients) and during pregnancy.

Occurrence: Polyomaviruses occur ubiquitously.

Prevention No preventive measures can be taken to avoid polyomavirus infection.

Treatment No treatment is available.

Section 3.9 Parvoviruses

Parvovirus B19 is the only known human pathogen among the parvoviruses.

General Features

- Parvoviruses are very **small** (18 to 26 nm in diameter) viruses.
- The virion is icosohedral and nonenveloped.
- The genome consists of linear, **single-stranded** DNA and codes for three structural proteins and one nonstructural protein.

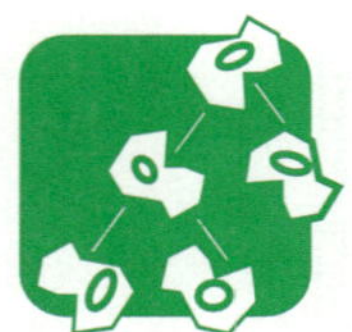

Replication

- Parvoviruses replicate only in mitotically active cells, (e.g., erythroid precursor cells).
- They replicate in the nucleus.
- Replication of viral DNA requires host factors that are present only in the S phase of the cell cycle.
- Members of the genus *Dependovirus* require a **helper virus** for their replication.

Laboratory Identification Parvovirus infection can be identified by detecting IgM antibodies.

Pathogenesis

- Parvoviruses replicate in the upper respiratory tract, followed by a viremic phase and subsequent infection of erythroid precursor cells in the bone marrow.
- Parvovirus infection in a host with chronic hemolytic anemia may lead to life-threatening reticulocytopenia (aplastic crisis).
- Infection of erythroid precursor cells shortens their life span and contributes to anemia.
- The characteristic symptom is an immune-mediated rash.

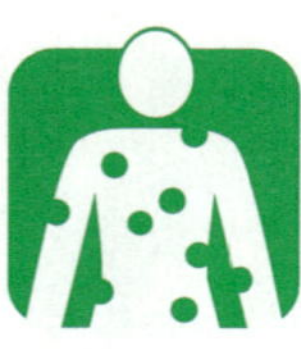

Diseases Caused by Parvovirus B19 (Fig. 3.23)

1. Erythema infectiosum ("fifth disease")
   - causes mild symptoms in normal children
   - initial phase consists of sore throat, myalgia, and a minor drop in hemoglobin levels from lytic virus infection
   - immune-mediated phase (**erythema infectiosum**) occurs 2 to 3 weeks later and is characterized by a rash and arthralgia
   - **rash** (slapped face appearance) appears on the face, spreads to the arms and legs, and lasts 1 to 2 weeks
   - relapses occur

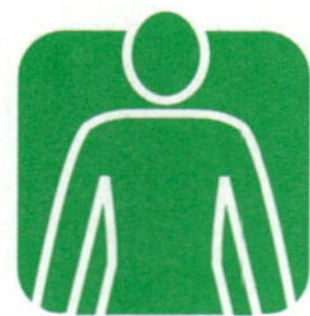

2. Arthritis
   - seen in adults
   - rash may not occur
   - arthritis present in knees, hands, wrists, and ankles

3. Aplastic crisis in chronic hemolytic anemia
   - transient reticulocytopenia (7 to 10 days)
   - decreased hemoglobin levels
   - symptoms include fever, malaise, itching, chills, possibly arthralgia, maculopapular rash, and joint swelling

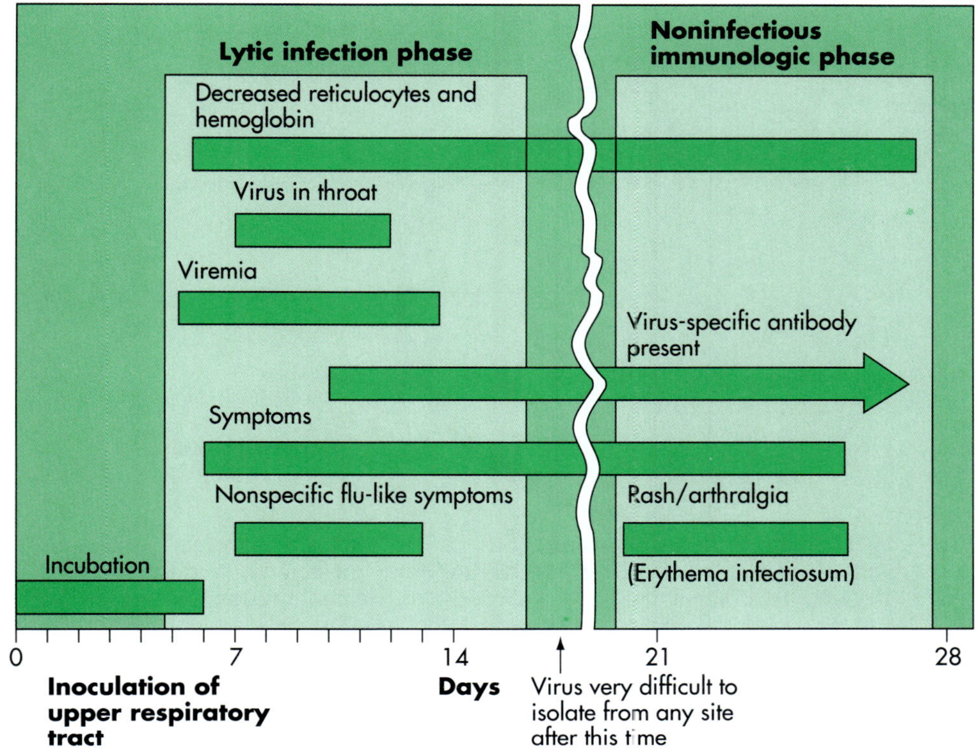

Fig. 3.23 Time course of parvovirus B19 infection. Parvovirus B19 causes a biphasic disease, an initial lytic infection phase, characterized by febrile, influenza-like symptoms, followed by a noninfectious immunologic phase characterized by a rash and arthralgia.

4. Fetal infection
   - results in stillbirth but not in congenital abnormalities

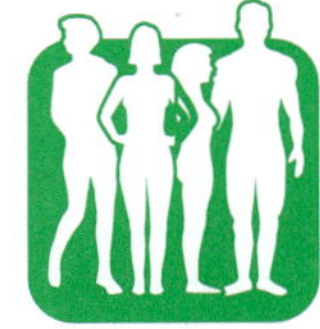

Epidemiology

Mode of spread: Parvoviruses are spread in respiratory droplets. They can cross the placenta, leading to intrauterine infections. Parenteral transmission can occur through administration of blood clotting factor.

Populations affected: Sixty-five percent of adults have antibodies to parvoviruses. Erythema infectiosum is most common in children 4 to 15 years of age.

Occurrence: Infections are most common in winter and spring.

Prevention Control of respiratory spread can help prevent infection.

Treatment No treatment is available for infections caused by parvoviruses.

Section 3.10 Poxviruses

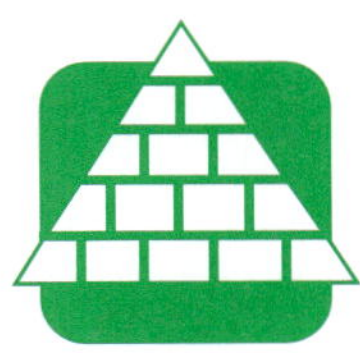

General Features (Fig. 3.24)

- Poxviruses are the largest and most complex of all the viruses (Table 3.17).
- The genome consists of linear, double-stranded DNA that is fused at the ends.
- The envelope surrounds the core, which contains DNA and protein and is surrounded by a core membrane and flanked by two lateral bodies.

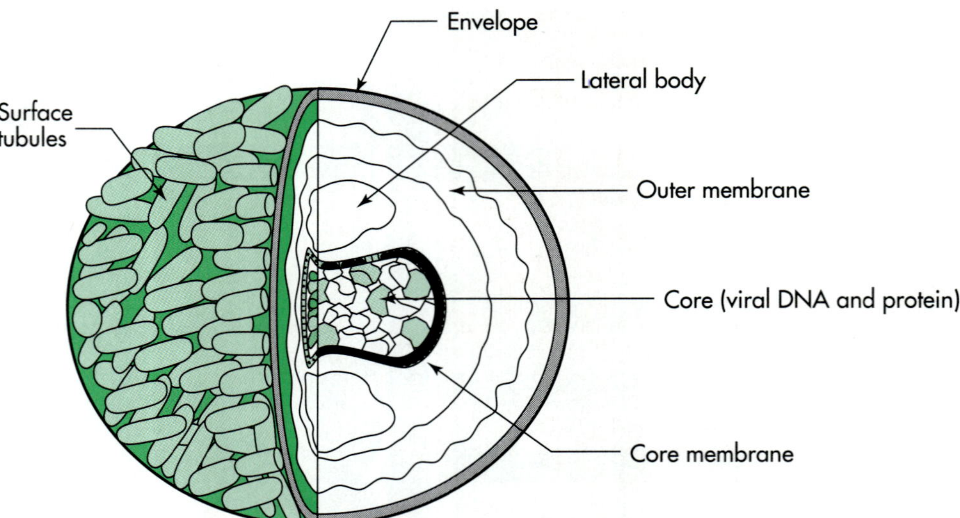

Fig. 3.24 Structure of the vaccinia virus. The viral DNA and several proteins within the core are organized as a "nucleosome." Within the virion, the core assumes the shape of a dumbbell because of the large lateral bodies. Virions released through the cytoplasmic membrane are enclosed within an envelope that contains host cell lipids and several virus-specific polypeptides, including the hemagglutinin; they are infectious. Most virions remain cell associated and are released by cellular disruption. These particles lack an envelope, so the outer membrane constitutes their surface; in similarity with the enveloped particles, they also are infectious.

Table 3.17 ***Diseases Associated with Poxviruses***

Virus	Disease	Source	Location
Variola	Smallpox (now extinct)	Humans	**EXTINCT**
Vaccinia	Used for smallpox vaccination	Laboratory product	—
Orf	Localized lesion	Zoonosis—sheep, goats	Worldwide
Cowpox	Localized lesion	Zoonosis—rodents, cats, cows	Europe
Molluscum contagiosum	Many skin lesions	Humans	Worldwide

Modified from Balows A, Hausler WJ Jr, and Lennette EH, editors: *Laboratory diagnosis of infectious diseases: principles and practice,* vol 2, New York, 1988, Springer-Verlag.

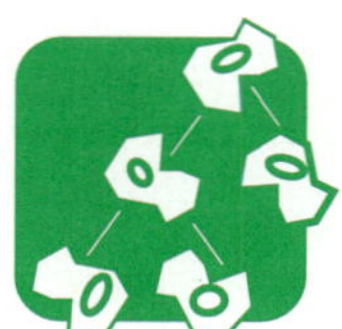

Replication

- The virus adsorbs to the cell membrane and penetration occurs within phagocytic vacuoles, where the outer membrane is uncoated by a viral enzyme (uncoatase).
- Early gene transcription takes place in the viral core. An uncoating protein is produced, which removes the core membrane, freeing the DNA into the cytoplasm.
- Viral DNA replication occurs in "viral factories" in the cytoplasm.
- Late mRNA and proteins are produced and processed before virions are assembled.
- The viral envelope is synthesized de novo in the cytoplasm and the virus is released primarily by cell lysis.
- Unlike other DNA viruses, poxviruses replicate in the cytoplasm and

Box 3.11

PROPERTIES OF SMALLPOX THAT LED TO ITS ERADICATION

Virus Characteristics

Exclusive human host range (no animal reservoirs or vectors)
Single serotype (immunization protects against all infections)
Animal and human poxviruses share antigenic determinants ("safe" live vaccines can be prepared from animal poxviruses)

Disease Characteristics

Smallpox disease *always* presents with visible pustular disease (identification of sources of contagion allows quarantine and vaccination of contacts)

Vaccine

Stable, inexpensive, easy to administer
Presence of a scar indicates successful vaccination

Public Health Service Efforts

Successful WHO worldwide program combining vaccination and quarantine

therefore must encode and carry both DNA and RNA polymerases in the virion.

■ **Variola Virus** Variola virus is the agent of smallpox, a disease that has been eradicated after a worldwide vaccination program and strict public health (quarantine) measures (Box 3.11).

● **Pathogenesis**

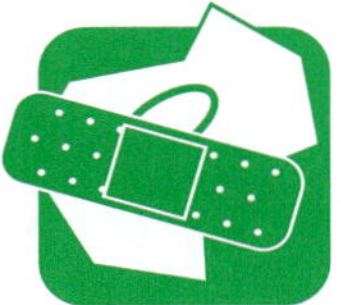

- Variola virus entered through the respiratory tract.
- Infected macrophages carried the virus to lymph nodes (primary viremia).
- Dissemination occurred via a *secondary viremia* and through the lymphatics, leading to infection of the skin and viscera.
- Only one serotype of variola existed.
- Lifetime immunity followed recovery.

● **Disease** Variola virus caused smallpox (both variola major and variola minor).

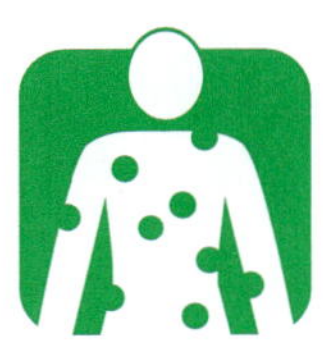

- Symptoms consisted of fever, headache, and backache associated with viremia.
- Vesicularpustular skin rash (pox) began on the face and spread to the shoulders, the chest, and other regions.
- Visceral organs, especially the spleen, liver, and lungs, were also infected.
- The incubation period ranged from 5 to 17 days (average 12 days), viremia continuing until day 28, with virus present in skin pocks up to day 42.

● **Epidemiology**

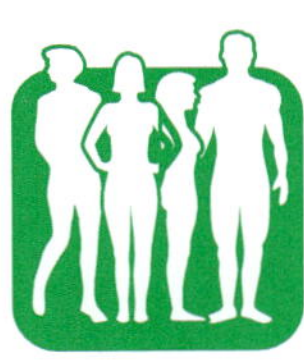

- The virus was spread mainly by the respiratory route, less often by contact with virus on clothing or objects.
- There were no asymptomatic carriers of the virus.

- Smallpox was declared **eradicated** by the World Health Organization in 1980, because of a worldwide vaccination program and the absence of animal reservoirs.

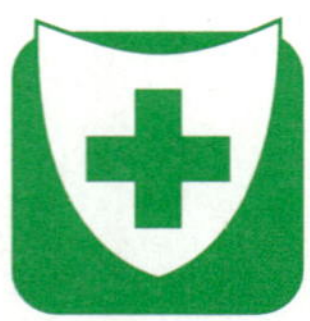

- **Prevention**
  - Quarantine of infected individuals curtailed the spread of disease.
  - Vaccination led to the eradication of smallpox.
  - The **vaccine** is no longer given because of the risk of side effects and because the disease has been eradicated.

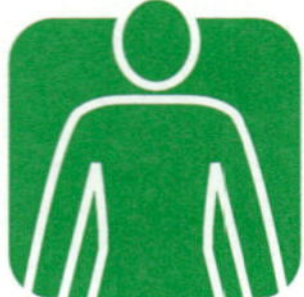

- **Virus of molluscum contagiosum**
  - Molluscum contagiosum is a common benign disease consisting of nodular or wartlike lesions on the trunk, genitals, and proximal extremities.
  - The virus has not been grown in culture but can be identified histologically by the presence of molluscum bodies (large eosinophilic inclusions in the cytoplasm of epithelial cells).
- **Vaccinia virus**
  - Vaccinia virus is used for vaccination against smallpox.
  - Serious side effects of vaccination included encephalitis and a progressive infection (vaccinia necrosum) in immunocompromised patients.
  - Vaccinia virus is used as a vector for recombinant vaccines.

- **Orf and cowpox viruses**
  - Orf and cowpox are diseases of sheep and cows, respectively, which can accidently infect humans upon direct contact.
  - Nodular lesions occur on the face and hands.
  - The viruses can be identified by growth in cell culture or by electron microscopy.

Section 3.11 Picornaviruses

The picornaviruses are an important group of viruses with over 100 viruses relevant to humans (Box 3.12).

General Features

- The enteroviruses are stable at a pH of 3.0 to 9.0. Optimal growth occurs at 35° C to 37° C.
- The rhinoviruses are acid labile. Optimal growth of rhinoviruses occurs at 33° C.

Box 3.12

PICORNAVIRIDAE
Enterovirus
Poliovirus types 1, 2, and 3
Coxsackie A virus types 1-22, 24
Coxsackie B virus types 1-6
Echovirus (ECHO virus) types 1-9, 11-27, 29-34
Enterovirus 68-72 (72 is hepatitis A virus)
Rhinovirus Types 1-100+
Cardiovirus
Aphthovirus

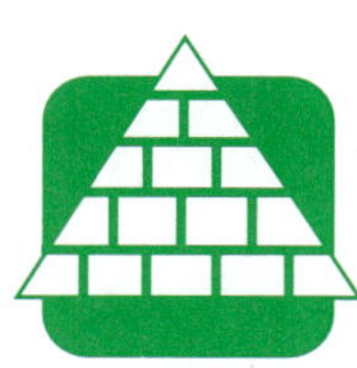

Structure

- Picornaviruses have a **small, naked** icosahedral capsid, 25 to 30 nm in diameter.
- The structural proteins consist of VP 1-4.
- The genome is linear single-stranded **(+) RNA** that encodes eight proteins. The VPg protein is attached to the 5′ end.
- As a (+) RNA virus, picornaviruses encode but do not carry a polymerase.
- The enteroviruses are extremely resistant to acids, detergents, and harsh treatments, thus being able to survive in the GI tract and sewage systems.

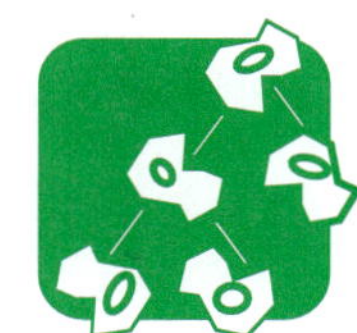

Replication (Fig. 3.25)

- The virus binds to a tissue-specific cellular receptor, via a canyon in VP1.
- The virus enters the cell by endocytosis.
- The virus replicates in the cytoplasm.
- **Polyprotein** is produced, which is cleaved to produce individual proteins.
- Virally encoded RNA-dependent RNA polymerase generates a (−) RNA template and then a (+) genomic RNA.
- The virion is assembled as follows:
  - VPO, VP1, and VP3 associate into protomers.
  - Three protomer units associate into a capsomere.
  - Twelve capsomeres assemble into a procapsid.
  - The RNA is inserted, VPO is cleaved into VP2 and VP4 to produce capsid.
- The virion is released by cell lysis.

Enteroviruses The enteroviruses important as agents of human disease are poliovirus, coxsackievirus A, coxsackievirus B, echovirus, and enterovirus.

Laboratory identification

- Many of the viruses are readily isolated from feces and will grow in appropriate cell culture systems.
- Serologic tests are used to detect a virus-specific IgM antibody or a fourfold increase in specific IgG antibody.

Pathogenesis

- The tissue tropism of the virus determines the symptoms of disease (Fig. 3.26). Poliovirus binds receptors in muscle and neurons and causes disease in the CNS.
- Coxsackieviruses and echoviruses have a broader tissue tropism, causing disease in the CNS, lungs, heart, pancreas, and other tissues.
- The virus enters through the oropharynx, the upper respiratory tract, or the intestinal tract.
- The virus replicates in the mucosa and lymphoid tissues of the pharynx and tonsils, and subsequently in the intestinal tract.
- The virus is resistant to stomach acid, digestive enzymes, and bile.
- The virus spreads to target tissue by viremia.

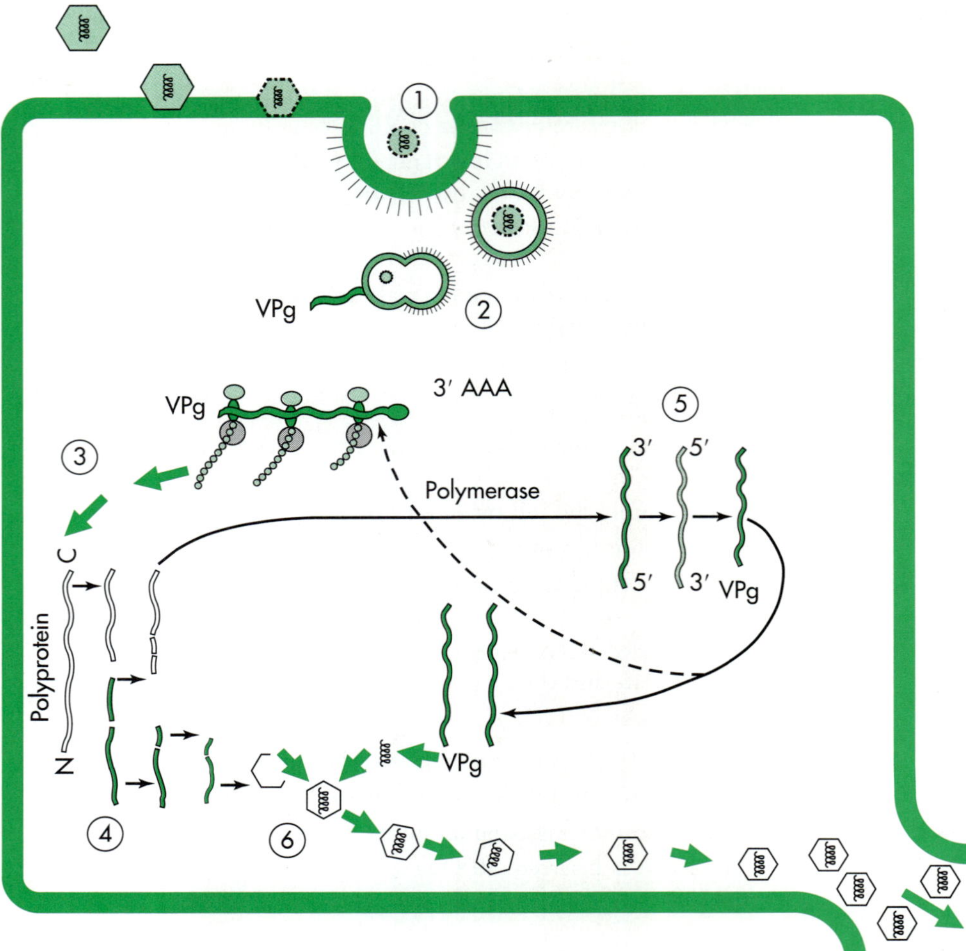

Fig. 3.25 Replication of picornavirus, a simple (+) RNA virus. (1) Interaction of the picornaviruses with receptors on the cell surface defines the target cell and weakens the capsid. (2) The virion is endocytosed, and the genome is released and used as an mRNA for protein synthesis. (3) One large polyprotein is translated from the virion genome. (4) This polyprotein is proteolytically cleaved into individual proteins, including an RNA-dependent RNA polymerase. (5) The polymerase makes a (–) strand template from the genome and replicates the genome. A protein (VPg) is covalently attached to the 5′ end of the viral genome. (6) The structural proteins associate into the capsid structure, the genome is inserted, and the virions are released upon cell lysis.

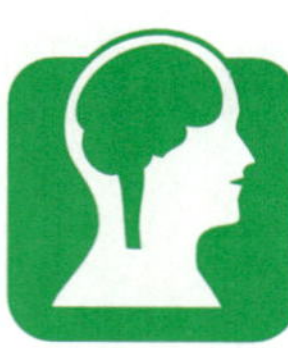

- Most enteroviruses are cytolytic, causing direct tissue damage.
- **Antibody** is protective.

● **Diseases** The enteroviruses cause a wide range of diseases (Table 3.18).

1. Poliomyelitis
   - caused by poliovirus
   - three types: asymptomatic, abortive poliomyelitis (minor illness); nonparalytic poliomyelitis (aseptic meningitis); or paralytic poliomyelitis (major illness), typified by flaccid paralysis
2. Herpangina and hand-foot-and-mouth disease

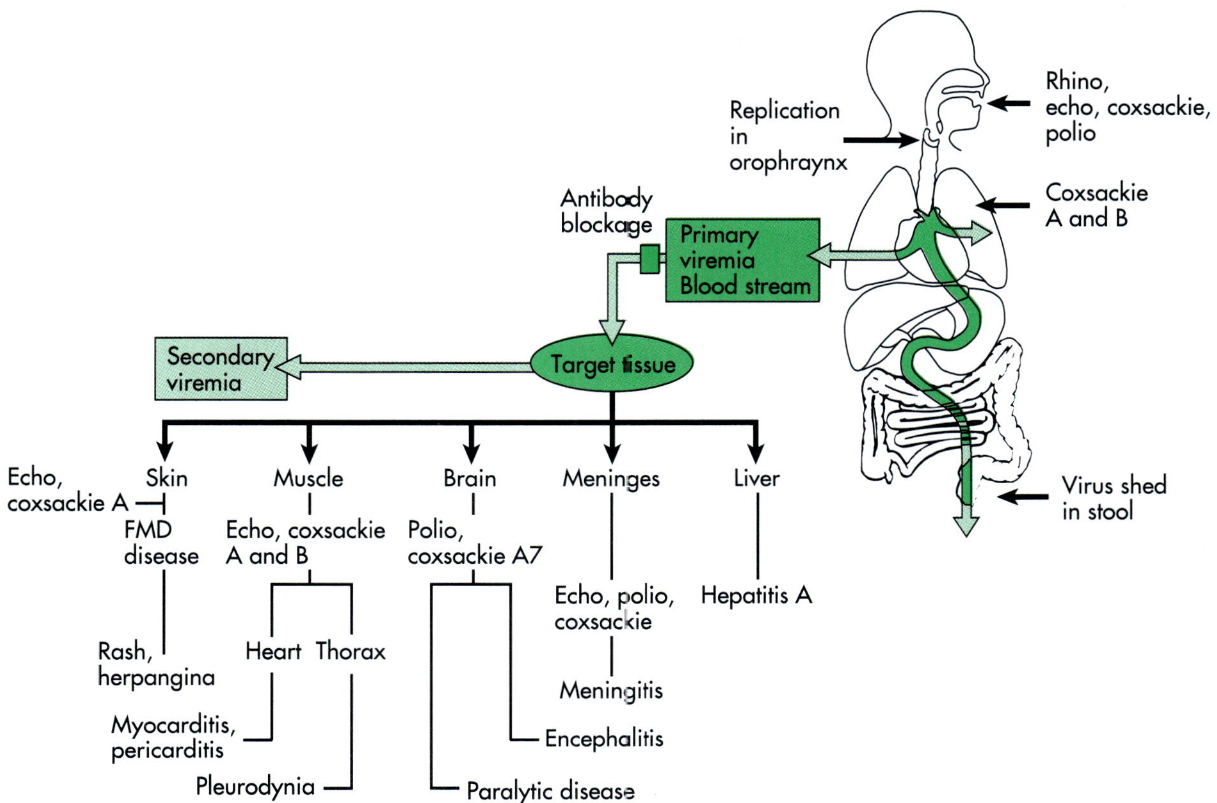

Fig. 3.26 Pathogenesis of picornaviruses. All of the enteroviruses are spread by the fecal-oral route but can cause different diseases depending on the target tissue. In addition to the rhinoviruses, some of the enteroviruses can also be spread by respiratory means and cause the symptoms of common cold. *FMD,* hand-foot-and-mouth disease.

Table 3.18 ***Summary of Clinical Syndromes Associated With Major Enterovirus Groups***

Syndrome	Occurrence	Polioviruses	Coxsackie A Viruses	Coxsackie B Viruses	Echoviruses
Paralytic disease	Sporadic	+	+	+	+
Encephalitis, meningitis	Outbreaks	+	+	+	+
Carditis	Sporadic		+	+	+
Neonatal disease	Outbreaks			+	+
Pleurodynia	Outbreaks			+	
Herpangina	Common		+		
Hand-foot-and-mouth disease	Common		+		
Rash	Common		+	+	+
Acute hemorrhagic conjunctivitis	Epidemics		+		
Respiratory infections	Common	+	+	+	+
Undifferentiated fever	Common	+	+	+	+
Diarrhea, gastrointestinal disease	Uncommon				+
Diabetes, pancreatitis	Uncommon			+	
Orchitis	Uncommon			+	
Disease in immunodeficient patients	—	+	+		+
Congenital anomalies	Uncommon		+	+	

- caused by coxsackievirus A; hand-foot-and-mouth disease is associated with coxsackievirus A16
- diseases consist of vesicular lesions with mild fever

3. Pleurodynia or Bornholm disease
   - caused by coxsackievirus B
   - symptoms consist of severe chest pain with fever; acute benign pericarditis (chest pain) is usually seen in young adults

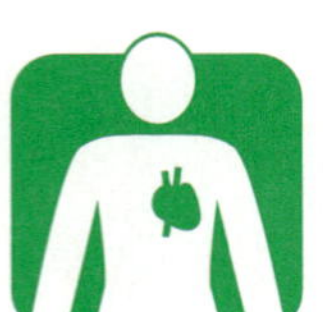

4. Myocardial
   - and pericardial infections caused by coxsackievirus B
   - can be life threatening in newborns
5. Aseptic meningitis with possible skin rash
   - caused by coxsackieviruses and echoviruses
6. Fevers and rashes can result from echovirus infection
7. Severe disseminated disease of newborns
   - caused by echoviruses
8. Acute hemorrhagic conjunctivitis
   - caused by enterovirus 70 and coxsackievirus A24 variant
   - very contagious, lasts 1 to 2 weeks

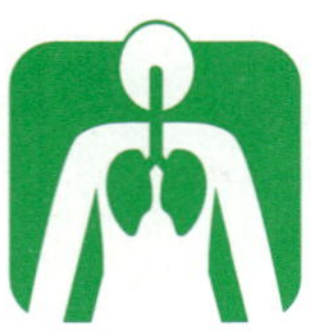

9. Respiratory infections
   - caused by coxsackieviruses and enteroviruses
10. Hepatitis A
    - caused by enterovirus 72

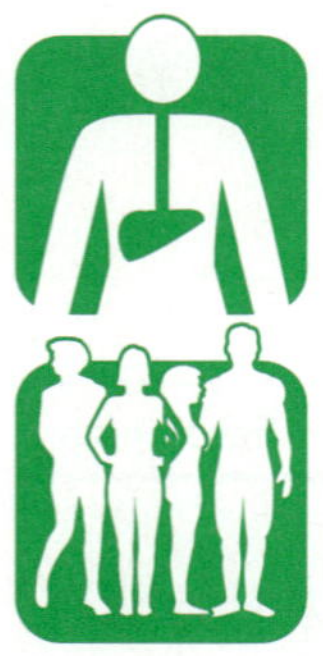

11. Diabetes
    - can be caused by coxsackievirus B
    - results from destruction of the islets of Langerhans

Epidemiology

Mode of spread: Enteroviruses are spread by the fecal-oral route and by aerosols. Transmission is increased by poor sanitation and crowding.

Populations affected: Poliovirus infection is often a mild or asymptomatic infection in early childhood. Paralytic polio is more common where good sanitation prevents exposure until late childhood or adulthood. Coxsackie B virus infection is serious in infants.

Occurrence: Natural polio has been eliminated from the Western Hemisphere by vaccination.

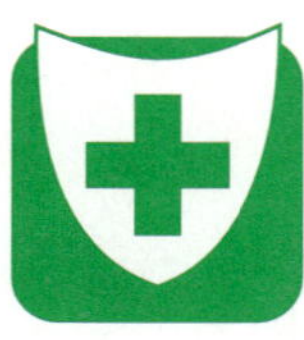

Prevention

- Polio can be prevented by vaccination. There are two types of vaccine. The formalin-inactivated polio vaccine (IPV; Salk vaccine) and the oral polio vaccine (OPV; Sabin vaccine). Immunocompromised individuals are at risk with live vaccine.
- A combined regimen of killed, then live vaccines is currently recommended.
- A killed vaccine was approved for hepatitis A virus in 1995.
- No vaccines are available for the other enteroviruses.
- Good hygiene may reduce transmission of enteroviruses.

- **Treatment** No antiviral therapy is available.

Rhinoviruses

Rhinoviruses Eighty-nine serotypes of the rhinoviruses have been identified.

- **Laboratory identification**
  - Laboratory identification is generally not done for the rhinoviruses.
  - The virus may be isolated from nasal washings and grown in primate cells at 33° C.
  - Rhinoviruses can be distinguished by acid lability and CPE.

- **Pathogenesis**
  - Eighty percent of the rhinoviruses bind the ICAM-1 cellular receptor (present on epithelial cells, fibroblasts, and B-lymphoblastoid cells).
  - Replication occurs in the nasal mucosa, causing edema of subepithelial tissue.
  - Secretory IgA and interferons may help limit infection.

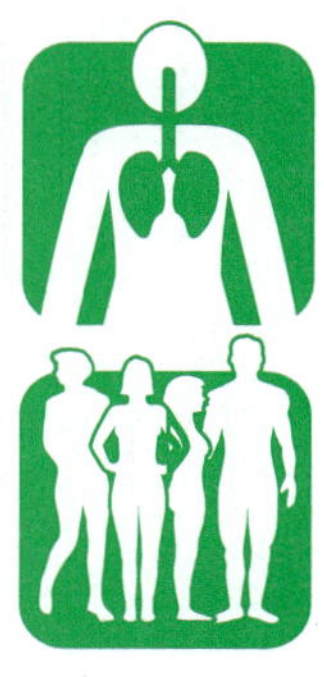

- **Diseases** Rhinoviruses cause upper respiratory tract infections that are characterized by sneezing, rhinorrhea (runny nose), headache, malaise, and rigors. The infection peaks in 3 to 4 days, but cough and nasal symptoms may last for 7 to 10 days.
- **Epidemiology**

  Mode of spread: Transmission is by respiratory droplets and by direct contact, especially via the hands.

  Populations affected: Active illness is seen in 50% of those infected, but those with asymptomatic disease can spread the infection. The highest infection rates occur in infants and children.

  Occurrence: In temperate climates, rhinovirus colds are most common in early fall and late spring.
- **Prevention** Hand washing and disinfecting objects may decrease spread of the viruses.
- **Treatment** Treatment of rhinoviral infection is symptomatic.

SECTION 3.12 ORTHOMYXOVIRUSES

General Features

- Influenza viruses A and B are the agents of influenza and have caused epidemics and pandemics throughout history.
- Many new strains of influenza virus A originate in the Orient where close proximity of humans, pigs, and birds (e.g., ducks) promotes mixed infections and the production of hybrid viruses by **reassortment** of genome segments.

Structure (Fig. 3.27)

- The influenza virus has a medium-sized virion that is enveloped and has a helical nucleocapsid.
- The genome contains segmented single-stranded (−) RNA.
- Eight RNA segments encode 10 proteins (Table 3.19).
- The glycoproteins are the major antigens of influenza virus:
  - **Hemagglutinin** (HA; viral attachment protein) binds sialic acid-containing cellular receptors. It undergoes antigenic drift and antigenic shift. HA also binds erythrocytes.

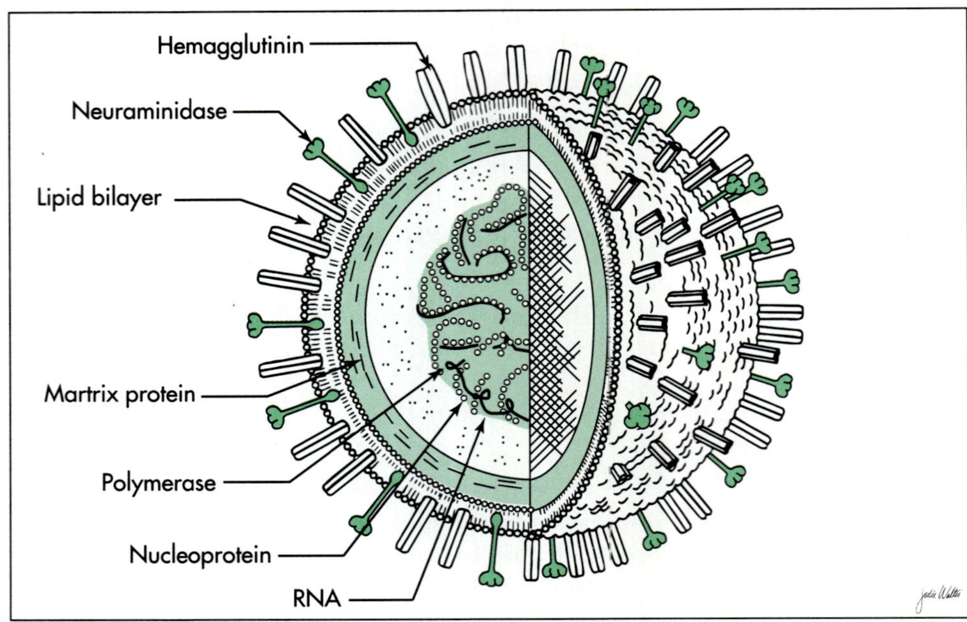

Fig. 3.27 General schematic of the influenza virus. The segmented, (–) RNA genome is associated with the nucleoprotein (elements of the RNA-dependent RNA polymerase) forming the nucleocapsid. This associates with the matrix proteins that line the inside of the membrane envelope. The envelope contains the hemagglutinin (HA) and neuraminidase (NA) glycoproteins.

Table 3.19 ***Products of Influenza Gene Segments***

Segment*	Proteins	Function
1	PB2	Polymerase component
2	PB1	Polymerase component
3	PA	Polymerase component
4	HA	Hemagglutinin, viral attachment protein, fusion protein, *target of neutralizing antibody*
5	NP	Nucleocapsid
6	NA	Neuraminidase: cleaves sialic acid and promotes virus release
7†	M_1	Matrix protein: virion structural protein, interacts with nucleocapsid and envelope, promotes assembly
	M_2	Membrane protein, forms membrane pore, *target for amantadine,* facilitates active HA production
8†	NS_1	Nonstructural protein, important but unknown function
	NS_2	Nonstructural protein, important but unknown function

*Listed in decreasing order of size.
†Encodes two mRNA.

- **Neuraminidase** (NA; enzyme) removes sialic acid and also undergoes antigenic drift and antigenic shift.
- Virions must carry an RNA-dependent RNA polymerase.
- Reassortment of the segmented genome yields new strains.
- Matrix protein lines the virion and is involved in virion assembly.

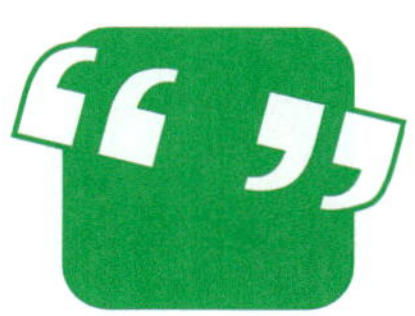

Classification Influenza viruses are classified according to the type (A, B, or C), the place of original isolation, the date of original isolation, and the antigen type of hemagglutinin (H) and neuraminidase (N). Examples of virus designation are A/Bangkok/1/79/(H3N2) and B/Singapore/3/64. (No mention of HA or NA type is necessary for influenza B.)

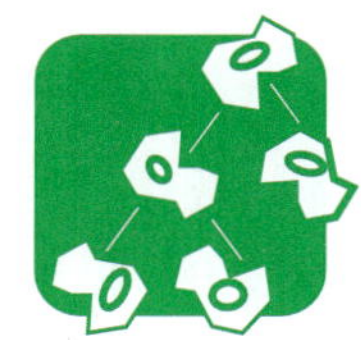

Replication

- The virus binds sialic acid-containing receptors through HA.
- The virus enters the cell by endocytosis in coated vesicles.
- Acidification of endosome promotes fusion of the virion envelope and vesicle.
- *Transcription and replication occur in the nucleus.*
- The virus is assembled near the cell membrane and is released by budding.

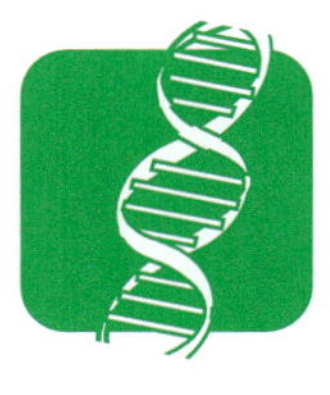

Genetics

Antigenic drift refers to a mutation in the genes for HA or NA, which alters the antigenicity.

Antigenic shift refers to the creation of new strains, usually by reassortment of genome segments.

Reassortment refers to the random mixing and packaging of segments into virions that occurs after co-infection with two strains of viruses, producing new hybrid viruses. For example, mixing of swine influenza virus (genome segments $S_{1\text{-}8}$), duck influenza virus ($D_{1\text{-}8}$), and human influenza virus ($H_{1\text{-}8}$) would create a new strain (e.g., $S_{1,2}D_{3\text{-}6}H_{7,8}$)—a new, antigenically distinct hybrid influenza virus capable of infecting humans.

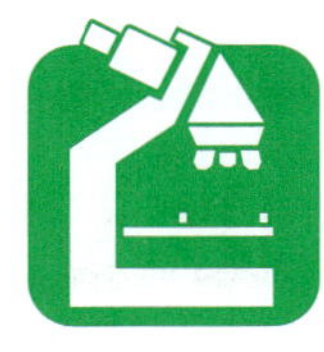

Laboratory Identification

- Influenza virus can be identified in nasal secretions.
- Immunologic techniques, such as ELISA, may be used for direct detection of virus in respiratory secretions.
- The virus can be grown in primary monkey kidney cells, but produces poor CPE.
- **Hemadsorption** (binding of erythrocytes to hemagglutinin expressed on the surface of infected cells to erythrocytes) and **hemagglutination** (virus-induced aggregation of erythrocytes) can be used to detect the virus.
- Serologic tests, such as **hemagglutination inhibition** (HI) (antibody blocking of hemagglutination) can also be used to type the strain of virus.

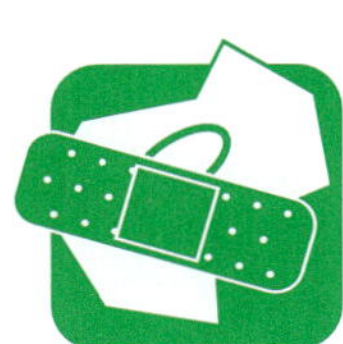

Pathogenesis

- The virus replicates in the respiratory tract, causing loss of ciliated and mucus-secreting cells.
- The virus inhibits T cell responses, leukocyte chemotaxis, and macrophage activity.
- Influenza-like symptoms are caused primarily by an interferon produced in response to infection.
- Secondary bacterial infections are common after influenza.
- Virus-induced or bacteria-induced tissue damage can cause pneumonia.
- Recovery from influenza can be attributed to interferons and to cell-mediated and antibody-mediated immunity.
- Antigenic shift and antigenic drift of the HA and NA limits antibody protection.

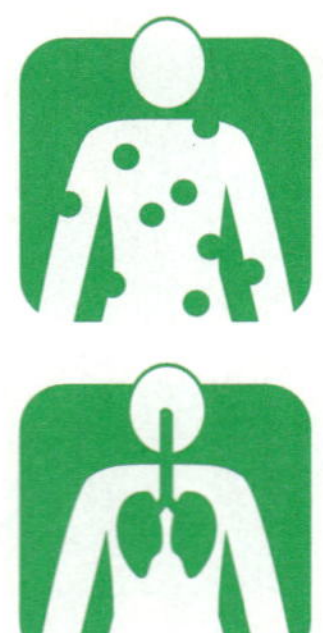

■ **Diseases** Influenza is caused primarily by influenza virus A, and less often by influenza virus B.

1. Classic influenza
   - prodrome of malaise and headache, followed by myalgia, fever, and nonproductive cough
   - incubation period is 1 to 3 days; prodromal period is 3 to 24 hours; disease lasts for up to 1 week
   - secondary bacterial infection (e.g., sore throat) may occur in the second week
   - disease may be asymptomatic to severe, depending on the presence of immunity to the virus strain
   - severe illness occurs in pregnant women and in patients with immunodeficiencies or cardiorespiratory disease
2. Croup, otitis media, bronchiolitis, and febrile convulsions (rare)
   - occur in young children
   - complications include *bacterial pneumonia,* myositis, encephalopathy, and Reye's syndrome
3. Gastrointestinal symptoms
   - predominate in influenza virus B infections

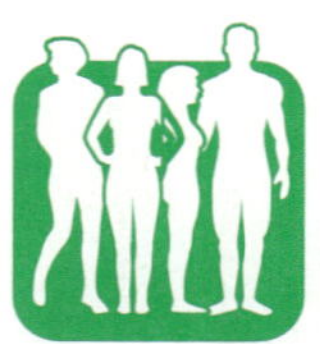

■ **Epidemiology**

Mode of spread: Infection is spread by respiratory droplets.

Populations affected: Nonimmune individuals are at risk. Antigenic drift (mutation), or minor antigenic changes, occurs every few years, resulting in local outbreaks. Antigenic shift, or major antigenic changes (reassortment), occur approximately every 10 years and are responsible for pandemics.

Occurrence: Influenza infections occur annually, especially in the winter, in temperate climates. Outbreaks last for 4 to 6 weeks.

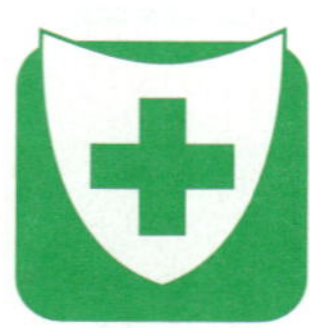

■ **Prevention**

- A formalin-killed **vaccine** consisting of the current strains is produced each year. Immunization is recommended for the elderly and those with cardiorespiratory disease.
- Reduction of contacts with infected individuals during an outbreak can help prevent disease.

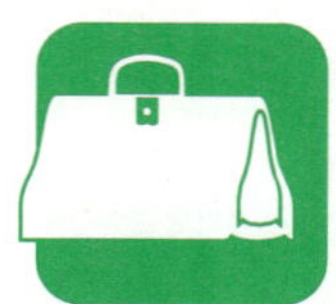

■ **Treatment**

- Acetaminophen can be taken to reduce symptoms of influenza.
- **Amantadine** and **rimantadine** block an early step in viral replication and may be used for prophylaxis in unimmunized individuals.
- Treatment must start before or within 24 to 48 hours of the appearance of symptoms.

Section 3.13 Paramyxoviruses

■ **General Features (Fig. 3.28)**

- Paramyxoviruses are large, **enveloped viruses** with a helical nucleocapsid.
- The genome is single-stranded (−) **RNA.**
- The important proteins are (a) the envelope glycoproteins: The viral attachment proteins HN, H, or G (depending on virus), and the fusion (F) protein;

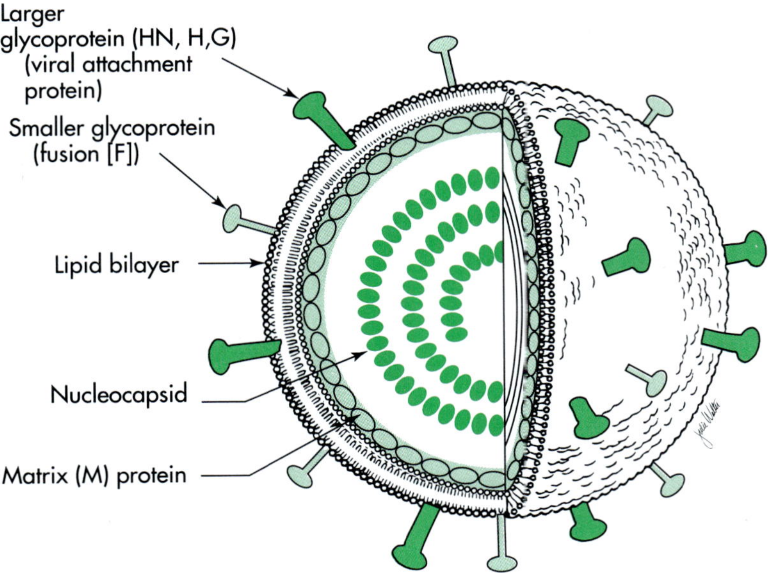

Fig. 3.28 General schematic of the paramyxovirus. The helical nucleocapsid, consisting of (−)ss RNA and the N, NP, and L proteins (polymerase elements) associate with the matrix protein (M) at the inner surface of the envelope membrane. The envelope contains the viral attachment glycoprotein HN (paramyxovirus), H (measles), or G (respiratory syncytial virus) and the fusion glycoprotein (F).

(b) the matrix protein: M protein; and (c) the nucleocapsid proteins associated with the genome: L (polymerase), NP, and P proteins.

- The virion must carry RNA-dependent RNA polymerase.

Replication (Fig. 3.29)

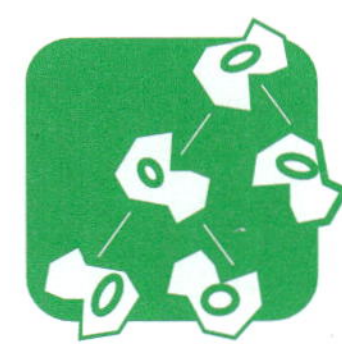

- The viral attachment proteins (HN [paramyxovirus], H [morbillivirus], or G [pneumovirus]) bind to sialic acid on glycoproteins or glycolipids.
- The F protein promotes fusion with the cell membrane and viral penetration.
- Transcription, replication, and assembly occur in the cytoplasm.
- The RNA polymerase carried in the nucleocapsid transcribes individual (+) mRNAs and a full-length (+) RNA template. Translation and replication follow.
- The newly formed genome combines with the L, N, and NP proteins to form the nucleocapsid, which then associates with the matrix protein on viral glycoprotein-modified cell membranes.
- Virions bud from the host cell membrane.

Measles Virus

Laboratory identification Measles virus infection is usually diagnosed clinically.

Pathogenesis

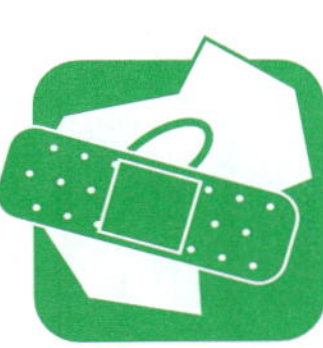

- Measles virus causes cell fusion, which results in the formation of multinucleated cells and allows the virus to evade the antibody response of the host.

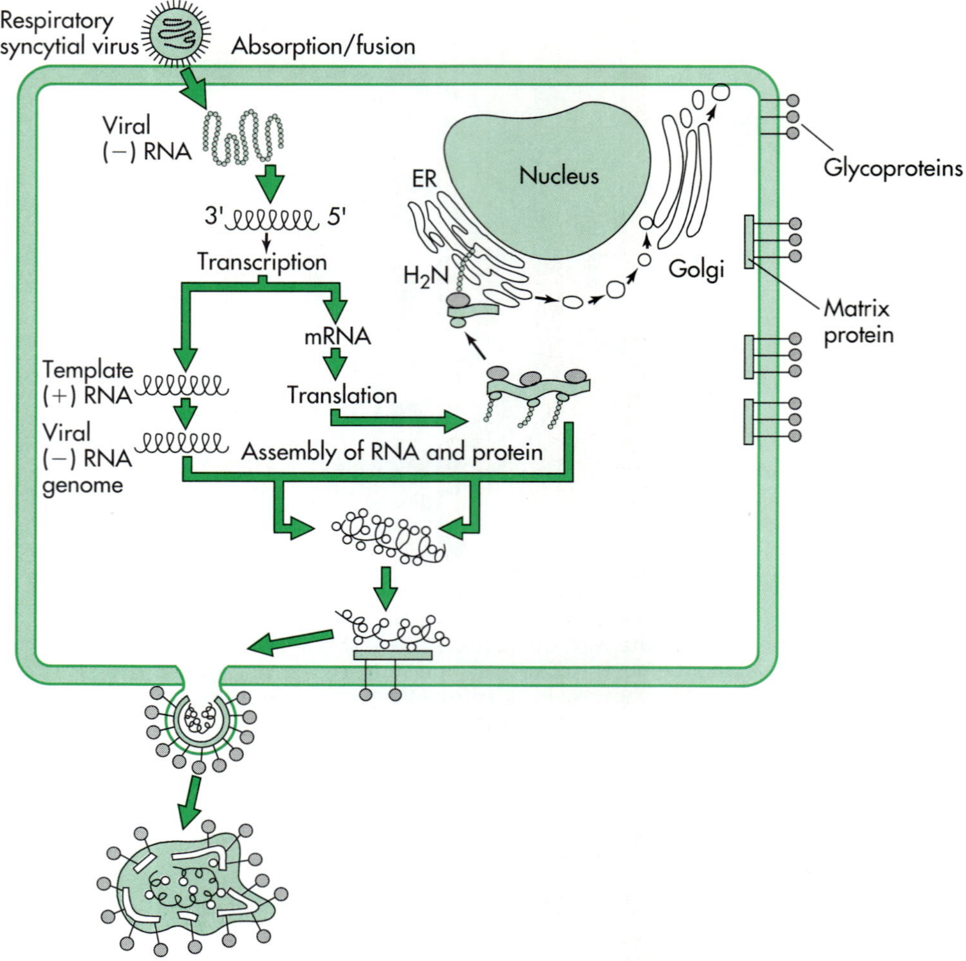

Fig. 3.29 Replication of paramyxoviruses. The virus binds to glycolipids and fuses with the cell surface. Individual mRNAs for each protein and a full-length template are transcribed from the genome. Replication occurs in the cytoplasm. The nucleocapsid associates with matrix and glycoprotein-modified plasma membranes and leaves the cell by budding. *(Redrawn from Balows A et al.:* Laboratory diagnosis of infectious diseases: principles and practice, *New York, 1988, Springer-Verlag.)*

- The infection is usually lytic but can become persistent in some cell types (e.g., brain).
- Initial replication occurs in the respiratory tract, after which there is lymphatic spread, viremia, and widespread dissemination of the virus to the conjunctiva, respiratory tract, urinary tract, small blood vessels, and CNS.
- Control of infection occurs by cell-mediated immunity.
- The measles rash is due to the T cell response.
- Immune-mediated postinfectious encephalitis may occur.
- Measles virus is a strictly human virus with only one serotype.
- Lifetime immunity is conferred after infection.

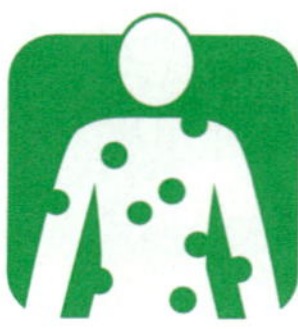

- **Diseases**
  1. Measles
     - serious febrile illness

- incubation period of 7 to 13 days is followed by prodrome marked by high fever, cough, coryza, conjunctivitis, and photophobia
- diagnostic Koplik's spots appear after 2 days and last for 1 to 2 days; spots occur on buccal membrane; lesions are small and have the appearance of a grain of salt surrounded by a red halo
- extensive maculopapular rash appears 12 to 24 hours after the Koplik's spots; starts below the ears and spreads over the body

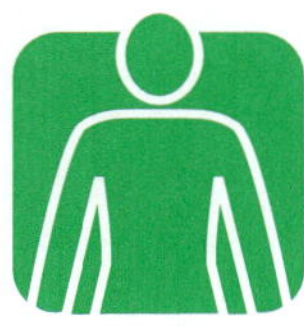

2. Complications of measles:
   a. Encephalitis
      - occurs in 0.5% of cases with a 15% mortality

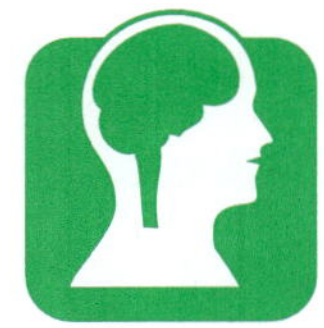

   b. Pneumonia
      - causes 60% of the deaths from measles
      - bacterial superinfection is common after measles infection

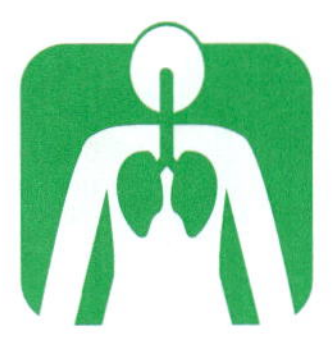

   c. Giant-cell pneumonia
      - occurs in children lacking T cell immunity
   d. Atypical measles syndrome
      - abrupt and more intense illness
      - occurs in patients with partial immunity (e.g., recipients of the original inactivated measles virus vaccine, which is no longer used)

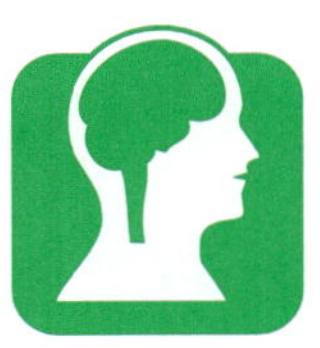

   e. Subacute sclerosing panencephalitis (SSPE)
      - slow virus infection
      - occurs months to years after measles infection
      - caused by defective measles virus in the brain
      - symptoms include changes in personality, behavior, and memory, followed by myoclonic jerks, blindness, and spasticity
      - high levels of measles antibodies are found
      - virtually eliminated due to vaccine

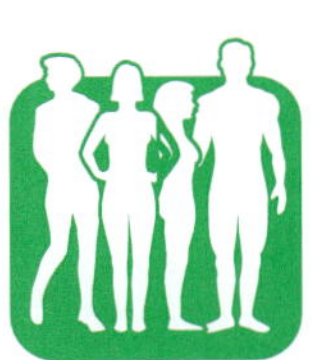

● **Epidemiology**

Mode of spread: Measles virus is spread by respiratory droplets, which are contagious before symptoms appear.

Populations affected: Unvaccinated individuals are at risk. The illness is more serious in immunocompromised individuals.

Occurrence: Measles is prevalent worldwide. Endemic fall to spring, possibly due to crowding indoors.

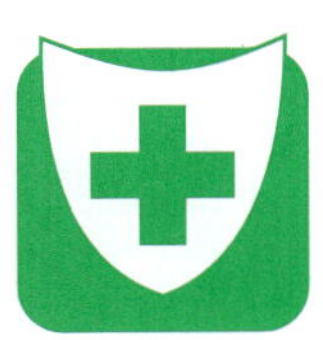

● **Prevention**

- A live, attenuated **vaccine**, is given at 15 months of age and at 11 to 12 years of age as part of the **measles-mumps-rubella (MMR)** triple vaccine.
- The success of the vaccine is because of the **single serotype** and strict human host range of the virus, the development of long-term immunity, and the presence of recognizable symptoms of disease.

● **Treatment** Immune serum globulin is effective in protecting unvaccinated immunocompromised children following exposure to measles.

■ **Mumps Virus** A **single serotype** of mumps virus exists.

- **Laboratory diagnosis**
    - The virus can be isolated from saliva (or from swabs taken from the pharynx and Stensen's duct), urine, or cerebrospinal fluid (CSF).
    - The virus replicates and causes CPE (syncytia formation) in monkey kidney cells.
    - Hemagglutination inhibition (HI), ELISA, and IF are used to detect the virus, viral antigens, and antibodies to the virus.

- **Pathogenesis**
    - Mumps virus sets up a lytic infection.
    - Local infection of the respiratory tract is followed by viremia and systemic infection of the parotid gland, testes, ovaries, thyroid, pancreas, and CNS (in 50% of the cases).
    - Cell-mediated immunity contributes to symptoms and recovery.

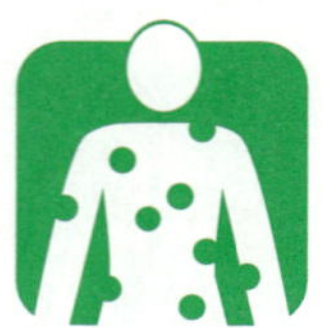

- **Diseases** Infection with mumps virus is often asymptomatic.
    1. Parotitis (swollen glands)
        - symptoms consist of fever, sudden onset of bilateral swelling of the parotid glands, redness and swelling of the ostium of Stensen's duct. Orchitis, oophoritis, and pancreatitis, and meningoencephalitis may occur after a few days
    2. Orchitis
        - may result in sterility
    3. Infection of the CNS
        - occurs in 50% of the cases; 10% of these show clinical illness, aseptic meningitis, or less often, encephalitis

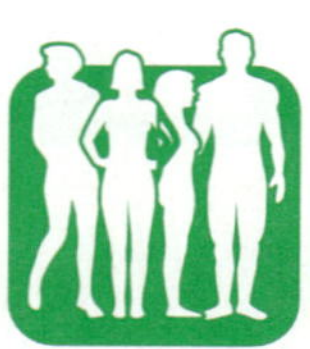

- **Epidemiology**

    Mode of spread: Mumps virus is spread by respiratory droplets and by direct contact. Mumps is a very contagious infection and the period of contagion precedes illness. Asymptomatic shedding may occur.

    Populations affected: Unvaccinated individuals are at risk. Immunocompromised individuals have a more serious outcome.

    Occurrence: The disease occurs worldwide. It is endemic in late winter and early spring.

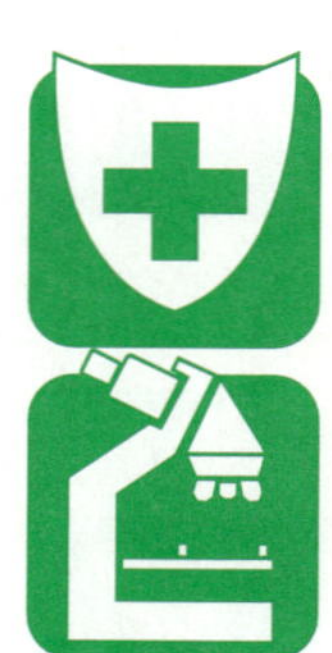

- **Prevention** A live attenuated **vaccine** is administered as part of the **MMR** vaccine.
- **Treatment** Treatment is symptomatic.

Parainfluenza Virus

Parainfluenza Virus There are four serotypes of parainfluenza virus.

- **Laboratory identification**
    - The virus can be isolated from nasal washings.
    - Immunofluorescence is used to identify the virus on tissue culture cells or in cell aspirates.
    - The virus causes the formation of syncytia in infected cells.
    - Hemagglutination
    - The viral serotype can be identified by HI.

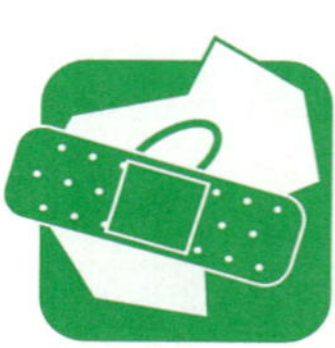

- **Pathogenesis**
    - Parainfluenza virus infects cells of the upper respiratory tract, replicates quickly, and causes giant cell formation.

- In 25% of the cases, the virus spreads to the lower respiratory tract causing serious problems.
- Cell-mediated immune responses are responsible for both cell damage and protection.
- Reinfection with other serotypes occurs, but infection is mild, suggesting that partial immunity occurs.

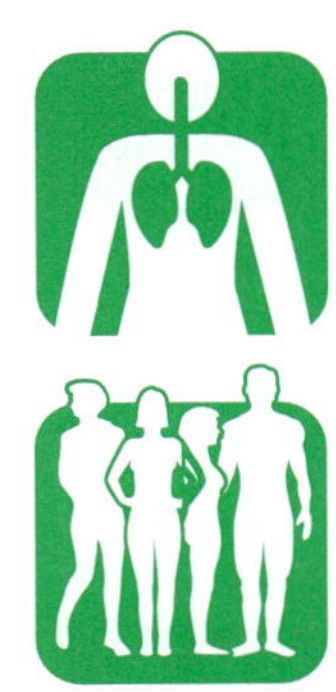

- **Diseases**
  1. Respiratory syndromes (mild colds in the upper respiratory tract)
  2. Infections of the lower respiratory tract—bronchiolitis, pneumonia, or **croup** *(laryngotracheobronchitis)*
     - characterized by a "seal bark" cough and subglottal swelling that may block the airway
- **Epidemiology**
  Mode of spread: The virus is transmitted by respiratory droplets and by direct contact.
  Populations affected: Parainfluenza viruses cause primary infections in children under 5 years of age. The elderly are at risk for pneumonia. Reinfections may occur.
  Occurrence:
  - Parainfluenza viruses are ubiquitous. They spread quickly in hospitals, causing outbreaks in nurseries and pediatric wards.
  - Infections with parainfluenza viruses 1 and 2 (e.g., croup) occur in the fall. Parainfluenza virus 3 infection occurs all year round.
- **Prevention** No preventive measures can be taken for parainfluenza virus infections.
- **Treatment** Treatment is symptomatic and consists of nebulized air or hot steam therapy, monitoring of the upper airway, and, rarely, intubation.

Respiratory Syncytial Virus (RSV)

RSV has no HA or NA activities.

- **Laboratory identification**
  - The virus can be detected in nasal wash samples.
  - Immunofluorescence and enzyme immunoassay can identify viruses in infected cells.
  - Seroconversion is identified by serologic methods.

- **Pathogenesis**
  - RSV causes a localized infection of the respiratory epithelium.
  - Cell-to-cell spread occurs via syncytium formation.
  - Pneumonia is the result of a direct CPE of the virus.
  - Bronchiolitis is immune mediated.
  - Necrosis of bronchi and bronchioles can lead to airway obstruction, especially in infants.
  - Maternal antibody is not protective.
  - Reinfection can occur.

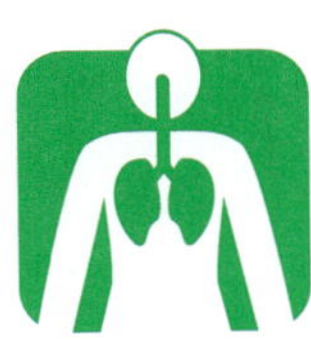

- **Diseases**
  1. Upper respiratory infections—common cold with rhinorrhea
  2. Bronchiolitis
     - a more severe lower respiratory tract infection of infants

- there is trapping of air, decreased ventilation, low-grade fever, tachycardia, and respiratory wheezes over the lungs
- disease is generally self-limiting
- disease is fatal in immunocompromised or premature infants with lung disease

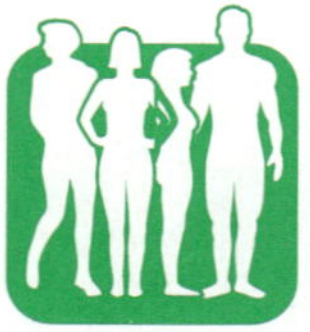

- **Epidemiology**

Mode of spread: Transmission occurs through aerosol droplets and by direct contact. The disease is very contagious with the virus being shed for many days. Contagion precedes symptoms and may occur in the absence of symptoms.

Populations affected: Infants are at risk for lower respiratory tract infections (such as pneumonia and bronchiolitis). In children the infection may range from a mild cold to pneumonia. Reinfection of adults causes milder symptoms. Most children are infected by 4 years of age.

Occurrence: The virus is ubiquitous. Annual epidermics occur in winter.

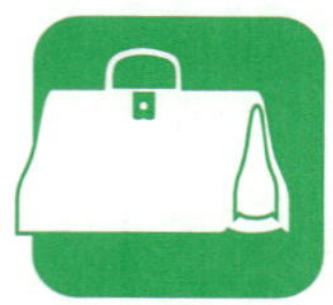

- **Prevention** Transmission to children in hospitals can be controlled by measures such as hand-washing and wearing masks and gowns.
- **Treatment**
  - Supportive treatment is administered in normal children.
  - The antiviral drug **Ribavarin,** a guanosine analogue, may be administered in aerosol form in severe cases.

Section 3.14 Rhabdoviruses

General Features (Fig. 3.30)

- Rhabdoviruses are **bullet-shaped, enveloped (−) RNA** viruses.
- Rabies virus is the most significant pathogen in this group of viruses.
- The viral genome encodes five proteins: glycoprotein (G protein), nucleoprotein (N protein), large RNA-dependent RNA polymerase (L protein), nonstructural protein (NS protein), and matrix protein (M protein).
- The nucleocapsid consists of (−) RNA, L, N, and NS proteins in a helical coil giving it a striated appearance.
- The virion must carry RNA polymerase.

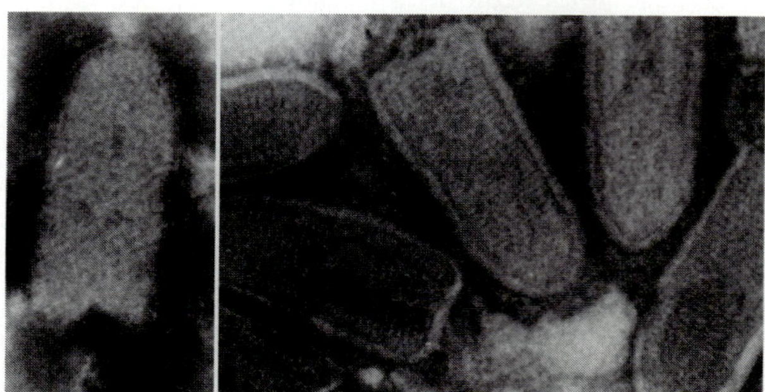

Fig. 3.30 Rhabdoviruses seen by electron microscopy: rabies virus *(left)* and vesicular stomatitis virus *(right)*.
(From Fields BN: Virology, *New York, 1985, Raven Press.)*

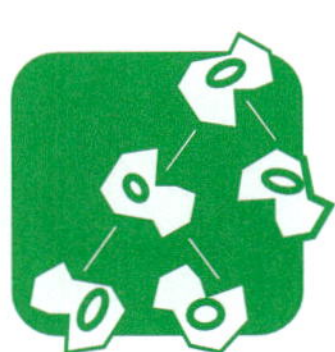

Replication (Fig. 3.31)

- Vesicular stomatitis virus (VSV) is the prototype for (–) RNA virus replication.
- The virus attaches via the G glycoprotein.
- The virus enters the cell by endocytosis.
- The endosome is acidified, the viral envelope fuses with the endosome membrane, and the nucleocapsid is released into the cytoplasm.
- Transcription and replication occur in the cytoplasm.
- The 5 viral proteins are translated from 5 separate mRNAs.
- Full length (+) template RNA is used to replicate the genome.
- The G protein is glycosylated by the cell and transported to the cell membrane, where the M protein associates with it.
- The nucleocapsid assembled in the cytoplasm associates with modified membrane and buds from the cell.

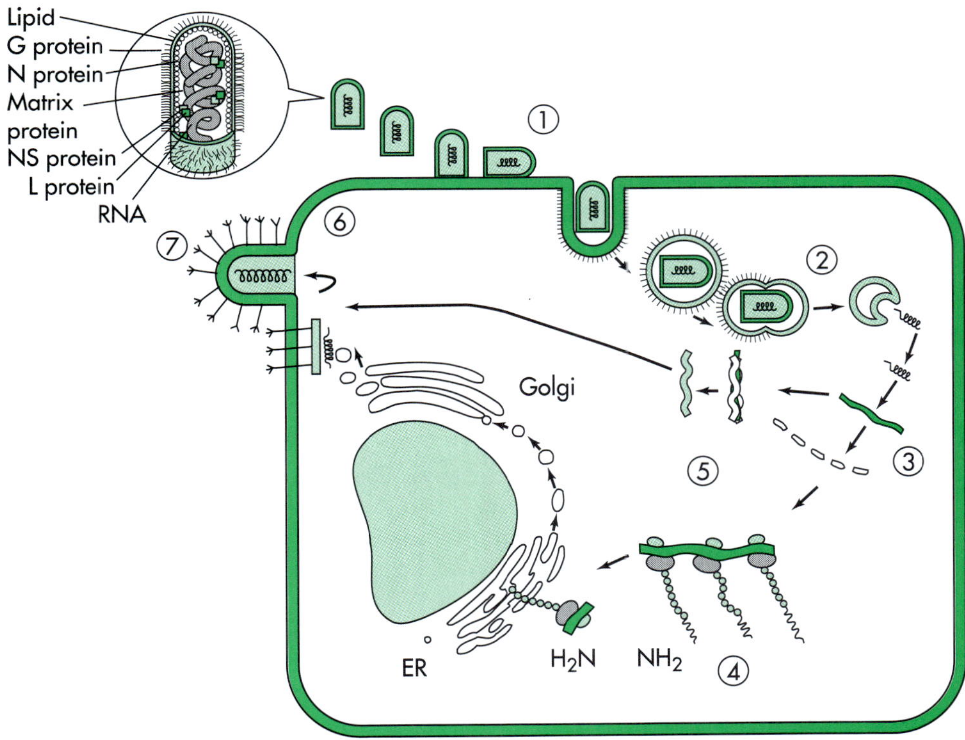

Fig. 3.31 Replication of rhabdoviruses; simple enveloped (–) RNA viruses. (1) Rhabdoviruses bind to the cell surface. (2) The viruses are endocytosed. The envelope fuses with the endosome vesicle membrane to deliver the nucleocapsid to the cytoplasm. (3) The virion must carry a polymerase and produce five individual mRNAs and a full-length (+) RNA template. (4) Proteins are translated from the mRNAs, including one glycoprotein (G), which is co-translationally glycosylated in the endoplasmic reticulum, processed in the Golgi apparatus, and delivered to the cell membrane. (5) The genome is replicated from the (+) RNA template, and the N, L, and NS proteins associate with the genome to form the nucleocapsid. (6) The matrix protein associates with the G protein-modified membrane, which is followed by assembly of the nucleocapsid. (7) The virus buds from the cell in a bullet-shaped virion.

Rabies Virus

Laboratory identification

- The diagnosis of rabies is based on a history of an animal bite and on neurologic symptoms.
- Laboratory tests are used to confirm the diagnosis.
- Viral antigen can be detected in CNS or in skin by immunofluorescence and *Negri bodies* (intracytoplasmic viral inclusions) are found in 70% to 90% of infected brains (animal or human).
- Antibody can be detected in the serum and the CSF during the terminal stages of disease.

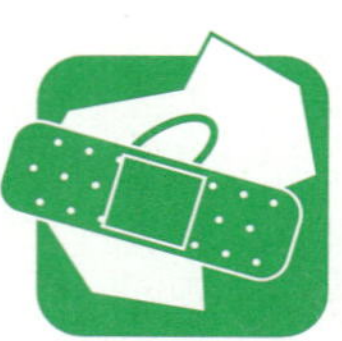

Pathogenesis

- Rabies virus is usually transmitted in the saliva after a bite from a rabid animal.
- The virus remains cell associated and produces little cell damage.
- During the incubation phase the virus replicates in the muscle at the site of the bite. The length of the incubation phase (may be weeks to months) depends on the dose of virus received and the proximity of the bite to the CNS.
- During the prodrome phase the virus infects peripheral nerves and travels to the CNS.
- During the neurologic phase the virus spreads to the glands, skin, and other organs. The virus is excreted from the salivary glands. Infection of the brain leads to the classic symptoms of rabies, coma, and death.
- The antibody response is apparent only in the late stages when the virus has infected the CNS and other sites.
- Treatment with antibody can block progression to the CNS.

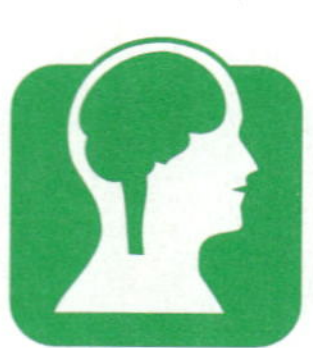

Diseases

- The characteristics of human rabies are presented in Table 3.20.
- Rabies is always fatal unless the vaccine is given.

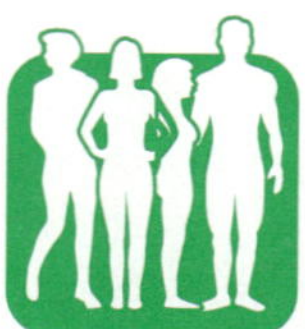

Epidemiology

Mode of spread: Rabies is a zoonosis. The reservoir for urban rabies is unvaccinated dogs. In nature, sylvatic rabies is endemic in wild animals. The important vectors for human infection are wild animals and unvaccinated dogs and cats. Transmission occurs by an animal bite or by aerosols, in caves harboring infected bats.

Populations affected: Veterinarians and animal handlers are occupationally at risk along with people in countries with no rabies vaccination program.

Occurrence: Rabies occurs worldwide, except for a few islands. It is especially prevalent in areas of the world that have no vaccination program (e.g., India and Latin America).

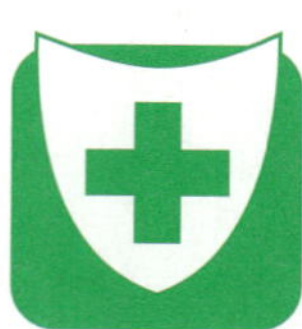

Prevention

- Vaccination of pets and high-risk personnel is recommended.

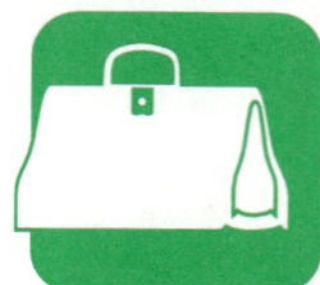

Treatment

- The human vaccine is prepared from infected diploid human tissue culture cells and killed by formaldehyde.
- Once symptoms have begun, death is inevitable.

Table 3.20 *Progression of Rabies Disease*

Disease Phase	Symptoms	Time	Viral Status	Immunological Status
Incubation phase	Asymptomatic	60-365 days after bite	Low titer Virus in muscle	
Prodrome phase	Fever, nausea, vomiting Loss of appetite Headache Lethargy Pain at site of bite	2-10 days	Low titer Virus in CNS and brain	
Neurologic phase	Hydrophobia, pharyngeal spasms Hyperactivity, anxiety, depression CNS symptoms: loss of coordination, paralysis, confusion, delirium	2-7 days	High titer Virus in brain and other sites	Detectable antibody in serum and CNS
Coma	Coma: Cardiac arrest Hypotension Hypoventilation Secondary infections Death	0-14 days	High titer Virus in brain and other sites	

• Postexposure prophylaxis can prevent disease in infected persons. This consists of immediate cleaning of the wound, vaccination with killed rabies vaccine, and administration of equine antirabies vaccine (ARS) or human rabies immune globulin (HRIG).

Section 3.15 Reoviruses

General Features

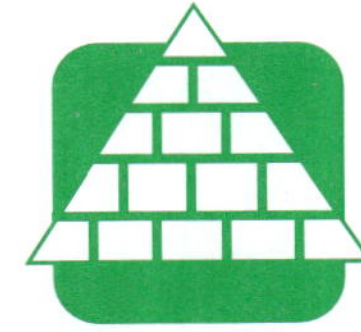

• Reoviruses are medium-sized viruses, with icosahedral symmetry and a **double capsid** virion.

• The genome consists of 10 to 12 **double-stranded RNA segments**; reassortment can occur.

• The virion is resistant to environmental conditions and to conditions in the GI tract.

• The inner capsid contains the complete transcription system, including the RNA-dependent RNA polymerase and enzymes for 5′ capping and for poly A addition.

Replication (Fig. 3.32)

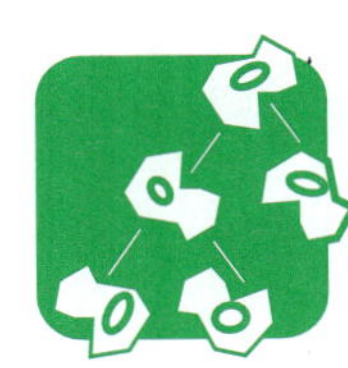

- The virion is partially digested in the GI tract and is activated by proteolytic cleavage of external capsid proteins.
- The σ1 /VP4 at the vertices of the virion binds receptors (reovirus binds β-adrenergic receptor).
- The virus penetrates the cell and the core is released into the cytoplasm.
- Transcription occurs in two phases, early and late.
- Viral proteins and (+) RNA aggregate to form cytoplasmic inclusions.
- In the new cores (–) RNA is made from the (+) RNA, forming double-stranded genomic RNA.
- Reovirus assembly involves the association of the outer capsid proteins with the core.

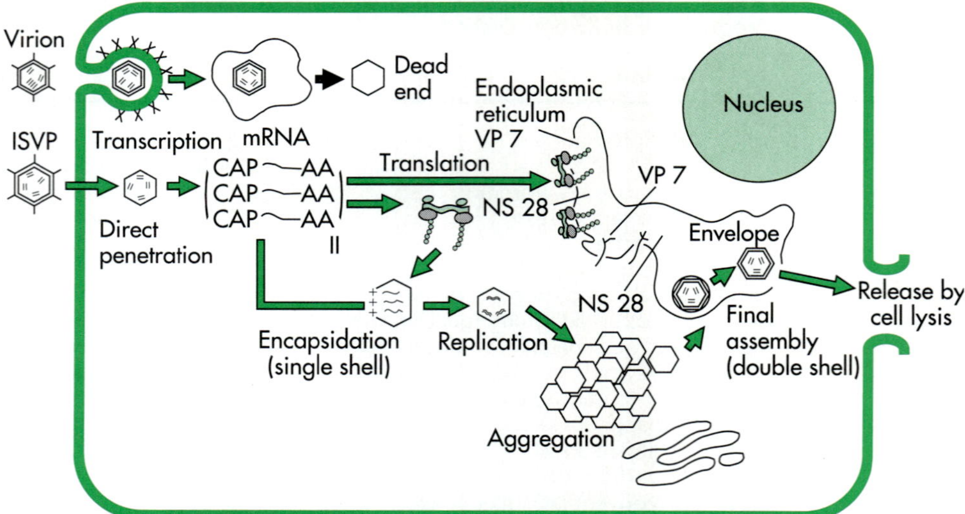

Fig. 3.32 Replication of rotavirus. Rotavirus virions are activated by protease (e.g., in the GI tract) to an ISVP. The ISVP binds, penetrates the cell, and loses its outer capsid. The inner capsid contains the enzymes for mRNA transcription using the (–) strand as a template. Some mRNA segments are transcribed early, others later. The VP7 and NS28 are synthesized as glycoproteins and are expressed in the endoplasmic reticulum. (+) RNA are mRNA and are also enclosed into inner capsids as templates to replicate the ± segmented genome. The capsids aggregate and then dock onto the NS28 protein in the ER, budding into the ER, acquiring VP7 and its outer capsid and an envelope. The virus loses the envelope and is released from the cell upon cell lysis.

- The virus is released by cell lysis.
- Rotavirus cores acquire outer capsid proteins in the endoplasmic reticulum.

■ **Rotaviruses** Rotavirus infection can cause life-threatening diarrhea to children of drought-stricken countries.

● **Laboratory diagnosis**

- ELISA or latex agglutination tests are used to detect viral antigens in stool specimens.
- The virus can be detected in stools by electron microscopy.

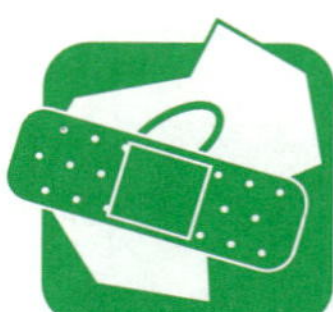

● **Pathogenesis**

- Rotavirus sets up a cytolytic infection of the intestinal epithelium that causes loss of electrolytes and stops reabsorption of water.
- Large quantities of the virus are shed during diarrhea.
- Immunity to rotavirus infection is conferred by IgA antibodies in the intestine.

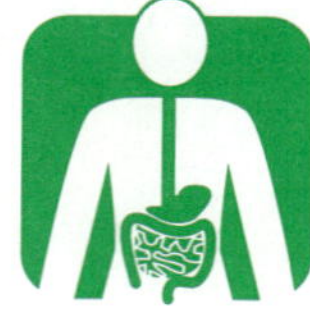

● **Diseases**

- Rotavirus causes gastroenteritis with diarrhea, vomiting, fever, and dehydration.
- The incubation period is 48 hours.
- The disease is self-limited and complete recovery occurs.

● **Epidemiology**

Mode of spread: The virus is spread by the fecal-oral route, especially in daycare centers. Transmission may potentially occur by the respiratory route.

Populations affected: Type A rotavirus infections occur in infants and children up to 24 months of age and result in infantile gastroenteritis and possible dehydration. Older children and adults develop mild diarrhea. Undernourished children in underdeveloped countries can develop diarrhea, dehydration, and death. Type B rotavirus infections occur in China and cause severe gastroenteritis in individuals of all ages.

Occurrence: Rotavirus occurs worldwide. Infections are more common in spring, winter, and fall.

- **Prevention** Frequent hand-washing can help prevent spread of rotavirus.
- **Treatment** Fluid replacement therapy can reduce mortality.

Orthoreoviruses

- Orthoreoviruses are mammalian reoviruses with very stable virions.
- There are three serotypes.
- The viruses are ubiquitous in mammals but do not cause significant human illness. They have served as a model of viral pathogenesis in mice.

Orbiviruses

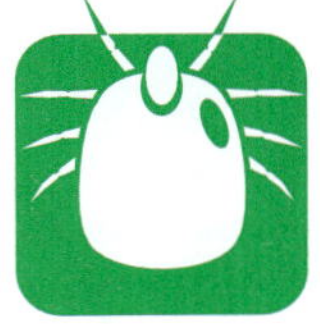
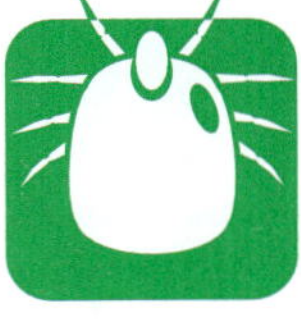

- The orbivirus group includes the Colorado tick fever virus. It is found in the western and northwestern United States and Canada.
- The virus is spread by wood ticks.

Section 3.16 Togaviruses and Flaviviruses

Overview

- *Togaviruses* are subdivided into four genera of which two contain viruses of significance to humans.
  - *Rubivirus:* Rubella virus (agent of German measles) is the only species in this genus.
  - *Alphavirus:* Members of the genus *Alphavirus* are arboviruses and consist of viruses, such as Eastern equine encephalitis (EEE) virus, Western EE virus, Venezuelan EE virus, Sindbis virus, and Semliki Forest virus.
- *Flavivirus:* yellow fever virus, dengue virus, St. Louis encephalitis virus, and hepatitis C virus.
- Most of the alphaviruses and flaviviruses are arboviruses and will be discussed together. Rubella will be discussed separately. Hepatitis C will be discussed with the other hepatitis viruses.

General Features

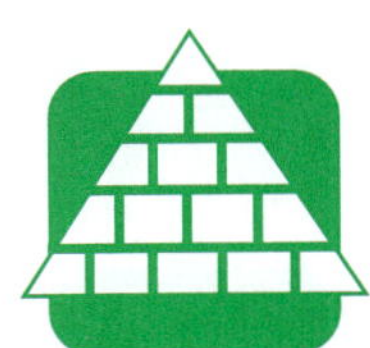

- The togaviruses and flaviviruses are small, enveloped viruses with an icosahedral capsid.
- The genome consists of single-stranded (+) RNA.
- Togaviruses produce early and late proteins.
- The arboviruses have a very broad host range infecting many species (e.g., insects, birds, and humans).

Replication

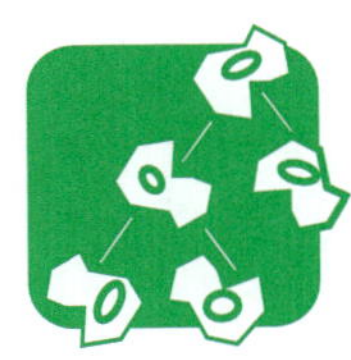

- Alphaviruses and flaviviruses can bind to animal, human, and insect cells.
- Penetration is by receptor-mediated endocytosis.

- The endosome is acidified, the virion envelope fuses with the cell membrane, and the capsid and genome are released into the cytoplasm.
- The RNA genome binds to ribosomes and is translated.
- Togavirus proteins are translated in early and late phases. Polyproteins are produced, which are cleaved by proteases.
- Virally encoded polymerase makes a (–) RNA template and the genome is replicated.
- Late mRNA is synthesized from the template.
- Nucleocapsids are assembled in the cytoplasm.
- The envelope is acquired by budding.
- Flaviviruses produce a polyprotein, but then no early and late phases of protein synthesis.
- Flavi virus buds into intracellular membranes (vesicles) and is released primarily by cell lysis (it remains more cell associated).

Rubella Virus

Laboratory identification

- Rubella virus infection is identified by the presence of anti-rubella IgM antibodies or a fourfold increase in IgG antibodies in serum.
- Antibodies are assayed in early pregnancy to determine the immune status of the mother.

Pathogenesis

- The virus is not cytolytic.
- The virus infects the upper respiratory tract and then spreads via the reticuloendothelial system.
- The virus spreads to the skin (causes a rash) and other tissues by viremia.
- The virus is shed during the 2-week prodromal period and during the 2 weeks of the rash.
- In pregnant women, the virus replicates in the placenta, is transferred to the fetus via the blood, and replicates in fetal tissues.
- Replication of the virus in the fetus alters growth, mitosis, and chromosome structure, leading to **teratogenic effects.**
- Antiviral antibody blocks viremia and infection of the placenta and fetus.

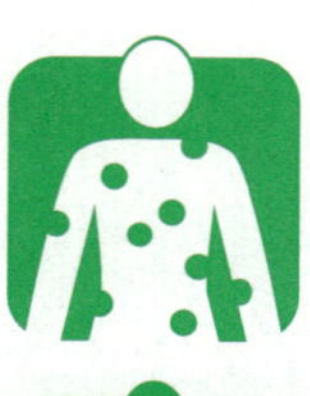

Diseases

1. German measles
   - infection in children is benign, consisting of swollen glands and a 3-day rash
   - infection in adults is more severe, with arthralgia, arthritis, thrombocytopenia (rare), and postinfectious encephalitis (from the immune response)
2. Congenital rubella
   - fetus is most at risk until the 20th week of gestation
   - leads to cataracts, mental retardation, and deafness

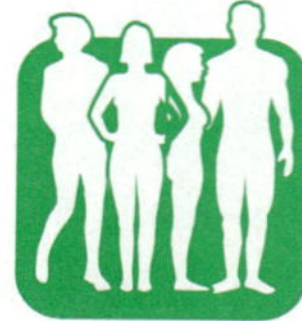

Epidemiology

Mode of spread: Rubella virus is transmitted by the respiratory route.

Table 3.21 *Disease Mechanisms of Togaviruses and Flaviviruses*

	Flu-like Syndrome	Encephalitis	Hepatitis	Hemorrhage	Shock
Flaviviruses					
Dengue	+		+	+	+
Yellow fever	+		+	+	+
St. Louis encephalitis	+	+			
Japanese encephalitis	+	+			
Togaviruses					
Venezuelan encephalitis	+	+			
Western equine encephalitis	+	+			
Eastern equine encephalitis	+	+			

Populations affected: Children and neonates less than 20 weeks of age are susceptible to infection.

Occurrence: The virus is present worldwide.

- **Prevention** Routine immunization is done with a live attenuated virus as part of the **MMR vaccine.**

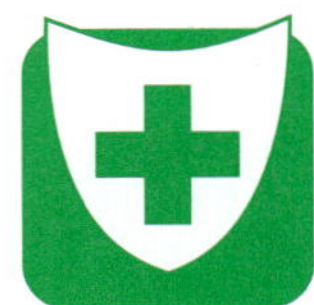

- **Treatment** No specific treatment is available.

Alphaviruses and Flaviviruses

- **Laboratory identification**

  - Blood samples are used for isolation of the virus.
  - The viruses are difficult to isolate. They can be grown in vertabrate and mosquito cell lines.
  - Viruses are identified by CPE, immunofluorescence, and hemadsorption.
  - Seroconversion is identified by serologic methods.

- **Pathogenesis**

  - These viruses are arboviruses.
  - The mosquito injects the virus into blood, and a viremia is initiated.
  - The viruses are cytolytic.
  - The viruses are good inducers of interferons, causing influenza-like symptoms with the disease.
  - The flaviviruses infect cells of the macrophage-monocyte lineage.
  - Flavivirus infection of macrophages is promoted by interaction of antibody with Fc receptors.
  - Antibodies block the spread of the virus.

- **Diseases** The characteristics of alphavirus and flavivirus infections are presented in Table 3.21.

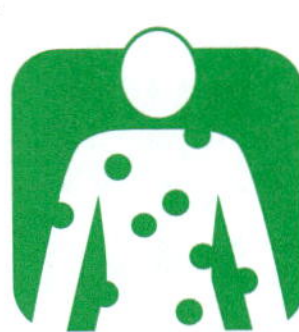

  - Most infections start with and may be limited to influenza-like symptoms caused by viremia and interferon induction.
  - The nature of the disease is determined by the target tissue. For example, the encephalitis viruses infect the brain, whereas the dengue and yellow fever viruses infect the liver, other organs, and vasculature.

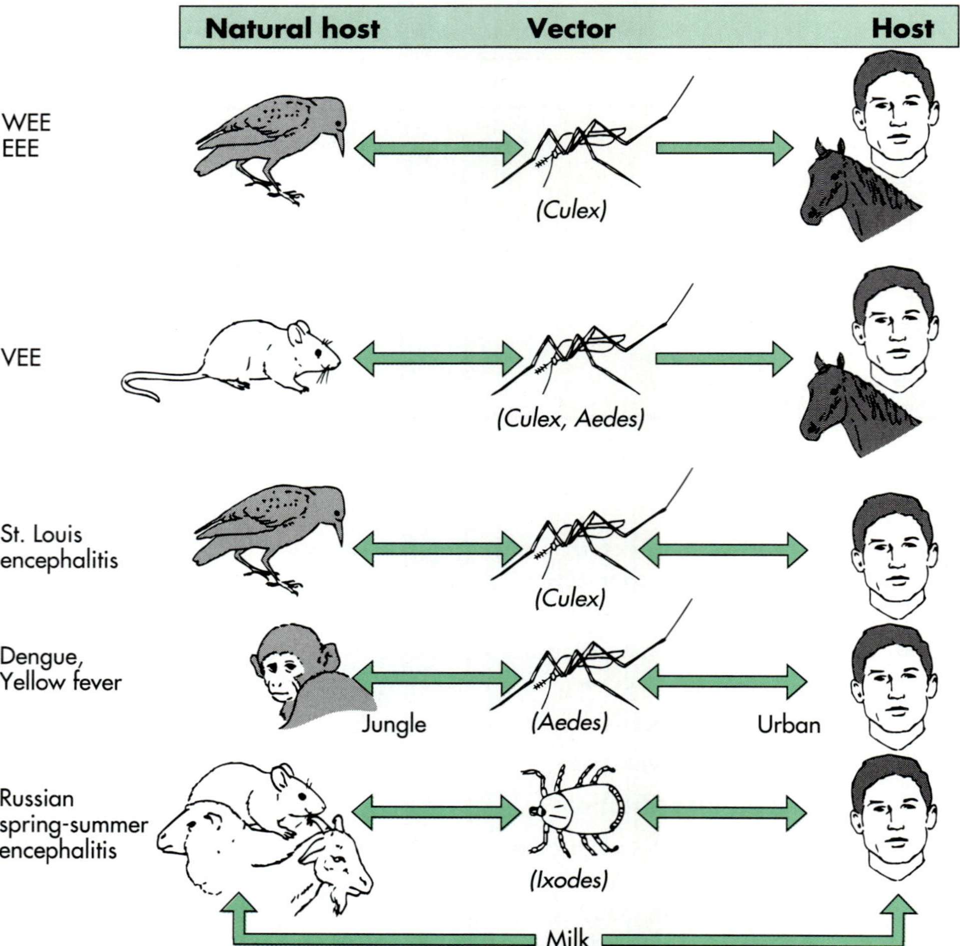

Fig. 3.33 Patterns of alphavirus and flavivirus transmission. The cycle of arbovirus transmission maintains and amplifies the virus in the environment. Host-vector relationships that can provide this cycle are indicated by the double arrow. "Dead-end" infections with no transmission of the virus back to the vector are indicated by the single arrow. For St. Louis encephalitis, yellow fever, and dengue virus, humans are not dead-end hosts but support an urban cycle. The Russian spring-summer encephalitis virus can be transmitted to humans by a tick bite and in milk from infected goats.

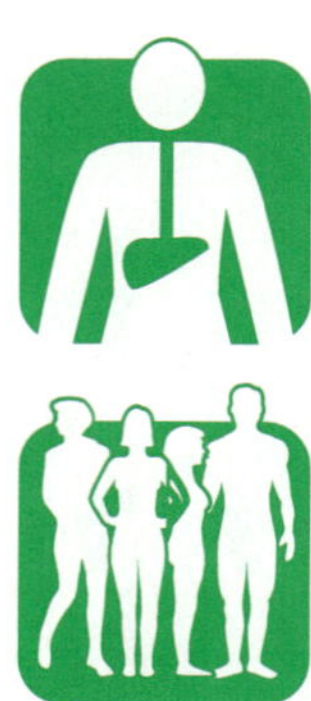

1. Dengue
   - rechallenge with dengue virus can result in severe hemorrhagic disease and shock (dengue hemorhagic fever [DHF] or dengue shock syndrome [DSS])
2. Yellow fever
   - severe systemic disease, with degeneration of the liver resulting in jaundice, degeneration of the kidneys and heart, and hemorrhage of blood vessels; "black vomit" results from GI tract hemorrhage
   - mortality is 50%

- **Epidemiology (Fig. 3.33)**

  Mode of spread: The viruses are transmitted by the bite of specific arthropods (mosquitos). Different mosquitos transmit different viruses.

Populations affected: People coming in contact with the arthropods are at risk.

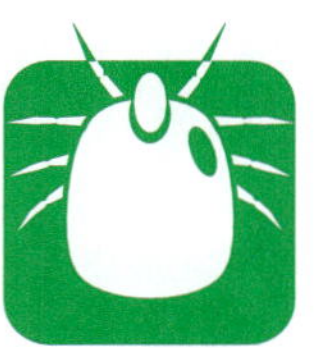

Occurrence: Endemic regions are determined by the habitat of the arthropod vector (usually the mosquito). The genus *Aedes* is found near pools of water and transmits dengue and yellow fever to urban populations. The *Culex* mosquito breeds in forests and causes urban outbreaks of St. Louis encephalitis. Outbreaks are common in summer.

- **Prevention**

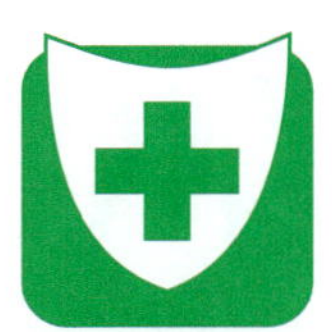

  - Elimination of mosquitoes can control arboviral diseases.
  - A live attenuated vaccine is available for yellow fever and Japanese encephalitis.

- **Treatment** Treatment consists of supportive care.

Section 3.17 Bunyaviruses

The bunyaviruses constitute a supergroup consisting of five genera: *Bunyavirus, Phlebovirus, Nairovirus, Uukuvirus,* and *Hantavirus.* Bunyaviruses and Hantaviruses occur in the United States.

General Features

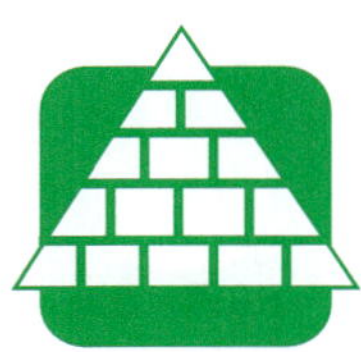

- Bunyaviruses are medium-sized, enveloped viruses with segmented (−) RNA.
- The nucleocapsid contains large (L), medium (M), and small (S) RNA molecules, RNA-dependent RNA polymerase (L), and two nonstructural proteins.
- More than 200 related viruses comprise the bunyavirus group.
- The viruses infect humans, animals (especially birds), and arthropods.

Replication

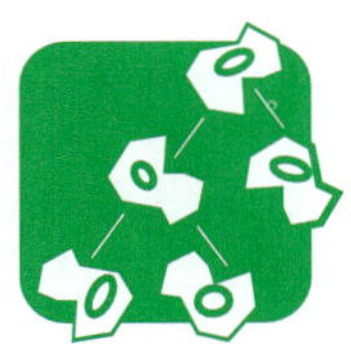

- The virus enters the cell by endocytosis.
- Transcription, translation, and genome replication occur in the cytoplasm.
- The virus buds into the endoplasmic reticulum (glycoproteins are not inserted into the plasma membrane).
- The virion is released by exocytosis or by cell lysis.

Laboratory Identification

Serologic tests, such as virus neutralization and ELISA, are employed for diagnosis.

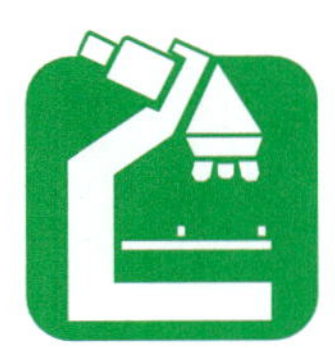

Pathogenesis

- The virus is injected into the skin by a bite from an arthropod (mosquito).
- A viremia is initiated causing influenza-like symptoms.
- A secondary viremia spreads the virus to the target organs (CNS, organs, and vascular endothelium).
- Encephalitis results from neuronal and glial cell damage and cerebral edema.
- *Rift Valley fever* causes hepatic necrosis.
- *Hantavirus* infection disrupts the vascular endothelium, causing hemorrhagic fever and respiratory distress.

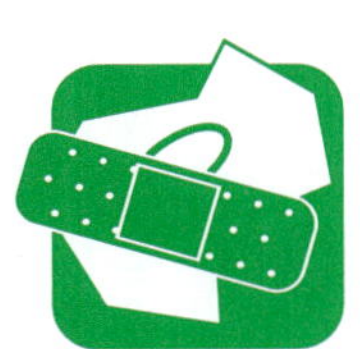

Diseases

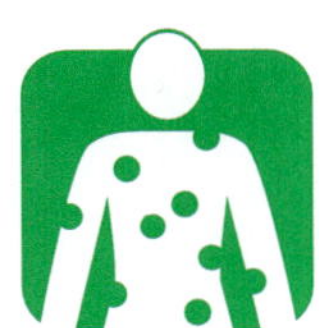

1. Nonspecific viral illness
   - associated with viremia
   - incubation period is 48 hours; illness lasts 3 days

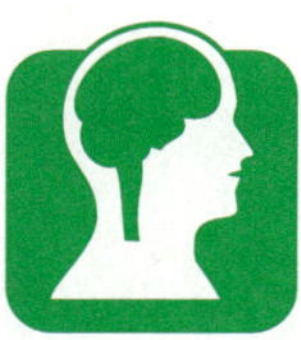

2. Encephalitis
   - example is California encephalitis caused by La Crosse virus
   - incubation period of 1 week with fever, headache, lethargy, vomiting, and seizures (in 50% of the cases)
   - fatality is less than 1%

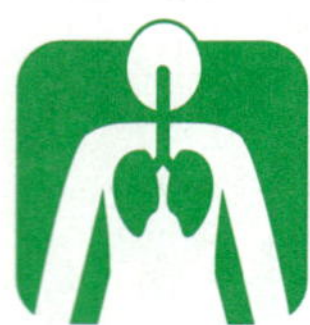

3. Hemorrhagic fevers
   - Rift Valley fever
   - fatality is 50%
4. Pulmonary syndrome
   - caused by hantavirus

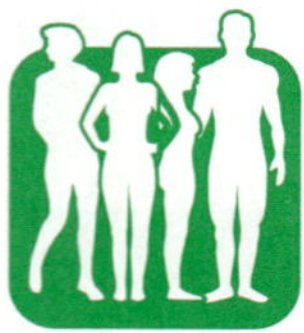

Epidemiology

Mode of spread: The California encephalitis group (including La Crosse virus) is transmitted by *Aedes* mosquitoes, which are daytime feeders, living in the forest and laying eggs in small pools of water. Infected rodents, birds, and larger animals act as reservoirs. Hantavirus spreads from mammal to mammal and can spread to humans in aerosols and rat feces.

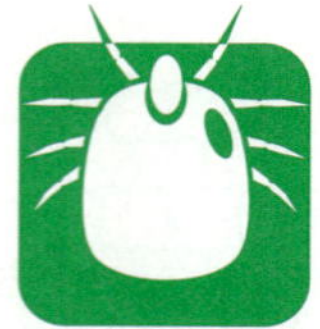

Populations at risk: People who enter the habitat of the arthropod vector are at risk. For example, campers, forest rangers, and woodsmen are at risk of acquiring California encephalitis.

Occurrence:

- The occurrence of disease correlates with the location of the vector.
- California encephalitis, La Crosse virus, and hantavirus outbreaks have occurred in the United States. Outbreaks are most common in summer (mosquito season).

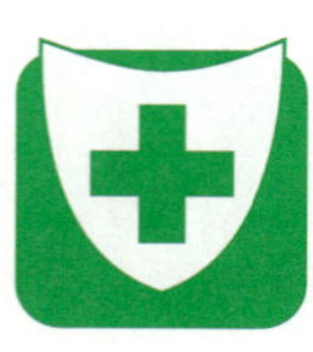

- **Prevention** Control of arthropod and mammalian vectors can reduce the incidence of disease.
- **Treatment** No treatment is available.

Section 3.18 Coronaviruses, Caliciviruses, Arenaviruses, and Filoviruses

Coronaviruses

General features

- Coronaviruses are medium-sized viruses with a corona-like appearance in electron micrographs.
- The viruses are enveloped with club-shaped projections (glycoproteins).
- The genome is (+) RNA and consists of early and late mRNA molecules.

Replication

- The enveloped virus enters by endocytosis.
- The (+) RNA is transcribed, polymerase is made, and a full length (–) RNA template is used for replication and to make individual late mRNAs (see Section 3.16).

- The virus is assembled on the rough endoplasmic reticulum.
- Release of virus occurs by exocytosis.

- **Laboratory identification** Coronaviruses are not routinely identified in the laboratory.

- **Pathogenesis**

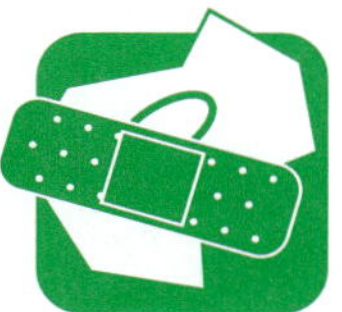

- Coronavirus infection is primarily localized to the respiratory tract epithelium, because the optimum temperature for viral growth is 33° C to 35° C.
- Antibody is elicited but does not prevent reinfection.
- Although enveloped, coronaviruses can be found in stools.

- **Diseases**

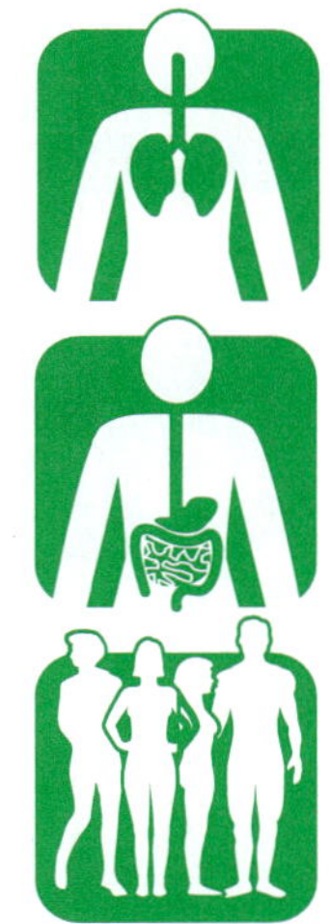

1. Common cold (most common presentation)
   - the disease is similar to that caused by rhinoviruses but with a longer incubation period (3 days)
2. Diarrhea and gastroenteritis
   - coronavirus-like particles seen in the stools of patients
3. Necrotizing enterocolitis
   - caused in infants
   - coronavirus-like particles seen in stools

- **Epidemiology**

Mode of spread: The viruses are spread by aerosol droplets.

Populations affected: The disease occurs mainly in infants and children. Antibodies are uniformly present in adults. Coronaviruses cause 10% to 15% of upper respiratory tract infections and pneumonias.

Occurrence: Occurrence is sporadic. Outbreaks may occur in winter and spring.

- **Treatment and prevention** No preventive measures or treatment exist for the disease.

Caliciviruses (Norwalk Agent and Other Small, Round Enteric Viruses)

- **General features**

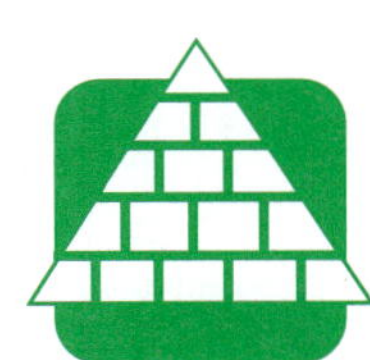

- Caliciviruses are small, naked capsid viruses with a single-stranded (+) RNA genome.
- They are resistant to environmental influences (e.g., detergents, drying, and acid).

- **Laboratory diagnosis** The viruses can be detected in feces by electron microscopy. Serologic tests can also aid in diagnosis.

- **Pathogenesis**

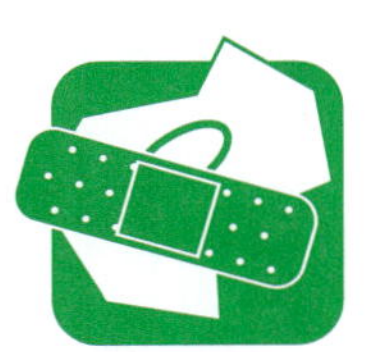

- Caliciviruses compromise the function of the brush border, preventing proper absorption of water and nutrients.
- Gastric emptying may be delayed, causing vomiting.

- **Diseases**

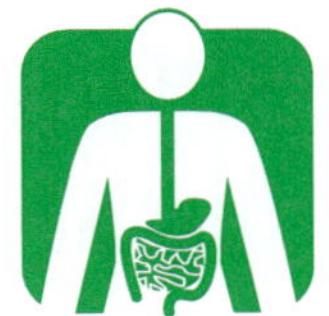

- Caliciviruses cause diarrhea with nausea and vomiting.
- Fever may be present in one third of the cases.
- The incubation period is very short (24 to 60 hours).
- The illness is short (12 to 60 hours) and self-limited.

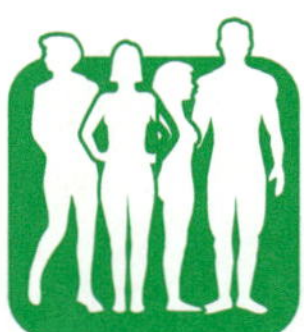

- **Epidemiology**
  - Transmission of caliciviruses occurs via the fecal-oral route through contaminated food and water.
  - Outbreaks occur year round, can be traced to a common source, and occur in contained environments, such as cruise ships and schools.
- **Prevention** No preventive measures can be taken.
- **Treatment** Bismuth salicylate may help reduce symptoms of gastroenteritis.

Arenaviruses Lymphocytic choriomeningitis (LCM) virus and the hemorrhagic fever viruses (Lassa fever virus, Junin virus, and Machupo virus)

- **General features**
  - Arenaviruses are medium-sized, enveloped viruses with circular RNA genomes (two circles) that carry a polymerase.
  - The viruses appear sandy on electron micrographs because of ribosomes in the virion.
  - The arenavirus RNA is ambisense.

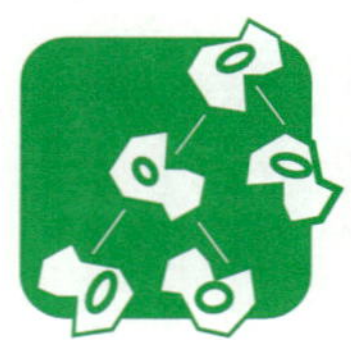

- **Replication**
  - The viruses replicate in the cytoplasm.
  - They acquire the envelope by budding through the cell membrane.
  - Persistent infection may result from inefficient transcription of the late glycoprotein gene.
- **Laboratory diagnosis**
  - Serologic tests are used for diagnosis.
  - The viruses are too dangerous to be isolated in routine laboratories.

- **Pathogenesis**
  - The viruses infect macrophages, possibly causing them to release mediators and cause vascular damage.
  - Disease is largely attributed to T cell immunopathogenesis.
  - Persistent infection in rodents results from neonatal infection and induction of immune tolerance.
  - LCM is studied as a classical example of immune tolerance and T cell response to viruses.

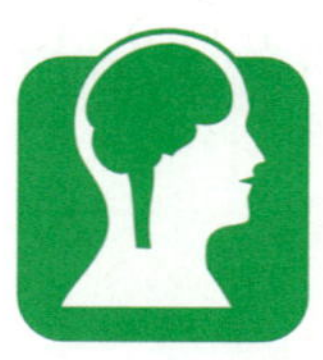

- **Diseases**
  1. Lymphocytic choriomeningitis
     - febrile illness with myalgia
     - CNS infection seen in 25% of cases
     - infection may be subacute and persist for months
  2. Lassa fever and other hemorrhagic fevers
     - clinical features include fever, coagulopathy, petechiae, liver and spleen necrosis, hemorrhage, shock, occasional cardiac and liver damage, pharyngitis, diarrhea, and vomiting
     - mortality to 50% for lassa fever, lower for other hemorrhagic fevers

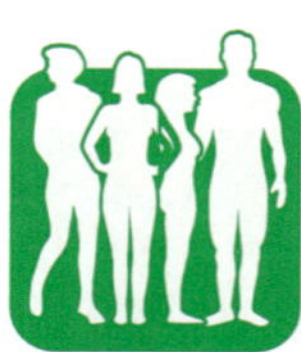

- **Epidemiology**

  Mode of spread: Chronically infected rodents (*Mastomys natalensis* for Lassa fever and house mice and hamsters in the United States for LCM) in endemic regions have viremia and shed virus. Viruses are transferred to humans by aerosols, food, and fomites. The Lassa fever virus can also spread from human to human via body fluids.

Populations affected: People in endemic regions and, in the United States, workers at rodent-breeding facilities are at risk.

Occurrence: The hemorrhagic fevers occur mainly in the tropical regions of Africa and South America.

- **Prevention** Limiting contact with the vector, practicing good hygiene, and trapping rodents can prevent disease.
- **Treatment**
  - The antiviral drug ribavarin, which is a guanosine analogue, can be used for treatment.
  - Supportive therapy is also used.

Filoviruses (Marburg Virus and Ebola Virus)

- **General features**
  - The filoviruses are filamentous viruses that resemble the rhabdoviruses in basic (not clinical) properties.
  - They are long, filamentlike and enveloped, with a (–) RNA genome.
  - The viruses replicate in the cytoplasm.
- **Laboratory identification** Filoviruses are too dangerous to be isolated. Specimens are handled with extreme care in level 4 containment facilities.

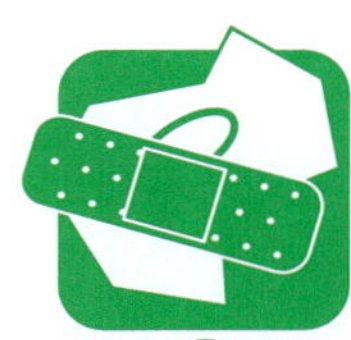

- **Pathogenesis**
  - The virus replicates efficiently causing extensive tissue necrosis in the parenchymal cells of the liver, lymph nodes, spleen, and lungs.
  - Widespread hemorrhage results in edema and hypovolemic shock.

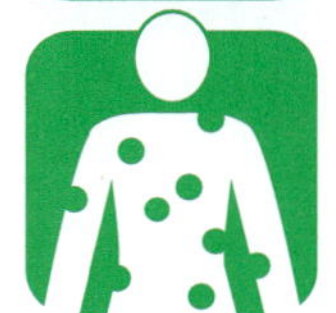

- **Diseases**
  - The viruses cause hemorrhagic diseases of the utmost severity.
  - The illness starts with influenza-like symptoms, and after a few days, nausea, vomiting, diarrhea, and possibly a rash develop.
  - Hemorrhage and death occur in 90% of the cases.

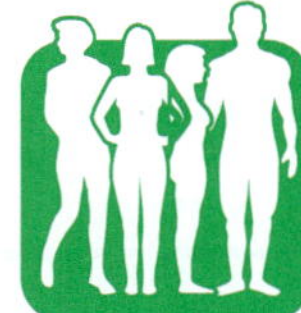

- **Epidemiology**

Mode of spread:

- The viruses may be endemic in monkeys and spread to humans.
- Transmission occurs by accidental injection or by close contact with body fluids.

Populations affected: Laboratory workers and travelers to and residents of central Africa are at risk. Subclinical infections may occur.

Occurrence: Ebola virus infections occur in central Africa. The Marburg virus causes rare cases of disease in Zimbabwe and Kenya.

- **Prevention** Control measures include quarantine of infected individuals and sacrifice of contaminated animals.
- **Treatment** Antibody-containing serum and interferons have been tried as treatments.

Section 3.19 Retroviruses

The retroviruses comprise the subfamilies oncovirus (human T-cell lymphotropic virus [HTLV-1, HTLV-2, and HTLV-5]), lentivirus (human immunodeficiency virus [HIV-1 and HIV-2]), and spumavirus (human foamy virus [does not cause clinical disease]) (Table 3.22).

General Features

- The first identified tumor virus was a C-type retrovirus (Rous sarcoma virus).
- The retroviruses are classified by disease, tissue tropism, and virion morphology (see Table 3.22).
- The morphology of the nucleocapsid core is used in classification (Fig. 3.34).
- The virus **integrates** into the host chromosome and becomes a "super gene" of the cell. It is transcribed into mRNA and this is also the means of replication.

Structure (Fig. 3.35)

Virion

- The virion is medium sized.
- It is enveloped and has a morphologically distinct nucleocapsid.
- The major envelope glycoprotein (in HIV, for example) has two parts: the fusion protein gp41 and the gp120 attachment protein.
- The virion contains two copies of the (+) RNA genome, reverse transcriptase, and integrase enzymes, and two tRNAs.

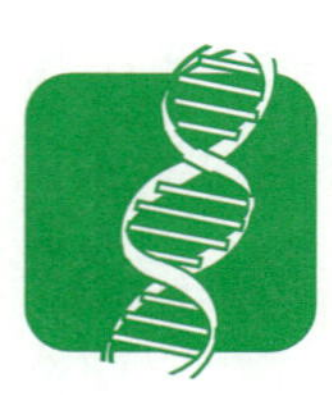

Genome

- The genome encodes three main polyproteins: *gag* (group antigen), *pol,* and *env.* The capsid is formed from cleavage of a polyprotein encoded by the gag gene. The pol gene encodes protease, integrase, and reverse transcriptase. The env gene encodes the viral envelope glycoproteins.
- Long terminal repeats (LTRs) are at each end of the genome.
- The LTR contains promoters, enhancers, and binding sites for cellular proteins.

Table 3.22 ***Classification of Retroviruses***

Subfamily	Characteristics	Examples
Oncovirus	Associated with cancer and neurologic disorders	
A	Intracytoplasmic precursor of B-type virus; double-membrane particles	
B	Eccentric nucleocapsid core in mature virion	Mouse mammary tumor virus
C	Centrally located nucleocapsid core in mature virion	Human T-lymphotropic virus (HTLV-1, HTLV-2, HTLV-5), Rous sarcoma virus (chickens)
D	Nucleocapsid core with cylindric form	Mason-Pfizer monkey virus
Lentivirus	Slow disease onset: causes neurologic disorders and immunosuppression; virus with D-type, cylindrical,nucleocapsid core	Human immunodeficiency virus (HIV-1, HIV-2), visna virus (sheep), Caprine arthritis/ encephalitis virus (goats)
Spumavirus	Causes no clinical disease but characteristic vacuolated "foamy" cytopathology	Human foamy virus

- The HIV (also HTLV) genome encodes regulatory proteins (e.g., tat protein, rev protein, and nef protein).
- Oncogenic retroviruses encode growth-stimulating genes captured from and resembling cellular genes (Table 3.23).

Replication (Fig. 3.36)

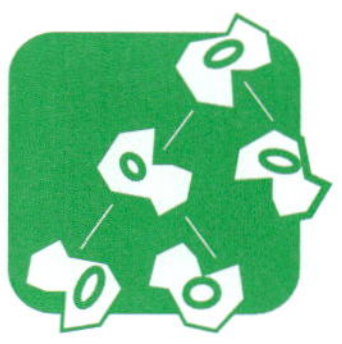

- The virus binds to specific cell receptors (major determinants of target specificity). For example, the HIV gp120 binds to CD4 found on T lymphocytes and cells of the macrophage lineage.
- Entry occurs by fusion of the virion envelope with the cell membrane.
- Reverse transcriptase synthesizes complementary negative-stranded DNA using virion tRNA as a primer, degrades the RNA, and synthesizes positive-stranded DNA (cDNA).
- The cDNA is integrated into the host DNA using viral integrase.
- The HIV reverse transcriptase is error prone, causing mutations.

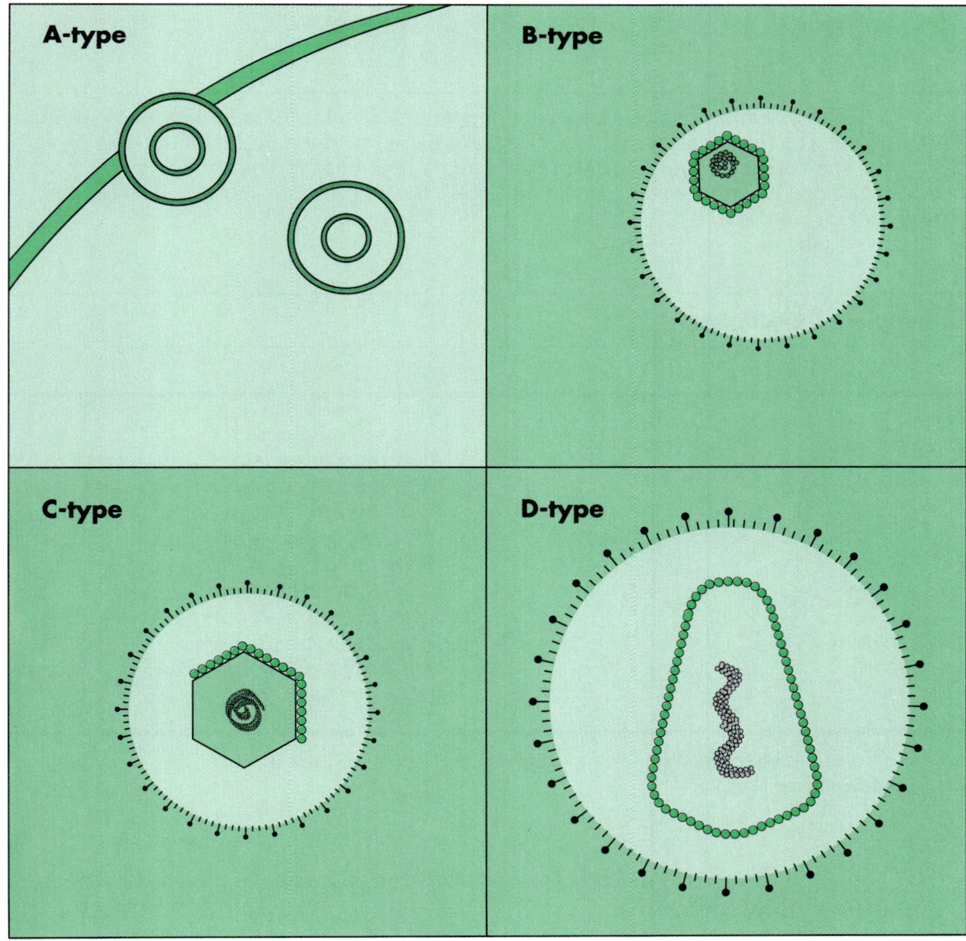

Fig. 3.34 Morphologic basis for classification of the retroviruses. The shape and position of the nucleocapsid core are the basis of classification. A-type particles are immature intracytoplasmic forms that bud through the plasma membrane into mature B-type particles. C-type particles (oncoviruses) and D-type particles (HIV) are mature virion forms.

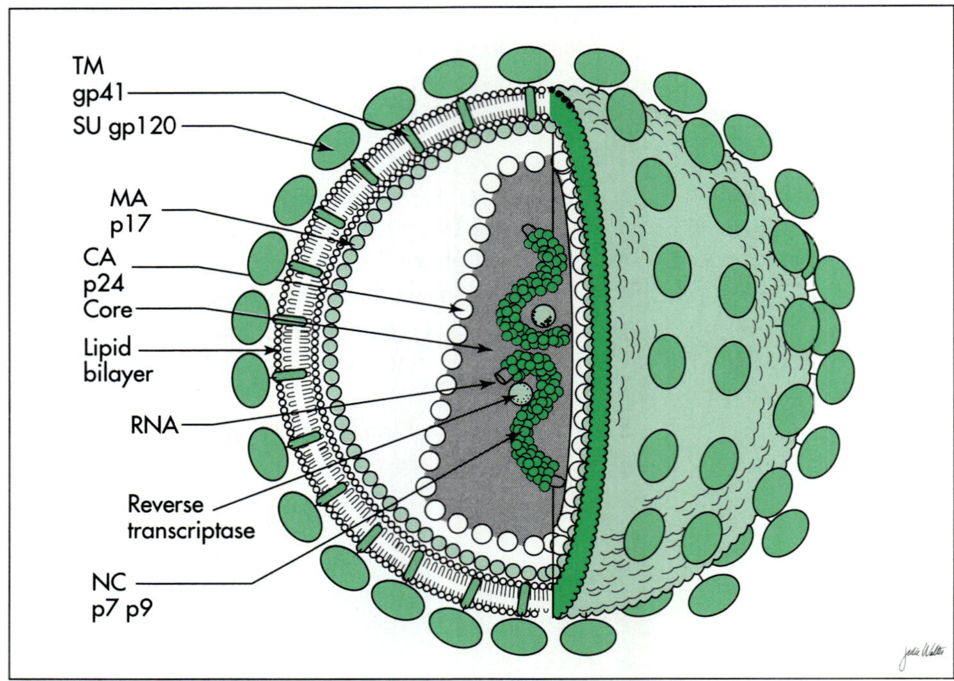

Fig. 3.35 Cross-section of HIV. The enveloped virion contains two identical RNA strands, RNA polymerase, integrase, and two tRNAs base-paired to the genome within the protein core. The core is surrounded by proteins and a lipid bilayer. The envelope spikes are made of the gp120 attachment protein and gp41 fusion protein. *(Redrawn from Gallo RC, Montagnier L:* Sci Am *259:41-51, 1988.)*

Table 3.23 ***Representative Examples of Oncogenes***

Function	Oncogene	Virus
Tyrosine kinase	src	Rous sarcoma virus
	abl	Abelson murine leukemia virus
	fes	ST feline sarcoma virus
Growth factor receptors	erb-B (EGF receptor)	Avian erythroblastosis virus
	erb-A (thyroid hormone receptor)	Avian erythroblastosis virus
GTP-binding proteins	Ha-ras	Harvey murine sarcoma virus
	Ki-ras	Kirsten murine sarcoma virus
Nuclear proteins	myc	Avian myelocytomatosis virus MC29
	myb	Avian myeloblastosis virus
	fos	Murine osteosarcoma virus FBJ
	jun	Avian sarcoma virus 17

Modified from Jawetz E, Melnick JL, Adelberg EA et al.: *Medical microbiology*, ed 18, Los Altos, Calif, 1989, Appleton & Lange. *GTP,* Guanosine triphosphate; *EGF,* epidermal growth factor.

- Integrated viral DNA (**provirus**) is transcribed as a cellular gene by host RNA polymerase.
- HIV replication is regulated by the viral proteins tat and rev (tax and rex proteins in HTLV-1).
- Gag, gag-pol, and env mRNA is translated into a polyprotein that is cleaved into functional proteins.

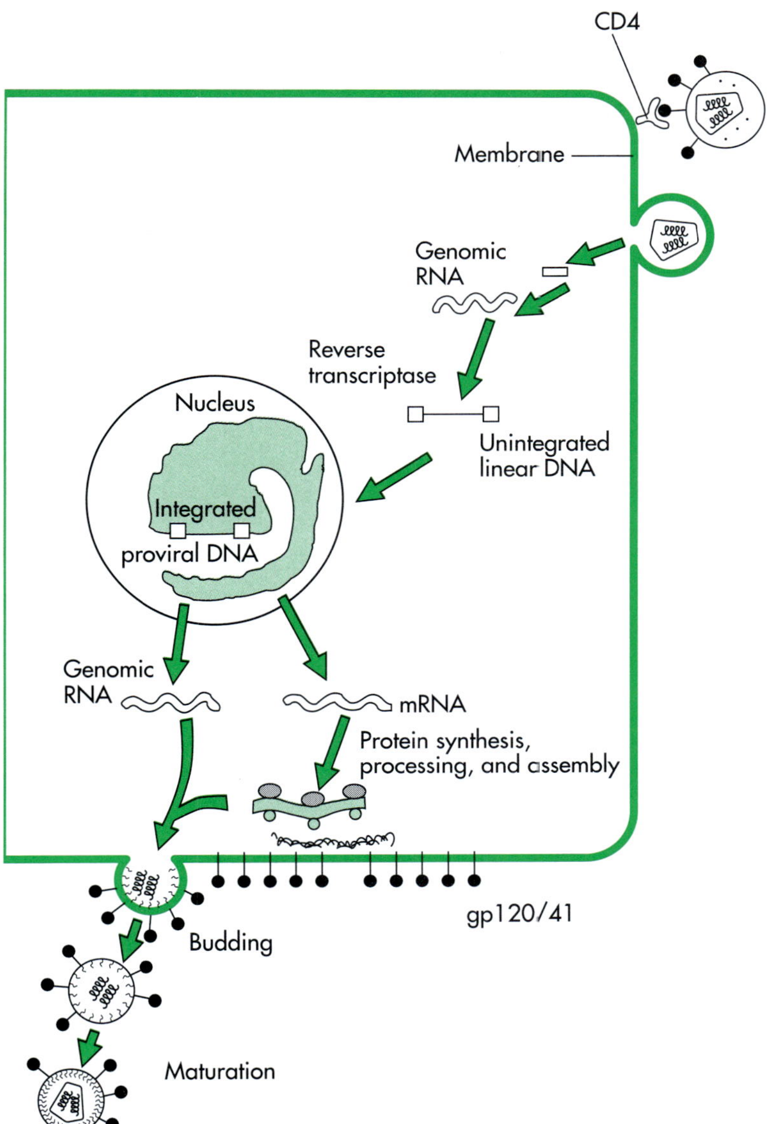

Fig. 3.36 The life cycle of HIV. HIV binds to CD4 molecules on cells and enters the cells by fusion. The genome is reverse transcribed into a cDNA in the cytoplasm and is integrated into the chromatin of the cell. The integrated genome is recognized as a host gene, and viral mRNA is transcribed by host machinery. Full-length transcripts become new genomes. The virus assembles at the plasma membrane and matures after budding from the cell. *(Redrawn from Fauci AS:* Science *239:617, 1988.)*

- Viral glycoproteins are synthesized and processed in the endoplasmic reticulum and golgi region.
- Gag and gag-pol proteins associate with the cell membrane with two copies of the viral genome and tRNA.
- Accessory proteins for HIV, the nef, vif, vpu, and vpr proteins, regulate replication and promote pathogenesis in the host.
- The virus buds from the cell and acquires its envelope.

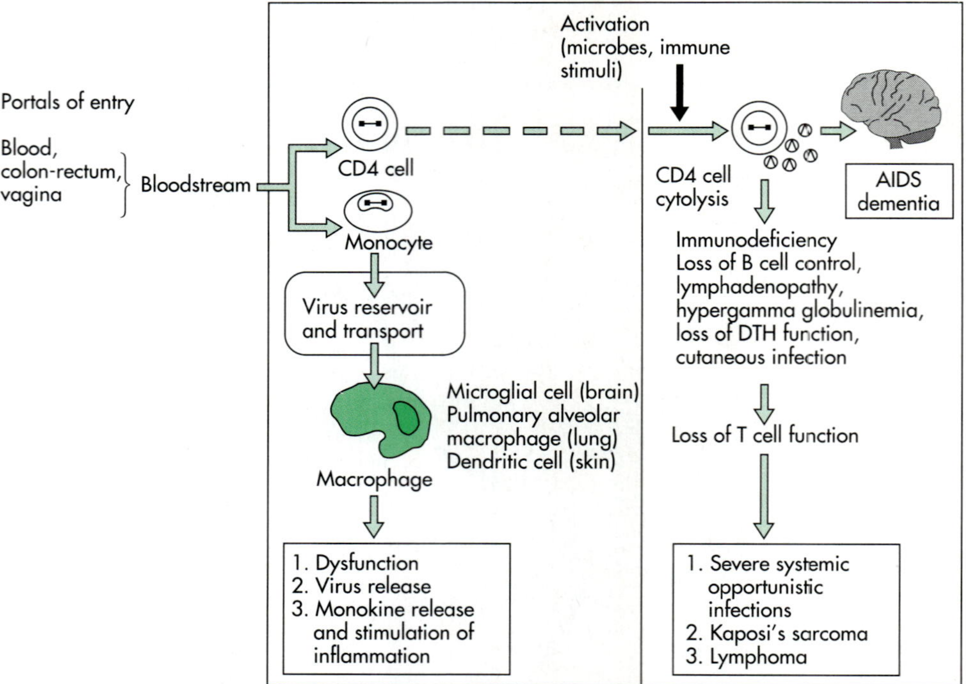

Fig. 3.37 Pathogenesis of HIV. HIV causes lytic and latent infection of $CD4^+$ T cells, persistent infection of cells of the monocyte/macrophage family, and disrupts neurons. The outcomes of these actions are immunodeficiency and AIDS dementia. *(Redrawn from Fauci AS:* Science *239:617, 1988.)*

- Virion protease cleaves polyproteins after the assembly of the virion to finish morphogenesis.
- HIV may spread from cell to cell by the formation of syncytia.
- The reverse transcriptase and the protease are targets for drug design.

Human Immunodeficiency Virus (HIV)

Laboratory diagnosis

- Serologic tests are used for initial screening (ELISA and latex agglutination) and for confirmation (Western blot).
- The *HIV p24 antigen* is an early marker of infection and active virus replication.
- A decrease in the CD4/CD8 T cell ratio correlates with progression of HIV disease.

Pathogenesis

- HIV establishes lytic infection (in T cells), latent infection (in T cells and macrophages), and persistent infections (in T cells and macrophages). Continuous killing of CD4 T cells depletes mature and stem cells leading to a decrease in CD4 and total T cell numbers and immunodeficiency.
- HIV infection is acquired from contaminated blood or semen.
- HIV enters the body by injection, through cuts in the skin, or passes across the musoca.
- The major pathogenic mechanism is the tropism of HIV for CD4-expressing T cells and macrophages (Fig. 3.37).

Table 3.24 ***Abnormalities in Immune Function Resulting from HIV Infection***

Cells	Abnormalities
T helper (CD4) lymphocytes	Decreased proliferative responses
	Decreased T-cell help and control
	Decreased cytotoxic T-cell activity against virus-infected cells
	Decreased DTH response
Monocytes	Decreased chemotaxis
	Decreased IL-1 production
	Decreased microbicidal activity
	Increased release of TNF and other cytokines
Natural killer cells	Decreased cytotoxic activity
B lymphocytes	Decreased antigen-specific humoral responses (antibody production)
	Uncontrolled production of antibody (hypergammaglobulinemia)

DTH, Delayed type hypersensitivity; *TNF,* tumor necrosis factor.

- HIV is cytolytic for T cells.
- Macrophages are persistently infected and may act as the major reservoir and distribution vehicle for the virus.
- HIV can cause neurologic abnormalities. Brain macrophages, microglial cells, and neurons can be infected.
- HIV incapacitates the immune system (Table 3.24).
- Resolution of the disease is prevented by the ability of the virus to inactivate the immune system, replicate in "privileged sites," and alter its antigenicity.

Diseases (Fig. 3.38)

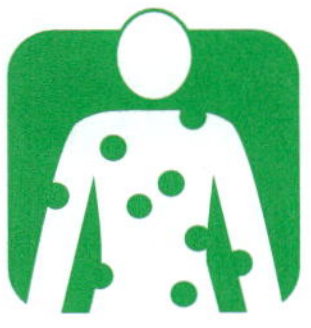

- HIV disease progresses from an asymptomatic infection to a condition with severe immunosuppression ("full-blown AIDS").
- Initial infection is asymptomatic or resembles mononucleosis with aseptic meningitis or a rash. The symptoms subside spontaneously.
- The virus persists in the host for months to years with limited symptoms.

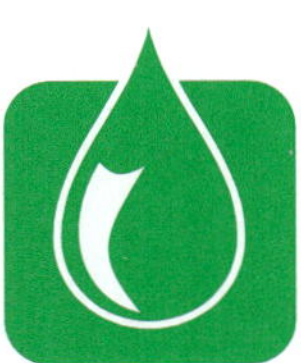

1. AIDS-related complex (ARC)
   - characterized by lymphadenopathy and fever, weight loss, malaise, opportunistic infections, diarrhea, night sweats, and fatigue
2. Full blown AIDS
   - defined by the presence of antibody to HIV, significant reduction in $CD4^{+}$ T cell levels to less than 500 cells per cubic millimeter, wasting syndrome for more than 1 month, opportunistic infections, and neoplastic malignancies (Box 3.13)
3. "Slim disease"

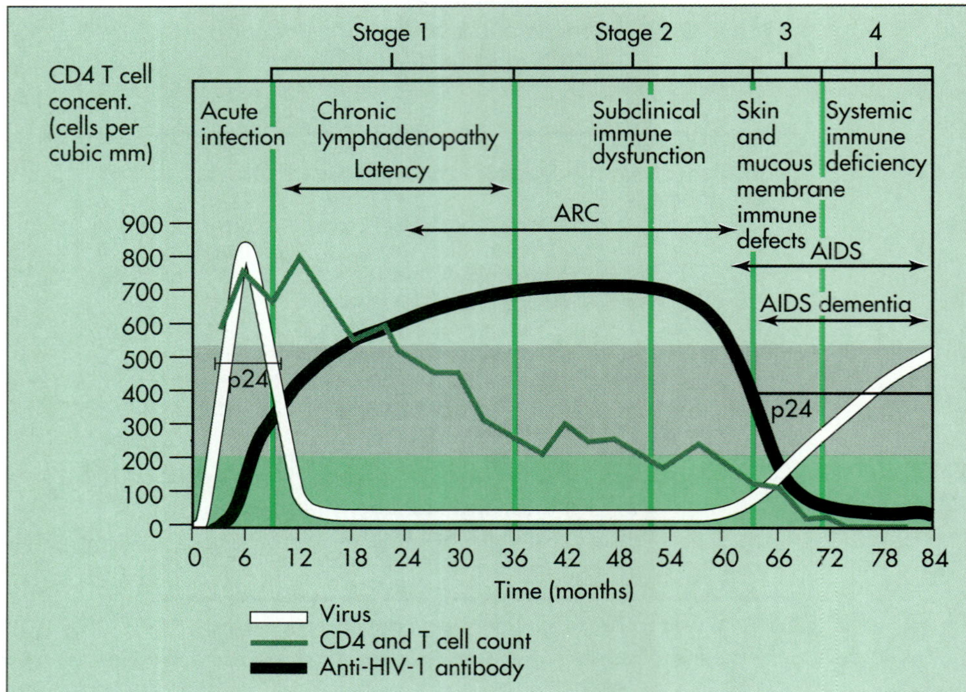

Fig. 3.38 Pathogenesis of HIV. HIV causes lytic and latent infection of $CD4^+$ T cells, persistent infection of cells of the monocyte/macrophage family, and disrupts neurons. Continuous HIV production, and the killing and turnover of CD4 T cells, depletes the numbers of these helper and delayed-type hypersensitivity mediating cells, leading to symptoms of immunodeficiency.

- common in Africa
- wasting, weight loss

4. AIDS-related dementia
   - slow deterioration of intellect and other neurologic disorders

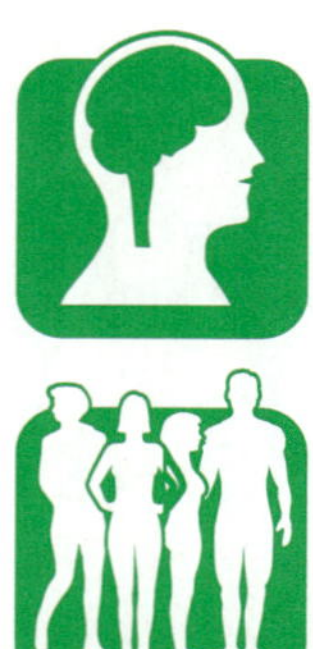

- **Epidemiology**

Mode of spread: HIV is transmitted by (a) inoculation with infected blood through transfusion of blood or blood products, sharing of needles by intravenous drug users, use of infected tatoo needles, accidental needle sticks, and contact with contaminated blood through open wounds and mucous membranes; (b) sexual contact (anal or vaginal intercourse); and (c) intrauterine or perinatal transmission or through breast milk.

Populations affected: Intravenous drug users, homosexuals and heterosexuals with multiple sex partners, prostitutes, newborns of HIV-positive mothers, and hemophiliacs, and other recipients of blood products and organ transplants before 1985 (when effective screening programs were instituted) are all at risk of contracting HIV infection.

Occurrence: HIV infection is prevalent in Africa and is an expanding epidemic worldwide. There is no seasonal incidence of disease.

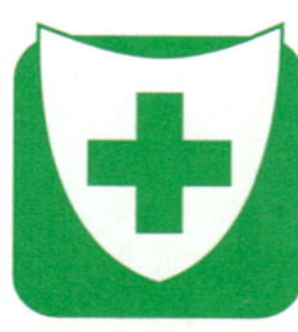

- **Prevention**

- Sexual transmission of HIV can be reduced by practicing safe monogamous sex.
- Use of sterile injection needles can also minimize spread.

Box 3.13

INDICATOR DISEASES OF ACQUIRED IMMUNODEFICIENCY SYNDROME (AIDS)*

Opportunistic Infections

Protozoal	Toxoplasmosis of the brain
	Cryptosporidiosis with diarrhea
	Isosporiasis with diarrhea
Fungal	Candidiasis of the esophagus, trachea, lungs
	Pneumocystis carinii pneumonia
	Cryptococcosis, extrapulmonary
	Histoplasmosis, disseminated
	Coccidioidomyocosis, disseminated
Viral	Cytomegalovirus disease
	Herpes simplex virus infection, persisting or disseminated
	Progressive multifocal leukoencephalopathy
Bacterial	*Mycobacterium avium* complex, disseminated
	Any "atypical" mycobacterial disease
	Extrapulmonary tuberculosis
	Salmonella septicemia, recurrent
	Multiple or recurrent pyogenic bacterial infections

Opportunistic Neoplasias

Kaposi's sarcoma
Primary lymphoma of the brain
Other non-Hodgkin's lymphomas

Others

HIV wasting syndrome
HIV encephalopathy
Lymphoid interstitial pneumonia

From Belshe RB, editor: *Textbook of human virology,* ed 2, St Louis, 1991, Mosby.
*Manifestations of human immunodeficiency virus (HIV) infection defining AIDS according to criteria of Centers for Disease Control.

- Screening of the blood supply, organ transplants, and clotting factors used by hemophiliacs for the presence of HIV has reduced transmission by these routes.
- Vaccines for prevention and treatment are in trials.

- **Treatment** Antiviral drugs, such as **azidothymidine** (AZT), dideoxyinosine (DDI), and dideoxycytidine (DDC), which are nucleotide analogues targeted at the reverse transcriptase, and saquinavir, targeted at the protease, delay the onset and severity of symptoms and decrease virus production and shedding. Resistance to single-drug therapy develops readily.

Human T-Lymphotropic Viruses (HTLV-1, HTLV-2, and HTLV-5) and Other Oncogenic Retroviruses

- **General features** Oncogenic retroviruses immortalize (transform) cells.

  The family members are differentiated from each other by the mechanism of transformation and thus the length of their latency period.

  1. The sarcoma viruses and acute leukemia viruses encode oncogenes that promote growth. They have a short latent period.
     - **Oncogenes** are growth promoting genes. The oncogene products resemble components of a growth factor cascade, for example, growth factor receptors, tyrosine kinases, or DNA binding proteins (see Table 3.22).

- These viruses are highly oncogenic.
- Many of these viruses are endogenous and can be transmitted vertically.
- There are no known human viruses that fit this description.

2. The leukemia viruses (HTLV) are replication competent and cannot transform cells in vitro.
   - There is a long latent period before cancer develops.
   - These viruses cause transformation by integrating into the host genome and turning on growth-stimulating genes.

- **Laboratory identification** Viral antigen is detected by immunologic methods.

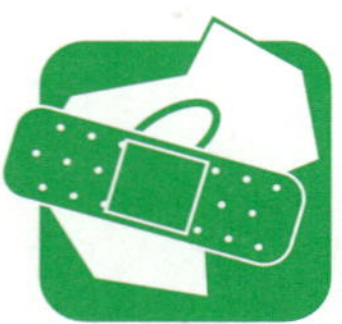

- **Human T-Lymphotropic virus 1 (HTLV-1)**

— ***Pathogenesis***

- The virus is cell associated.
- The virus is acquired by blood transfusion, sexual intercourse, or by breast feeding.
- The virus enters the blood stream and infects $CD4^+$ T helper and DTH cells.
- The virus may remain latent in T cells or replicate slowly for years.
- The viral tax protein transactivates the cellular genes for IL-2 and its receptor, thus promoting cell growth.
- Chromosomal aberrations and rearrangements during continued growth may produce leukemia.
- The virus also infects neurons.

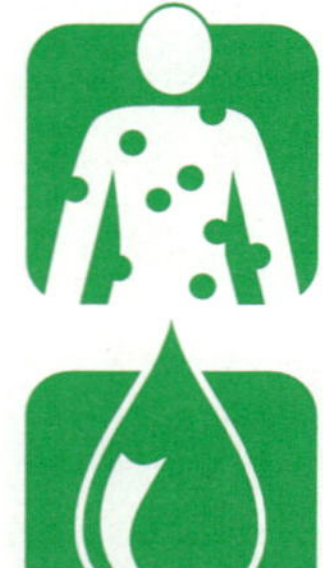

— ***Diseases*** HTLV-1 infection is usually asymptomatic but can progress to adult acute T-cell lymphocytic leukemia (ATLL).

1. ATLL
   - incubation period is long (30 years)
   - neoplasia of $CD4^+$ T helper cells, either acute or chronic
   - malignant cells resemble flowers (pleomorphic cells with lobulated nuclei)
   - elevated white cell count
   - skin rash occurs from T cells homing to the skin, similar to the Sezary syndrome
   - acute disease is usually fatal within 1 year of diagnosis

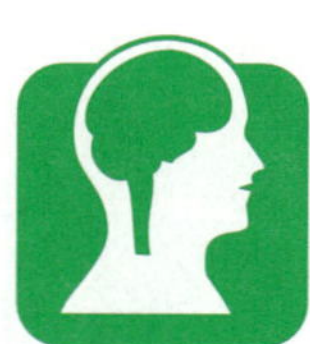

2. Tropical spastic paraparesis
   - a nononcologic neurologic disease

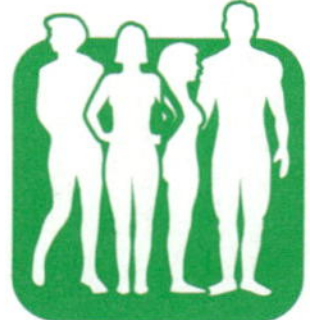

— ***Epidemiology***

Mode of spread: In Japan, transmission is by sexual contact in adults or through breast milk to children. In the United States, HTLV-1 is transmitted during IV drug use or by transfusion.

Occurrence: HTLV-1 disease is endemic in southern Japan, the Caribbean, and in the black population in the southeastern United States.

Table 3.25 *Comparative Features of Hepatitis Viruses*

	Hepatitis A	Hepatitis B	Hepatitis C	Hepatitis D	Hepatitis E
Common name	"Infectious"	"Serum"	"Non A Non B" post-transfusion	"Delta"	"Enteric Non A Non B"
Virus structure	Picornavirus Capsid, RNA	Hepadnavirus Envelope, DNA	Flavivirus Envelope, RNA	Envelope, circular RNA	Calicivirus-like Capsid, RNA
Transmission	Fecal-oral	Parenteral, sexual	Parenteral, sexual	Parenteral, sexual	Fecal-oral
Onset	Abrupt (varies)	Insidious (varies)	Insidious (varies)	Abrupt (varies)	Abrupt (varies)
Incubation period	15-50 days	45-160 days	14-180 days	15-64 days (*Requires HBV*)	15-50 days
Severity	Mild	Occasionally severe	Usually subclinical	*Co-infection* with HBV occasionally severe; *superinfection* with HBV often severe	Normal patients: mild; pregnant patients: severe
Mortality	<0.5%	1%-2%	0.5%-1%	High to very high	Normal patients: 1%-2%; pregnant patients: 20%
Chronicity/carrier state	No	Yes	Yes	Yes	No
Other disease associations	None	Primary hepatocellular carcinoma, cirrhosis	Primary hepatocellular carcinoma, cirrhosis	Cirrhosis, fulminant hepatitis	None
Laboratory diagnosis	Symptoms and anti-HAV IgM	Symptoms and serum levels of HBsAg, HBeAg, and anti-HBc IgM	Symptoms and anti-HCV ELISA	Anti-HDV ELISA	—

HAV, Hepatitis A virus; *HBsAg,* Hepatitis B surface antigen; *HBeAg;* hepatitis B e antigen; *anti-HBc,* anti-hepatitis B core; *HCV,* hepatitis C vius; *HDV,* hepatitis D virus.

— ***Prevention*** Practicing safe sex and screening the blood supply can help reduce infection.

— ***Treatment*** No treatment is available.

- **Endogenous retroviruses** Endogenous retroviruses are integrated in the host chromosome, are vertically transmitted, and are found in animals and humans. These incomplete retroviruses are part of the human chromosome.

Section 3.20 Hepatitis Viruses

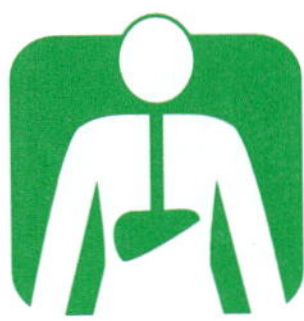

General Features (Table 3.25)

- The hepatitis viruses infect and damage the liver causing jaundice and release of liver enzymes.
- The specific nature of the virus and the disease differ for each virus.
- Hepatitis viruses A and E are transmitted by the fecal-oral route and cause acute disease.
- Hepatitis viruses B, C, and D are transmitted in blood and semen and have insidious onset of disease with the potential for chronic disease.

Hepatitis A Virus

General features

- Hepatitis A virus (HAV) is a picornavirus, renamed Enterovirus 72 (see Section 3.11 for structure and replication).
- It is extremely stable to environmental conditions and can persist in sewers and the GI tract.

Replication

- The virus interacts with a receptor on liver cells.
- It causes a slow steady-state infection with little or no CPE.

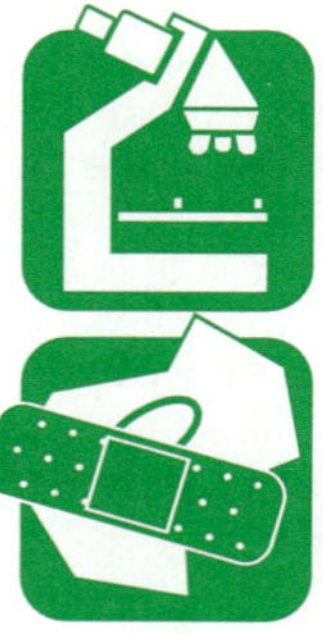

Laboratory diagnosis

- Hepatitis A virus infection is identified by the time course of symptoms and identification of the infected source.
- Anti-HAV IgM can be detected by ELISA or RIA in serum.

Pathogenesis

- HAV is ingested, probably replicates in the oropharynx and the intestinal epithelium, establishes a transient viremia, and infects hepatic parenchymal cells.
- The virus is produced, released into the bile, and shed into the stool 10 days before the start of symptoms.
- Liver damage probably results from immunopathologic mechanisms.

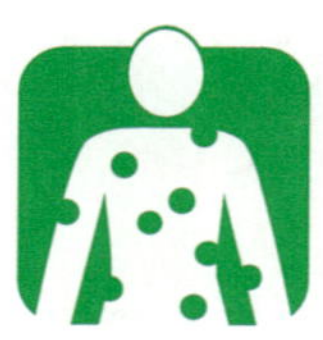

Disease (Infectious Hepatitis)

- Mild or asymptomatic infection occurs in children.
- *Sudden onset* hepatitis occurs in adults. The symptoms occur abruptly 15 to 50 days after exposure and increase for 4 to 6 days before the icteric (jaundice) phase.
- The symptoms wane during the jaundice phase.
- Complete recovery occurs in 99% of the cases.
- Fulminant hepatitis occurs in 1 to 3 persons per 1000 infected.

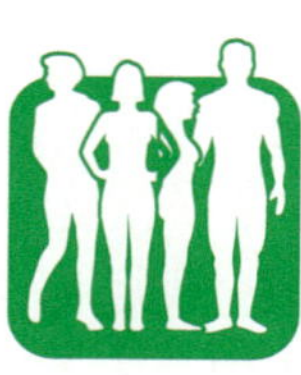

Epidemiology

Mode of spread: The virus is transmitted by the fecal-oral route through ingestion of contaminated water and food, especially shellfish (filter feeders concentrate the virus). The virus can be spread by food handlers, daycare workers, and children.

Populations affected: People living in overcrowded, unsanitary conditions are at risk. Daycare centers are a major source of spread of the virus.

Occurrence: The virus occurs worldwide and there is no seasonal incidence.

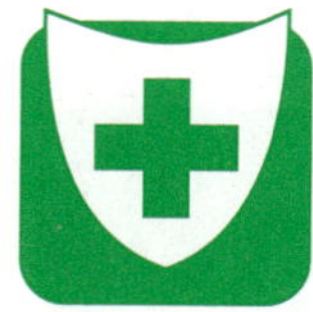

Prevention

- Good hygienic practices and avoidance of contaminated food and water, especially uncooked shellfish, can help prevent infection.
- Chlorine treatment of water kills the virus.
- A new inactivated vaccine was approved in 1995 for travelers to endemic regions.

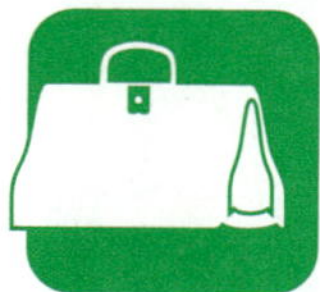

Treatment **Passive antibody** protects contacts.

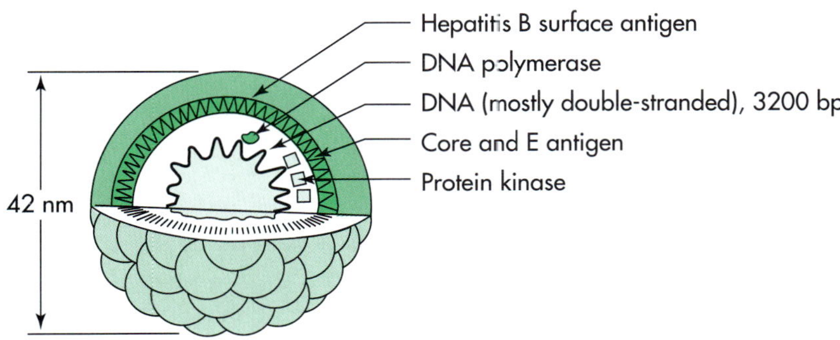

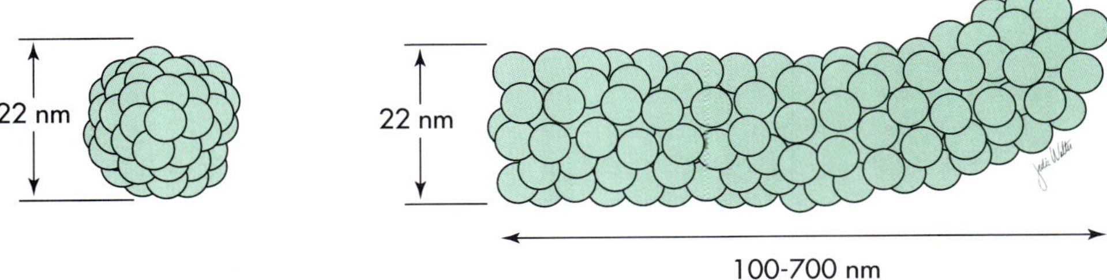

Fig. 3.39 Hepatitis B virus (Dane particle) *(above)* and HBsAg particles *(below)*. The HBsAg particles contain different forms of the hepatitis B surface antigen but no viral DNA and are not infectious. HBsAg particles were used as the first vaccine for hepatitis B.

Hepatitis B Virus (HBV)

General features (Fig. 3.39)

- HBV is a small, **enveloped DNA virus**. The genome is small (3200 bases), circular, and consists of partially double-stranded DNA.
- The virion (also called the **Dane particle**) is 42 nm in diameter and is very resistent to ether, low pH, and moderate heating.
- The virion contains reverse transcriptase and a protein kinase surrounded by the core antigen (**HBcAg**).
- The envelope contains the L, M, and S glycoprotein forms of the hepatitis B surface antigen (**HBsAg**).
- HBsAg is also present on spherical and filamentous particles.
- Presence of HBeAg in serum indicates the presence of an infectious virus.
- The hepatitis B e antigen (**HBeAg**) is a minor component of the virion.
- The virus replicates through an RNA intermediate using its reverse transcriptase.
- The genome can integrate into the host genome.
- The virus displays strict liver tropism.
- Infected cells release large amounts of HBsAg particles, which lack DNA.

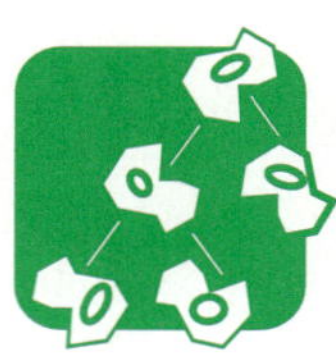

- **Replication (Fig. 3.40)**
    - The virus attaches to hepatocytes via HBsAg.
    - After penetration, the partial DNA strand is completed to form a circle and is delivered to the nucleus.
    - Transcription is controlled by cellular factors.
    - DNA is transcribed into three major and two minor classes of RNA.
    - Replication of the genome occurs in the cytoplasm.
    - A viral RNA that is longer than the complete full-length RNA is the template for reverse transcriptase production of an RNA-DNA circle.
    - The RNA-DNA genome is enveloped by HBsAg-containing membranes.
    - The RNA is degraded, yielding partially double-stranded DNA in the virion.
    - The virions are released by exocytosis.

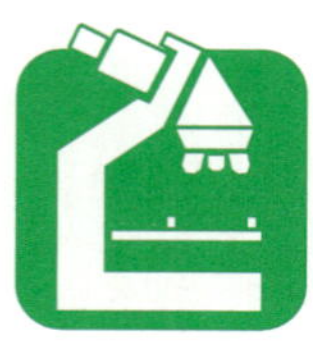

- **Laboratory identification (Fig. 3.41 and Table 3.26)** Hepatitis B virus infection is diagnosed by clinical symptoms and the presence of liver enzymes in the blood.

    Serology defines the course and nature of the disease. The presence of HBeAg is the best correlate for the presence of infectious virus. The continued presence of HBeAg or HBsAg and a lack of antibodies to these antigens signals a chronic infection. A recent acute infection is indicated by IgM antibodies to HBcAg.

- **Pathogenesis**
    - HBV is acquired from contaminated blood products, semen, vaginal secretions, and mother's milk.
    - The virus replicates in hepatocytes with little CPE and continues to do so for a long period without damage to the liver.
    - HBV integrates into host chromatin and can remain latent.
    - Antibody to HBV can block infection.
    - The incubation period is 45 days or longer and corresponds to the development of a cell-mediated immune response.
    - Cell-mediated immunity is responsible for both the symptoms and the resolution of the disease.
    - HBV can cause acute, chronic, or asymptomatic illness, depending on the T cell immune response.
    - A mild immune response results in mild symptoms with incomplete resolution of the disease and leads to chronic infection.
    - Infants with immature cell-mediated immunity have mild disease but become carriers.
    - HBsAg in the serum will bind antibody, form immune complexes that inactivate the antibody, and lead to hypersensitivity reactions.
    - Fulminant infection, activation of a chronic infection, or coinfection with the delta agent can cause permanent liver damage and cirrhosis.

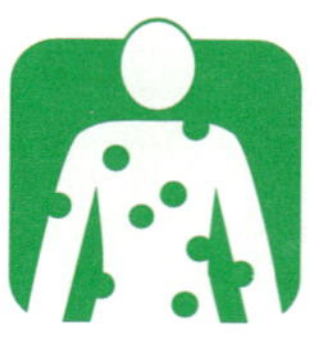

- **Diseases (Fig. 3.42) (Serum Hepatitis)** Acute infection in children is mild and asymptomatic. In adults, clinical illness occurs in 25% of the individuals infected.

    1. Acute hepatitis
        - It has a long incubation period (*insidious onset*).

Text continued on p. 234.

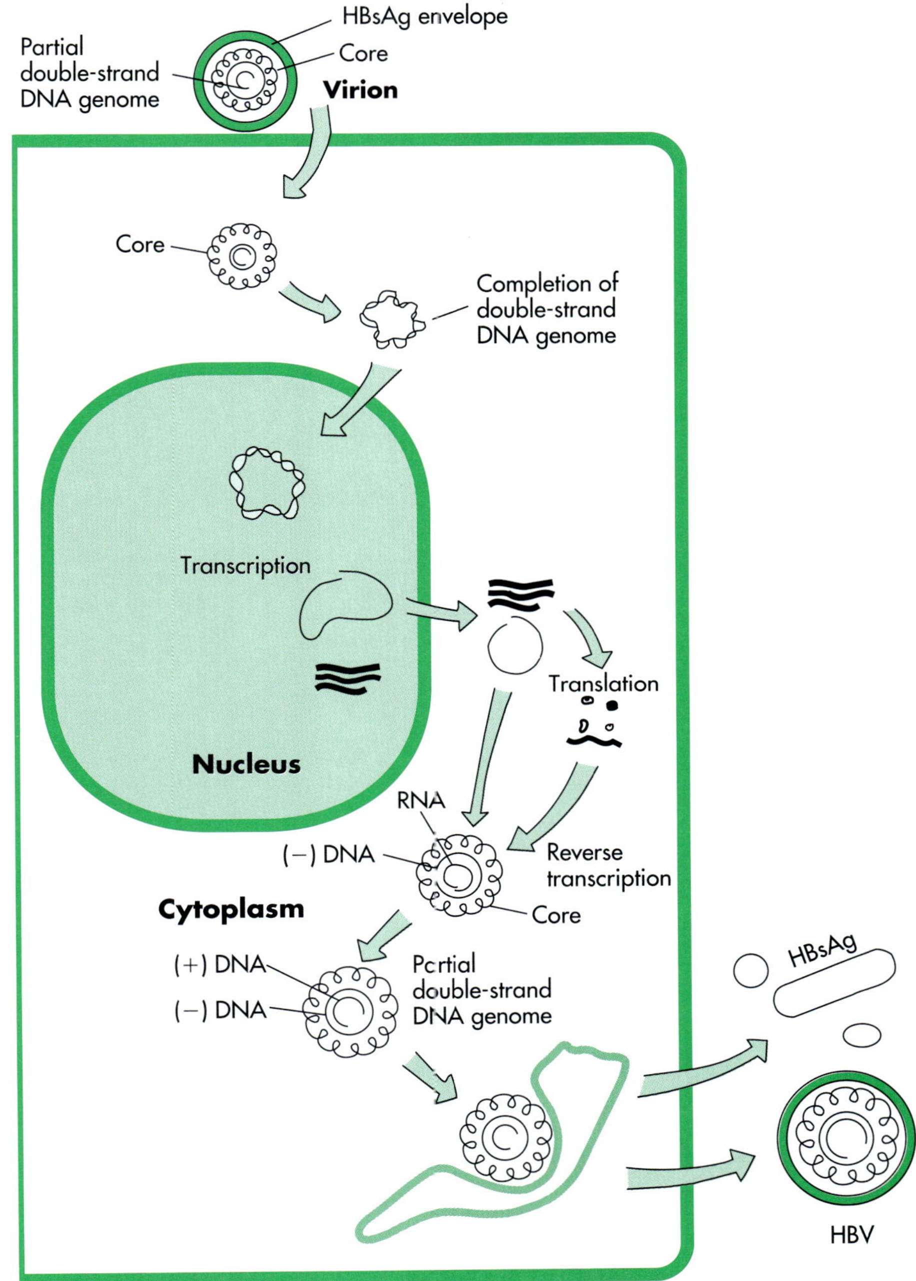

Fig. 3.40 Proposed pathway for replication of hepatitis B virus. After entry into the hepatocyte and uncoating of the nucleocapsid core, the partially double-stranded DNA genome is completed by enzymes in the core and then delivered to the nucleus. Transcription of the genome produces four mRNAs including an mRNA larger than the genome (3500 bases). The mRNA moves to the cytoplasm and is translated into protein. Core proteins assemble around the 3500-base mRNA and (–) DNA is synthesized by reverse transcriptase in the core. The RNA is then degraded as a (+) DNA strand is synthesized. The core is enveloped before completion of the (+) DNA and then released by exocytosis.

A

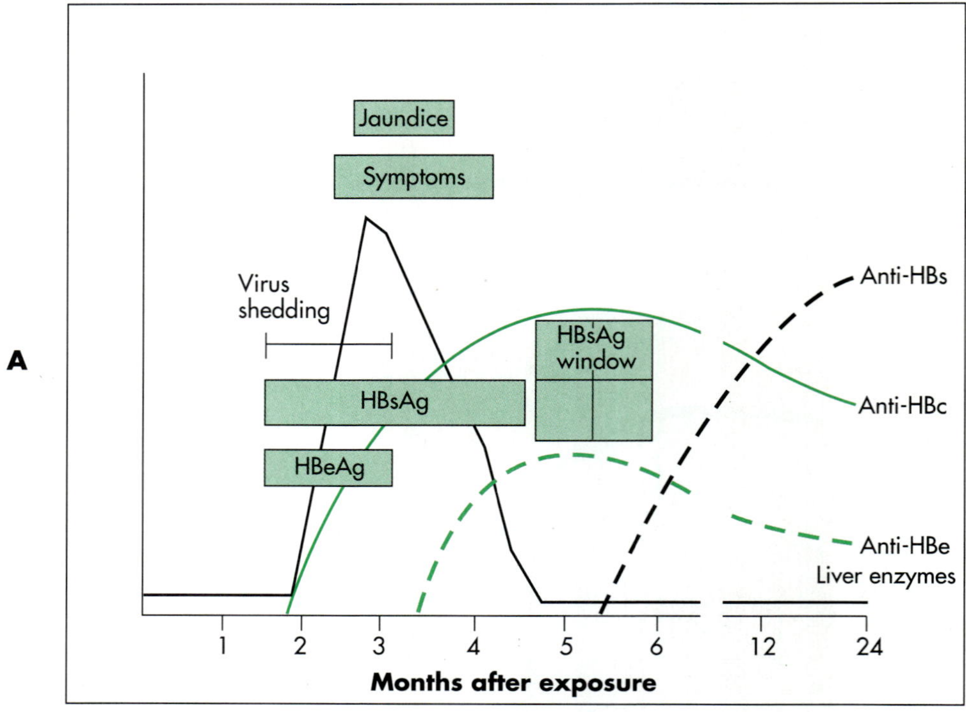

B

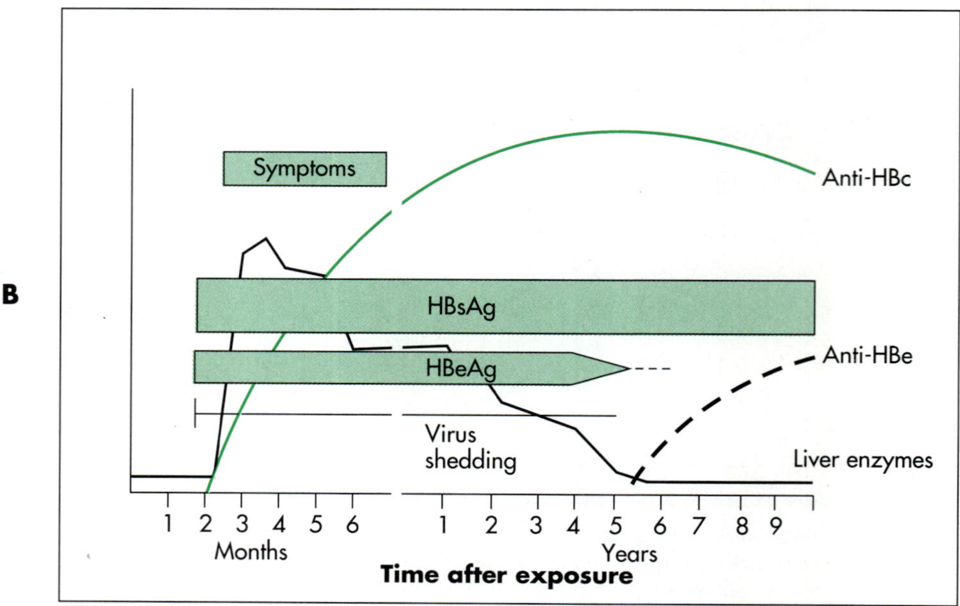

Fig. 3.41 **A,** The serologic events associated with a typical course of acute hepatitis B disease. HBeAg is present with virus. Antibodies to HBsAg or HBcAg will be detected when these antigens cease to be produced. The HBsAg window occurs with the decrease in HBsAg and before anti-HBsAg detection. *HBeAg,* Hepatitis B e antigen; *Anti-HBsAg,* antibody to HBsAg; *Anti-HBc,* antibody to hepatitis B core antigen; *Anti-HBe,* antibody to HBeAg. **B,** Development of the chronic hepatitis B virus carrier state. Note that HBsAg is continually synthesized and that anti-HBsAg is not detectable. Also, HBeAg and virus are present. (B *redrawn from* Hoofnagle JH: Ann Rev Med *32:1, 1981.)*

Table 3.26 *Expected Hepatitis B Virus Prevalence in Various Population Groups*

Group	Prevalence of Serologic Markers of HBV Infection	
	HBsAg (%) (Chronic)	All Markers (%)
High Risk		
Immigrants and refugees from areas of high HBV endemicity	13	80-85
Clients in institutions for mentally retarded persons	10-20	35-80
Users of illicit parenteral drugs	7	60-80
Homosexually active males	6	35-80
Household contacts of HBV carriers	3-6	30-60
Patients on hemodialysis units	3-10	20-80
Intermediate Risk		
Prisoners (male)	1-8	10-80
Staff of institutions for the mentally retarded	1	10-25
Health care workers with frequent blood contact	1-2	15-30
Low Risk		
Health care workes with no (or infrequent) blood contact	0-3	3-10
Healthy adults (volunteer blood donors)	0-3	3-5

From Hoofnagle JH: *Lab Med,* 14:705, 1983.

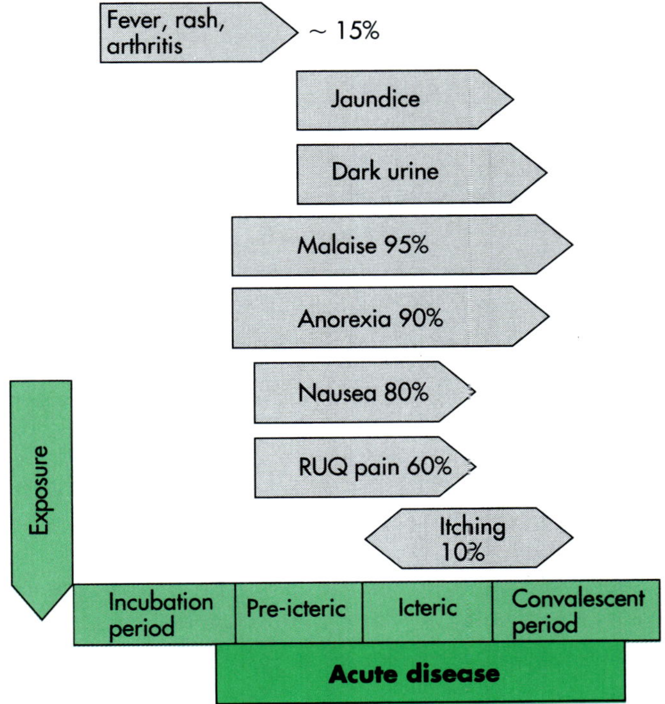

Fig. 3.42 Symptoms of typical acute viral hepatitis B infection are correlated with the four clinical periods of this disease. *(Redrawn from Hoofnagle JH:* Lab Med, *14:705, 1983.)*

- Prodrome consists of fever, malaise, and anorexia.
- Symptoms include nausea, vomiting, abdominal upset, fever, and chills, followed by the classic icteric signs of liver damage.
- Fulminant hepatitis occurs in 1% of the patients, with severe liver damage accompanied by ascites fluid and bleeding, and may be fatal. It is caused by coinfection or superinfection with hepatitis D virus.

2. Chronic hepatitis
   - 5% to 10% of HBV infections become chronic, usually after mild or asymptomatic infection.
   - 10% of these patients develop cirrhosis and liver damage.
   - Patients are at high risk for developing primary hepatocellular carcinoma.

3. Primary hepatocellular carcinoma (PHC)
   - HBV is a co-factor for PHC.
   - HBV is integrated into the neoplastic cells, and they express viral antigens.
   - Integration may stimulate cell growth.
   - The latent period between infection and appearance of cancer ranges from 9 to 35 years.
   - The disease is usually fatal.

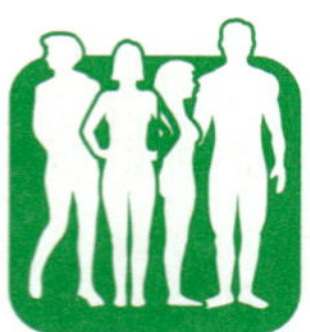

- **Epidemiology**

Mode of spread:

- The virus is shed during asymptomatic and chronic periods.
- HBV is less sensitive to detergents and disinfection than are other enveloped viruses.
- *The virus is present in blood, semen, vaginal secretions, saliva, and mother's milk*. The infection is transmitted via transfusions, sharing of needles, sexual contact, and by nursing of babies.

Populations affected: Groups at risk for acquiring HBV infection are household contacts of HBV carriers, sexual partners of carriers, hemodialysis patients, recipients of pooled plasma products, healthcare workers exposed to blood, and babies born to carriers.

Occurrence: The virus occurs worldwide. There is no seasonal incidence.

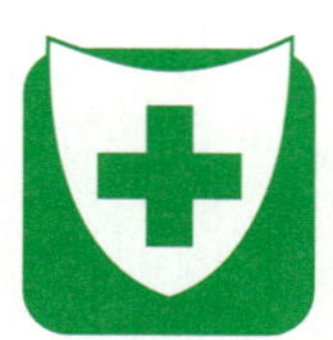

- **Prevention**
  - Avoidance of high-risk behavior can decrease the chances of infection.
  - Screening of the blood supply has decreased transmission through blood products.
  - **Vaccine:** A **subunit vaccine** consisting of HBsAg prepared by genetic engineering in yeast is now available.
- **Treatment** Supportive care is used to treat infections.

Hepatitis C Virus

- **General features**
  - Hepatitis C virus is a flavivirus with a (+) **RNA genome.**
  - *It causes 90% of the cases of non-A non-B hepatitis (NANBH).*
  - It is a major cause of **posttransfusion hepatitis.**

- **Laboratory identification**
  - Hepatitis C virus infection can be diagnosed by serology (ELISA). However, an antibody is not always present in viremic patients.
  - Virion RNA can be detected in the serum by PCR.

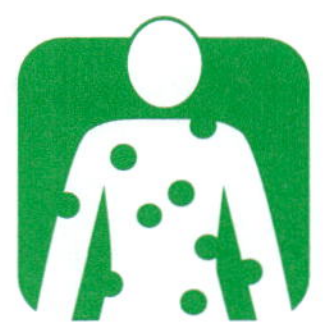

- **Diseases** Viremia is detected 1 to 3 weeks after transfusion with infected blood. Antibody is not protective.
  1. Acute infection
     - Viremia lasts 4 to 6 weeks.
     - Symptoms are similar to those of HAV or HBV infection.
     - The inflammatory response is less and symptoms are milder.
  2. Chronic infection
     - Viremia can last more than 10 years.
     - Chronic infection is common and leads to acute disease and cirrhosis.

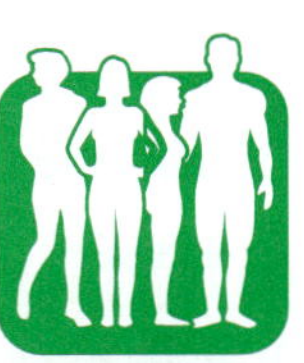

- **Epidemiology** The epidemiologic features of hepatitis C virus infection are the same as those for hepatitis B virus infection.
- **Prevention** Infection can be prevented by avoiding high-risk behavior. (See HBV.)

- **Treatment** Recombinant *alpha interferon* and supportive therapy are used for treatment.

Hepatitis D Virus (Delta Agent)

- **General features**
  - Fifteen million individuals are infected with hepatitis D virus worldwide.
  - The virus causes 40% of the cases of *fulminant hepatitis.*
  - It is a defective satellite virus that can replicate only in HBV-infected cells.
  - *HBsAg is needed for packaging the virus.*
  - Hepatitis D virus has a small, single-stranded circular RNA genome (1700 bases).
  - The virion is small and contains the genome and the small (predominant) or large form of the delta antigen, surrounded by an HBsAg-containing envelope.

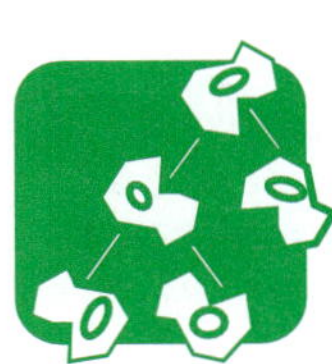

- **Replication**
  - Hepatitis D virus binds and enters hepatocytes similarly to HBV (because of the presence of HBsAg).
  - The genome is transcribed and replicated in the nucleus, using small delta agent protein (RNA-binding protein).
  - The delta antigen gene mutates, causing production of the large delta antigen, which limits virus replication and cell destruction.
  - The genome, delta antigen, and HBsAg combine and are released from the cell.

- **Laboratory identification** Detection of the delta antigen or antibodies to the delta antigen in serum using ELISA or RIA identifies hepatitis D virus infection.

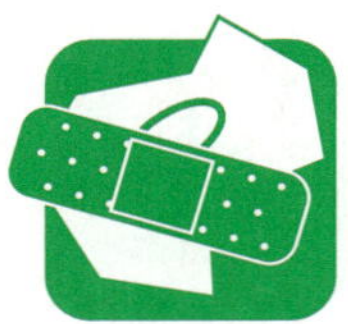

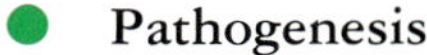

- **Pathogenesis**
  - HDV is acquired by the same means as HBV.
  - The virus replicates in liver cells with active HBV infection.
  - If HDV infects a cell already infected with HBV (*superinfection*), the progression is more rapid and severe than if there is *coinfection* with HBV.
  - Replication results in cytotoxicity and liver damage.
  - Persistent infection may occur in HBV carriers.

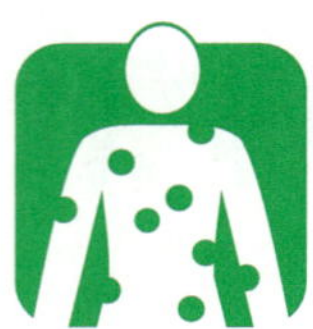

- **Diseases**
  - HDV increases the severity of HBV infections.
  - Fulminant hepatitis is more likely with HDV than with other hepatitis viruses.

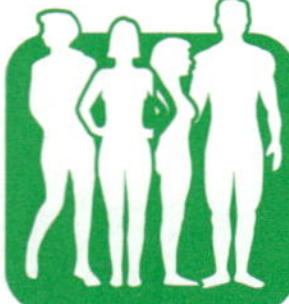

- **Epidemiology**
  - The epidemiologic features for HDV are similar to those for HBV.
  - The agent has worldwide distribution. It is endemic in southern Italy, the Amazon basin, Africa, and the Middle East.
  - Epidemics may occur in North America and Western Europe, especially in *intravenous drug users.*

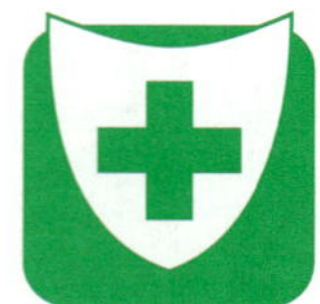

- **Prevention**
  - Immunization with HBV vaccine (preventing infection with the cofactor) reduces the incidence of HDV infection.
  - Limiting exposure to HDV results in less transmission.
- **Treatment** No treatment exists for HDV infection.

Hepatitis E Virus (HEV)

- Hepatitis E virus is spread by the fecal-oral route.
- It resembles calicivirus or Norwalk agent in size.
- It is most prevalent in the developing nations.
- HEV causes acute disease similar to HAV disease.
- The mortality from HEV infection is 1% to 2%, rising to 20% in pregnant women.

Section 3.21 Unconventional Slow Viruses (Prions)

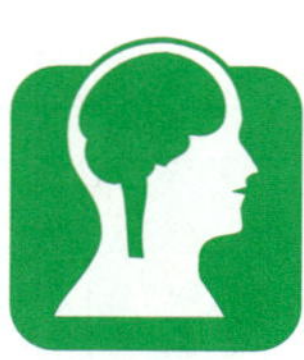

General Features

- Prions are filterable infectious agents that do not have a virion structure or a genome.
- They do not elicit an immune response.
- Prions are very resistant to inactivation by disinfectants, proteases, heat, and radiation.
- Prions consist of aggregates of protease-resistant glycoproteins.
- Scrapie-associated fibrils (SAF) in the brains of infected sheep contain prions and are infectious.
- The scrapie prion protein PrP^{Sc} is similar to a cellular protein PrP^{c}.

Laboratory Identification

- The diagnosis of a slow virus infection is made on the basis of clinical symptoms, and is confirmed by histopathology of the brain.

- Histologic examination of the brain at autopsy shows spongy, vesiculated cells with no inflammation.

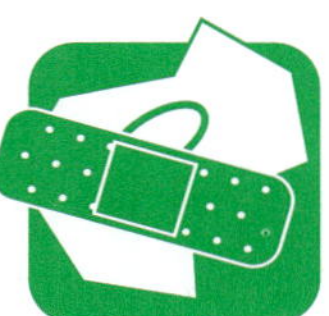

Pathogenesis

- Prions do not produce CPE in vitro.
- The diseases have a long incubation period.
- Prions cause vacuolation of neurons (spongiform), amyloid-like plaques, and gliosis.
- The agents are not antigenic, there is no inflammation, and no immune response is elicited.

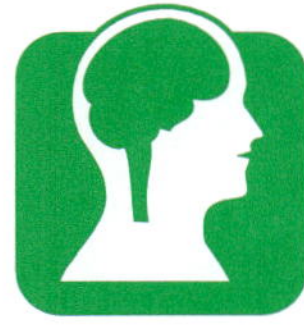

Diseases

- Slow viruses cause progressive degenerative neurologic disease.
- The incubation period is long (1 to 30 yrs), but death occurs rapidly after onset of symptoms (within 4 months).
- Symptoms include loss of muscle control, shivering, tremors, and dementia.
- Human slow virus diseases include kuru, Creutzfeldt-Jakob disease (CJD), and Gerstmann-Straussler-Scheinker syndrome (GSS).
- Animal diseases include scrapie (in sheep and mink).

Epidemiology

Mode of spread: CJD is transmitted by injection, transplantation of infected tissue, or by contact with contaminated medical devices. CJD and GSS *may be inherited.* Kuru is acquired by consumption of or contact with infected tissue.

Populations affected:

- Surgeons and patients undergoing transplant or brain surgery are at risk of acquiring CJD or GSS. Family members may inherit the disease.
- Women and children of the Fore tribe of New Guinea were afflicted with Kuru.

Occurrence: CJD and GSS occur worldwide. Kuru is confined to New Guinea.

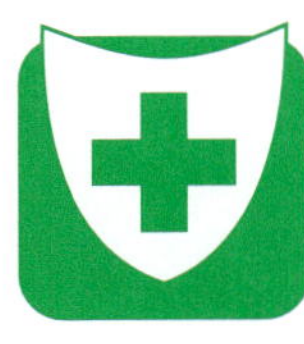

Prevention

- Disinfection of neurosurgical tools and electrodes in 5% hypochlorite solution (bleach) or 1.0 M sodium hydroxide or autoclaving at 15 psi for 1 hour can prevent transmission of GSS and CJD.
- Cessation of the cannibalistic ritual has caused Kuru to be almost extinct.

Treatment

No treatment is available.

Section 3.22 Summary of Viruses and Correlations

A summary of viruses and correlations is presented in Tables 3.27 through 3.30.

Table 3.27 *DNA Virus Replication*

Virus	Structure	Replication
Parvovirus	Naked capsid virion Single-stranded DNA	Dependent on host Requires growing cells Replicates in nucleus
Papovavirus	Naked capsid virion Circular DNA	Replicates in nucleus Early genes: growth-promoting proteins, e.g., T antigen of SV40 and E7 and E8 proteins of HPV 16 and HPV 18 Late genes: structural proteins
Adenovirus	Naked capsid virion with fibers Linear DNA with proteins at S'ends	Fiber proteins determine tissue tropism Replicates in nucleus Early genes: polymerase, growth-promoting proteins Late genes: structural proteins
Herpesvirus	Enveloped with icosadeltahedral nucleocapsid DNA	Glycoproteins define tissue tropism Replicates and acquires envelope in nucleus Immediate early genes: DNA-binding proteins Early genes: polymerase, scavenging enzymes, e.g., thymidine kinase Late genes: structural proteins Latency in specific cell types: HSV and VZV in neurons, EBV in B cells, CMV in monocytes and T cells
Poxvirus	Complex, enveloped Linear DNA	Replicates in cytoplasm Encodes DNA and RNA polymerase Complex structure

Table 3.28 *RNA Virus Replication**

Virus	Structure	Replication
Picornavirus	Naked capsid virion, (+) RNA	Canyon on capsid interacts with ICAM-like receptors Polyprotein translated from genome Polyprotein proteolytically cleaved to viral proteins (–) RNA template used to replicate virus Capsid assembled, then filled with genome Released by cell lysis
Togavirus	Enveloped (+) RNA Icosahedral capsid	Glycoproteins bind cell-surface receptors Enter by receptor-mediated endocytosis Early proteins (polymerase) translated from genome (–) RNA template used to replicate virus and transcribe, smaller late mRNA Late proteins: structural Virion assembled at plasma membrane, shed by budding
Flavivirus	Enveloped (+) RNA	Glycoproteins bind cell-surface receptors Antibody facilitates entry into macrophages Polyprotein translated from genome Virion assembles at cell membrane
Rhabdovirus	Enveloped (–) RNA Matrix protein Polymerase	Glycoprotein binds to cell receptor Receptor-mediated endocytosis Virion polymerase transcribes mRNAs from genome for each protein A (+) RNA template is used to replicate genome Polymerase components associate with genome forming the nucleocapsid Viral glycoprotein processed by host cell system Nucleocapsid associates with matrix proteins associated with glycoprotein on plasma membrane Virus buds from cell
Paramyxovirus	Enveloped (–) RNA Matrix protein Polymerase	Glycoproteins include viral attachment and fusion proteins Enters cell by fusion Replication similar to that of rhabdovirus
Orthomyxovirus	Enveloped (–) segmented RNA Matrix proteins Polymerase	HA binds to sialic acid on cell surface Receptor-mediated endocytosis Transcription and replication in nucleus Individual gene segments encode proteins Assembly in cytoplasm and at plasma membrane Budding releases virus
Reovirus	Double capsid Double-stranded RNA (segmented) Polymerase	Viral attachment protein binds specific receptor Receptor-mediated endocytosis Uncoating of outer capsid Transcription of (–) RNA strand by capsid proteins (+) RNAs coalesce and are enclosed in inner capsid (+/–) RNA produced Late proteins surround core capsid Cells lyse, virus released
Retrovirus	Enveloped Capsid contains 2 copies of (+) RNA, 2 tRNA, Reverse transcriptase	Glycoprotein binding to receptor determines tropism Fusion Reverse transcription of genome to cDNA cDNA is double-stranded and circularized Enters nucleus and integrates into chromosome Transcribed as host gene to produce viral mRNAs which produce polyproteins (gag, pol, env) Genome associates with gag polyproteins and glycoprotein-modified membrane Virus buds from cell surface Gag protein cleaved by viral protease to form nucleocapsid

*All RNA viruses encode an RNA-dependent RNA polymerase.
HA, Hemagglutinin.

Table 3.29 *DNA Viruses*

Classification			Structure		
Family	**DNA Viruses (Name)**	**Disease(s)**	**Size (S, M, L)**	**Enveloped or Naked**	**Genome**
Parvoviridae	B-19	(Fifth disease) Erythema infectiosum	S	Naked	SS DNA
Papovaviridae	Human papilloma virus	Warts; associated with cervical cancer	S	Naked	DS circular DNA
	JC virus	Progressive multifocal leukoencephalopathy	S	Naked	DS DNA
	SV-40	No human disease	S	Naked	DS DNA
Hepadnaviridae	Hepatitis B virus	"Serum" hepatitis	S	Enveloped	DS circular DNA, partial circle, RNA intermediate
Adenoviridae	Adenovirus Adenovirus	Respiratory conjunctivitis Diarrhea	M	Naked	DS linear DNA, proteins at 5′ ends
Herpesviridae	Herpes simplex virus-1	Gingivostomatitis, keratoconjunctivitis, encephalitis, disseminated neonatal disease (latent-recurrent)	L	Enveloped (w) Internal capsid (icosadeltahedral)	DS DNA
	Herpes simplex virus-2	Gingivostomatitis, keratoconjunctivitis, encephalitis, disseminated neonatal disease (latent-recurrent)	L	Enveloped (w) Internal capsid	DS DNA

Pathogenesis	Epidemiology		Means of Control		Laboratory Diagnosis
Target Organ	**Populations at Risk**	**Transmission**	**Vaccine (N = None, L = Live, K = Killed)**	**Antiviral Drug (N = None)**	
Erythroid precursors	Anemics in aplastic crisis	Respiratory spread	N	N	None
Skin, epithelium	Ubiquitous	By contact	N	N	DNA probe analysis
Respiratory organs; demyelination in CNS Prototype oncogenic virus in hamsters	Ubiquitous		N	N	DNA probe analysis
Liver	Blood and organ recipients, drug addicts, sexually active individuals, children of chronically infected mothers	Through blood and semen	Subunit vaccine (Hb_sAg)	N	Serology
Lungs, eyes	Ubiquitous	Respiratory route, contact, fecal-oral route	K	N	Antigen assays: ELISA, IF; cell culture isolation
Mucoepithelium: skin, mouth, oropharynx, eyes; CNS; genitalia	Mild disease: ubiquitous; serious disease: neonates and immunocompromised individuals	By contact	N	Acyclovir, famciclovir, valacyclovir Ara A	Cell culture isolation; CPE: syncytia, Cowdry type A inclusion bodies; IF, EIA, ELISA; DNA probe analysis
Mucoepithelium: skin, mouth, oropharynx, eyes; CNS; genitalia	Mild disease: ubiquitous; serious disease: neonates and immunocompromised individuals	By contact	N	Acyclovir, famciclovir, valacyclovir Ara A	Cell culture isolation; CPE: syncytia, Cowdry type A inclusion bodies; IF, EIA, ELISA; DNA probe analysis

Continued.

Table 3.29 *DNA Viruses—cont'd*

Classification			Structure		
Family	**DNA Viruses (Name)**	**Disease(s)**	**Size (S, M, L)**	**Enveloped or Naked**	**Genome**
	Varicella-zoster virus	Primary: chicken pox Recurrent: shingles (pneumonia)	L	Enveloped (w) Internal capsid	DS DNA
	Epstein-Barr virus	Infectious mononucleosis; associated with African Burkitt's lymphoma; nasopharyngeal carcinoma	L	Enveloped Internal capsid	DS DNA
	Cytomegalovirus	Cytomegalic inclusion disease; mononucleosis; opportunistic infection	L	Enveloped Internal capsid	DS DNA
	Human herpesvirus	Roseola (exanthem subitum)	L	Enveloped Internal capsid	DS DNA
Poxviridae	Poxvirus Variola virus	Smallpox	L	Enveloped complex virus	DS linear DNA
	Vaccinia virus	Vaccine virus Recombinant Vaccine vector	L		
	Molluscum contagiosum virus	Molluscum contagiosum	L		

Pathogenesis	Epidemiology		Means of Control		Laboratory Diagnosis
Target Organ	**Populations at Risk**	**Transmission**	**Vaccine (N = None, L = Live, K = Killed)**	**Antiviral Drug (N = None)**	
CNS, skin	Ubiquitous; mild disease in children; serious disease in adults	Respiratory spread	L Passive (VZIG)	Acyclovir, famciclovir valacyclovir	IF, EIA, ELISA
B Lymphocytes; oral epithelium	Mild disease in children; more severe disease in teens and adults; lymphoma/leukemialike disease in T cell immunocompromised individuals	By saliva	N	N	Heterophile antibody; Downey (Atypical) lymphocytes; serology for specific antigens
Lymphocytes, secretory organs, CNS, eye, GI tract	Neonates of infected mothers; transfusion and transplant patients; immunocompromised individuals	All body secretions	N	Ganciclovir, foscarnet	Cell culture isolation; owl's eye inclusion bodies; IF; ELISA DNA probe analysis
Lymphocytes	Children (ubiquitous)	Respiratory	N	N	From symptoms
Skin		Contact			
Skin	Animal handlers	Animal contact			

Table 3.30 *RNA Viruses*

Classification			Structure		
Family	**RNA Viruses (Name)**	**Disease(s)**	**Size (S, M, L)**	**Enveloped or Naked**	**Genome**
Picornaviridae	Poliovirus	Asymptomatic; aseptic meningitis; paralytic polio	S	Naked	(+) SS RNA
	Coxsackievirus A	Hand-foot-and-mouth disease, herpangina, aseptic meningitis, rash	S	Naked	(+) SS RNA
	Coxsackievirus B	Myocarditis of newborn, pleurodynia, Bornholm's disease	S	Naked	(+) SS RNA
	Echovirus	Aseptic meningitis, fever, rash	S	Naked	(+) SS RNA
	Rhinovirus	Common cold	S	Naked	(+) SS RNA
	Hepatitis A virus (enterovirus 72)	Infectious hepatitis	S	Naked	(+) SS RNA
Togaviridae	Rubella virus	German measles; teratogenic for neonate	S	Enveloped	(+) SS RNA
	Venezuelan equine encephalitis virus	Influenza-like; encephalitis	S	Enveloped	(+) SS RNA
	Eastern equine encephalitis virus	Influenza-like; encephalitis	S	Enveloped	(+) SS RNA
	Western equine encephalitis virus	Influenza-like; encephalitis	S	Enveloped	(+) SS RNA
Flaviviridae	Dengue virus	Dengue, DHF/DSS, breakbone fever	S	Enveloped	(+) SS RNA
	Yellow fever virus	Yellow fever	S	Enveloped	(+) SS RNA
	St. Louis encephalitis virus	Influenza-like; encephalitis	S	Enveloped	(+) SS RNA
Paramyxoviridae	Measles virus	Measles: rash and cough, conjunctivitis, coryza	L	Enveloped	(–) SS RNA
	Mumps virus	Mumps	L	Enveloped	(–) SS RNA
	Parainfluenza virus	Cold, croup, pneumonia, bronchiolitis	L	Enveloped	(–) SS RNA
	Respiratory syncytial virus	Cold, bronchiolitis, pneumonia (infants)	L	Enveloped	(–) SS RNA
Orthomyxoviridae	Influenza A virus	Influenza, pneumonia (viral and bacterial)	M	Enveloped	(–) segmented RNA
	Influenza B virus	Influenza	M	Enveloped	(–) segmented RNA
Rhabdoviridae	Rabies virus	Rabies	M	Enveloped	(–) SS RNA

Pathogenesis	Epidemiology		Means of Control		Laboratory Diagnosis
Target Organ	**Populations at Risk**	**Transmission**	**Vaccine (N = None, L = Live, K = Killed)**	**Antiviral Drug (N = None)**	
Oropharynx, CNS, muscle	Nonvaccinated individuals	Fecal-oral route	L: Sabin K: Salk	N	Isolation: cell culture (feces)
Oral mucosa, skin, CNS	Ubiquitous; children	Fecal-oral and respiratory routes	N	N	
Muscle, skin	Ubiquitous; children	Fecal-oral and respiratory routes	N	N	
	Ubiquitous; children and infants	Fecal-oral and respiratory routes			
Nose	All individuals	Respiratory route, contact	N	N	
Liver		Fecal-oral route	K	N	Serology
Viremia, CNS		*Aedes* and *Culex* mosquito; host: rodents	N	N	
Viremia, CNS		*Aedes* mosquito; host: birds	N	N	
Viremia, CNS		*Culex* mosquito; host: birds	N	N	
Viremia, skin, neonate	Children, neonates	Respiratory route	L: (MMR)	N	
Viremia, endothelium	Tropical regions	*Aedes* mosquito; host: humans, monkeys	N	N	
Viremia, liver	Tropical regions, urban and jungle	*Aedes* mosquito; host: humans, monkeys	L	N	
Viremia, CNS	Forest and city dwellers	*Culex* mosquito; host: birds	N	N	
Lung, skin, CNS	Nonvaccinated individuals	Respiratory route	L: (MMR)	N	
Glands	Nonvaccinated individuals	Respiratory route	L: (MMR)	N	
Lung	Young children	Respiratory route	N	N	Isolation; hemagglutination, IF
Lung	Infants, immunocompromised individuals	Respiratory route	N	Aerosol ribavirin	
Lung	Epidemics and pandemics; children and elderly	Respiratory route	K	Amantadine, rimantadine	Hemagglutination, ELISA
Lung	Epidemics	Respiratory route	K	N	
Brain		Animal bite	K Vaccine is used for treatment		IF on biopsy, Negri bodies

Continued.

Table 3.30 *RNA Viruses—cont'd*

Classification			Structure		
Family	**RNA Viruses (Name)**	**Disease(s)**	**Size (S, M, L)**	**Enveloped or Naked**	**Genome**
Filoviridae	Marburg virus	African hemorrhagic fever	M	Enveloped	(–) SS RNA
	Ebola virus	African hemorrhagic fever	M	Enveloped	(–) SS RNA
Miscellaneous hepatitis viruses	Hepatitis C virus	Hepatitis	S	Enveloped	(+) SS RNA
	Hepatitis D	Hepatitis	S	Hepatitis B surface antigen	RNA; requires HBV as cofactor
	Hepatitis E	Hepatitis	S	Naked capsid	(+) SS RNA
Reoviridae	Rotavirus	Gastroenteritis	M	Naked double capsid	DS segmented RNA
Retroviridae	Human T-lymphotropic virus-I (HTLV-I)	Adult T cell leukemia (ATL), spastic paraparesis, myelopathy	M	Enveloped capsid Reverse transcriptase	(+) SS RNA converted to cDNA and integrated
	Human immunodeficiency virus (HIV)	AIDS	M	Enveloped capsid Reverse transcriptase	(+) SS RNA converted to cDNA and integrated
	Oncoviruses (animal)				Encodes oncogene resembling cellular gene which promotes cell growth
Coronaviridae	Coronavirus	Colds	M	Enveloped	(+) SS RNA
Arenaviridae	Lymphocytic choriomeningitis virus	Meningitis	M	Enveloped	(–) SS segmented RNA
	Lassa fever virus	Mild influenza-like		Enveloped	(–) SS segmented RNA
Bunyaviridae	California encephalitis virus	Influenza-like symptoms, encephalitis	M	Enveloped	(–) SS RNA
	La Crosse virus	Influenza-like symptoms, encephalitis	M	Enveloped	(–) SS RNA
	Hantavirus	Adult respiratory distress syndrome or hemorrhagic fever	M	Enveloped	(–) SS RNA
Caliciviridae	Norwalk virus	Diarrhea with vomiting	S	Naked	(+) RNA
Prions	Agent of kuru, Creutzfeld-Jacob disease, and scrapie (in sheep and hamsters)	Spongiform encephalopathy; scrapie used as a model of prion disease		Prion: Infectious protein, very small, resistant to inactivation	

Pathogenesis	Epidemiology		Means of Control		Laboratory Diagnosis
Target Organ	**Populations at Risk**	**Transmission**	**Vaccine (N = None, L = Live, K = Killed)**	**Antiviral Drug (N = None)**	
	African jungle	Monkeys			
	African jungle	Monkeys			
Liver	Same as for HBV	Blood, semen; sexually transmitted	N	Interferon α	Serology
Liver	HBV-infected individuals; coinfection: less severe; superinfection: severe	Blood, semen; sexually transmitted disease	N	N	Serology
Liver	Pregnant women in third world countries	Fecal-oral route	N	N	
GI tract	Malnourished infants and children	Fecal-oral route; third world countries	N	N	ELISA
T lymphocytes, neurons	Sexually active individuals, blood and organ recipients, IV drug users, neonates of infected mothers	Blood; sexually transmitted	N	N	ELISA, serology
T lymphocytes, macrophages, neurons	Sexually active individuals, blood and organ recipients, IV drug users, neonates of infected mothers		N	Azidothymidine, dideoxyinosine, dideoxycytidine, saquinavir	ELISA, western blot
Lungs	Ubiquitous	Respiratory route	N	N	
Lungs, CNS	Slum dwellers	Rat feces	N	N	
	West Africans	Rodent feces and urine			
CNS	Forest dwellers	*Culex* mosquito	N	N	
CNS	Forest dwellers	*Culex* mosquito	N	N	
Lungs		Rodents	N	N	
GI tract	Sporadic outbreaks	Fecal-oral route	N	N	
Brain—no immune response	Neurosurgeons, neurosurgical patients, family members	Infected tissue, genetic?	N	N	No antibody; histology: vacuolization of brain cells

Multiple Choice Review Questions

1. A virus is detergent sensitive and its genome is infectious (microinjection of the genome is sufficient to infect a cell). Which of the following viruses share these properties?
   a. Adenovirus
   b. Influenza virus
   c. Yellow fever virus
   d. Mumps virus
   e. Papilloma virus

2. Which of the following statements regarding virus replication is *false?*
   a. SV40 papovavirus does not produce virus in SV40-transformed hamster cells.
   b. Rous sarcoma retrovirus (RSV) produces virus in RSV-transformed cells.
   c. Herpes simplex virus produces virus upon latent infection of the neuron.
   d. HBsAg of hepatitis B virus is produced during chronic infection.
   e. HIV virus is produced during persistent infection.

3-7. Match the genome structure with its properties. Each item may be used more than once or not at all. More than one answer may be correct.
Genome structure:
   a. Double stranded DNA
   b. (+) RNA
   c. (−) RNA
   d. (+)/(−) RNA
   e. Retrovirus

3. Naked genome is infectious and replicates in the nucleus
4. Utilizes a (+) RNA template for replication
5. Must be integrated into the host chromosome for replication
6. May utilize host polymerase for replication
7. Must carry an RNA-dependent RNA polymerase in the virion

8. Which of the following statements regarding viral immunopathology is *false?*
   a. $CD4^+$ T cells lyse infected cells in an MHC class I-restricted manner.
   b. Cell-mediated immunity is primarily responsible for the symptoms associated with measles infection.
   c. Interferon is responsible for the influenza-like symptoms associated with viremias.
   d. Immune complexes of antibody and HBsAg can lead to renal problems.
   e. Enveloped viruses are more likely to elicit inflammatory reactions leading to greater immunopathogenesis.

9. Which of the following statements is *false?*
   a. Acyclovir is a nucleotide analogue.
   b. Acyclovir is activated by the herpes simplex virus (HSV) thymidine kinase and then inhibits the viral polymerase.
   c. Foscarnet is a nucleotide analogue.
   d. Foscarnet inhibits herpesvirus polymerases.
   e. Ganciclovir is a nucleotide analogue.

10. Which of the following statements is *false?*
   a. Amantadine inhibits uncoating of influenza virus B.
   b. Amantadine is only effective if given within 3 days of infection.
   c. Ganciclovir is licensed for cytomegalovirus.
   d. Acyclovir is licenced for HSV and varicella-zoster virus.
   e. Azidothymidine (AZT), dideoxyinosine (DDI), and dideoxycytidine (DDC) are nucleotide analogues effective against HIV.

11. Which of the following is incorrectly associated with its site of latent infection?
   a. Herpes simplex virus: neuron
   b. Varicella-zoster virus: neuron
   c. Epstein-Barr virus:neuron
   d. Cytomegalovirus: monocyte

12. Which of the following is incorrectly associated with its clinical presentation?
   a. Herpes simplex virus: vesicle
   b. Varicella-zoster virus: petechial rash
   c. Epstein-Barr virus: swollen glands, sore throat, and fatigue
   d. Cytomegalovirus: retinitis and esophagitis in immunocompromised hosts
   e. Human herpes virus 6: high fever followed by rash

13. Which of the following statements is *false?*
   a. Papilloma virus types 16 and 18 are associated with human cervical carcinoma.
   b. JC polyoma virus is associated with a slow virus disease, progressive multifocal leukoencephalopathy.
   c. Papilloma virus is readily isolated and grown from warts.

d. JC virus and BK virus are ubiquitous.

14-18. Match the virus with the appropriate statements. More than one answer may be correct and the viruses may be used more than once.

a. Poliovirus
b. Coxsackievirus type A
c. Coxsackievirus type B
d. Echovirus
e. Rhinovirus
f. All of the above

14. Causes symptoms of the common cold
15. Causes pleruodynia (Bornholm disease)
16. Associated with vesicular disease
17. Associated with severe neonatal disease
18. Preventable by vaccine

19. Which of the following statements is *false?*

a. Influenza virus is an enveloped virus with a segmented (–) RNA genome.
b. Influenza virus mRNA and genome synthesis occurs in the nucleus.
c. Influenza virus type A is sensitive to the antiviral drugs amantadine and rimantadine.
d. Influenza undergoes antigenic shift and drift by recombination of the genomes.
e. The hemagglutinin of influenza is the viral attachment protein and elicits protective antibody.

20-23. Match the most appropriate virus with its symptoms. More than one answer may be correct.

a. Measles virus
b. Parainfluenza virus
c. Mumps virus
d. Respiratory syncytial virus

20. Croup
21. Koplik's spots
22. Orchitis
23. Pneumonia

24-27. Match the virus with the statements below. More than one answer may be correct.

a. Rubella virus
b. St. Louis encephalitis virus
c. Dengue virus
d. Yellow fever virus
e. All of the above

24. Undergoes both an urban and a forest transmission cycle
25. German measles
26. Hemorrhagic fever
27. Prodrome of influenza-like symptoms

28. Which of the following statements is *false?*

a. All oncogenic retroviruses encode an oncogene that resembles a host growth control gene.
b. HTLV-1 encodes a transactivator protein (tax), which also activates transcription of the IL-2 and IL2-receptor genes.
c. The retrovirus genome is transcribed like host mRNA.
d. Retroviral mRNA produce polyproteins that are subsequently cleaved to individual proteins.
e. Final morphogenesis of the HIV virion occurs after envelopment by proteolytic cleavage of the gag-pol gene products.

29. Which of the following statements about HIV is *false?*

a. HIV establishes lytic, persistent, and latent infection of $CD4^+$ T cells and also infects macrophages and neurons.
b. HIV infection of $CD4^+$ T cells induces cytolytic syncytia.
c. Mutation of HIV within an individual promotes escape from immune control.
d. HIV p24 is an indicator of virus replication.
e. Major anti-HIV drug targets are the reverse transcriptase, protease, and src gene product.

30. A blood donor was screened for hepatitis B infection to determine whether he would be eligible to be a donor. Which of the following serologic profiles would be considered safe and appropriate for donating blood?

	Anti-HBc	Anti-HBe	Anti-HBsAg	HBsAg
a.	+	–	–	+
b.	–	–	+	–
c.	+	–	–	+
d.	–	–	–	+
e.	–	–	+	+

Chapter 4

Mycology

Section 4.1 Introduction to Mycology

Fungi are defined as yeasts or moulds based on their morphology and means of reproduction.

- **Classification** Fungi are differentiated by the types of structures produced during sexual reproduction (Table 4.1).
- **Fungal Biology and Taxonomy**
  - Morphology
    - *Cell structure (Fig. 4.1)*

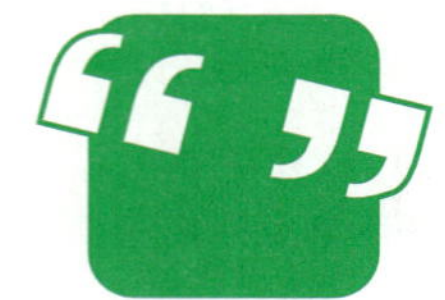

1. Filamentous fungi, called **moulds,** are made up of **hyphae.** Hyphae are branching, threadlike tubular filaments that elongate at their tips.

- Hyphae are made up of one of two types of cells:
  - **Septate** cells are divided into individual walled-off cells containing nuclei.
  - **Aseptate** (coenocytic) cells are hollow.

Table 4.1 *Taxonomic Classification of the Fungi Kingdom*

Organism	Characteristics	Medially Important Genera
Phylum Zygomycota	Sexual reproduction produces a **zygote.** Asexual reproduction is by spores inside sporangia (sporangiospore).	Agents causing zygomycosis
Phylum Dikaryomycota	**Septate** hyphae.	
Subphylum Ascomycotina	Sexual reproduction occurs in a sac called an ascus, and the resultant spores are called **ascospores.**	Agents causing ringworm, histoplasmosis, and blastomycosis
Subphylum Basidiomycotina	Sexual reproduction takes place in a sac called a basidium. The haploid progeny are called **basidiospores.**	Agent causing cryptococcosis
Form-class Deuteromycotina (Fungi imperfecti)	Septate hyphae, dimorphic. **No sexual stage** has been observed in these fungi.	*Candida, Trichosporon, Torulopsis, Pityrosporum, Epidermophyton, Coccidioides, Paracoccidioides*

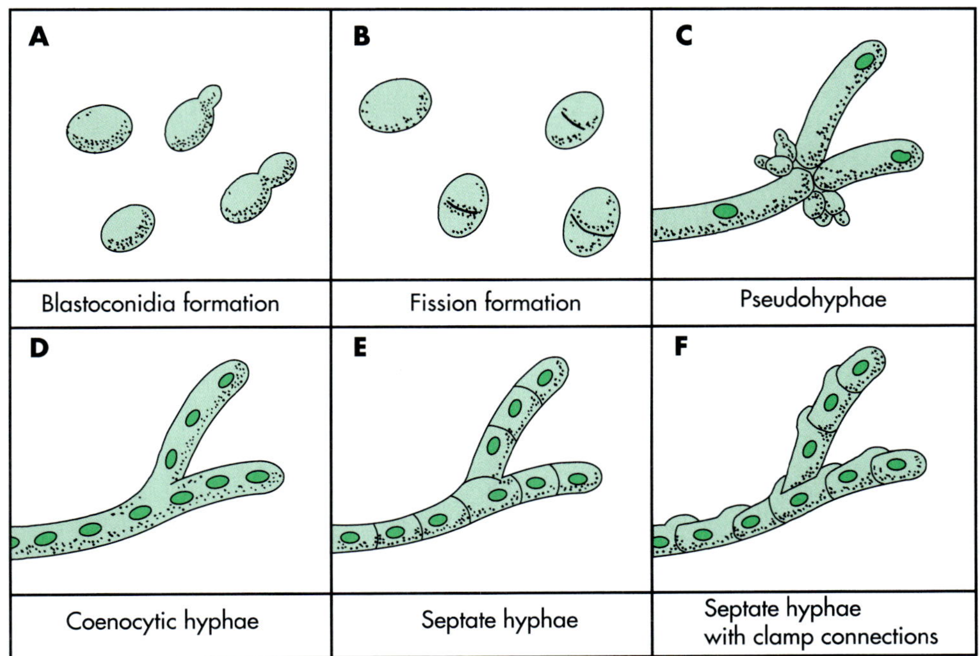

Fig. 4.1 Fungal cell morphology. **A,** Yeast cells reproducing by blastoconidia formation. **B,** Yeast cells dividing by fission. **C,** Pseudohyphal development. **D,** Coenocytic (not separated) hyphae. **E,** Septate hyphae. **F,** Septate hyphae with clamp connections.

- Vegetative hyphae (feeding or "invading" hyphae) absorb nutrients from the environment.
- Aerial hyphae stick up into the air from the medium and often serve a reproductive function.

2. Yeasts are often unicellular.

- **Reproduction (asexual and sexual) (Fig. 4.2)**
  - In moulds the vegetative and the reproductive stages are different.
  - Yeasts reproduce asexually by production of blastoconidia (budding) or by fission.
  - Both moulds and yeasts may have asexual and sexual modes of reproduction (see Table 4.1).

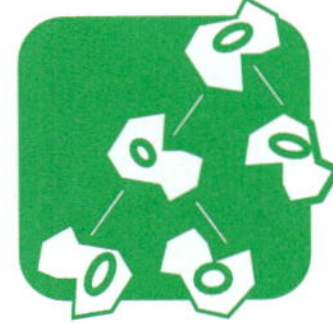

— ***Asexual reproduction*** The phase of asexual reproduction is called the anamorph stage and, clinically, is the *most commonly encountered stage.*

1. **Moulds** produce threadlike mats called hyphae. The total mass of hyphae making up the mould is called the **mycelium** (Fig. 4.3). Aerial hyphae (if reproductive) produce conidia, which are "naked" spores that push out from the hyphae or sporangia, which are protected endospores within a sporangium (see Fig. 4.2).

2. **Yeasts** are often single cells that reproduce by **fission** or by blastoconidia (blastospore) formation (**budding** or pinching off of the reproductive element).

3. **Dimorphic** fungi are fungi that may appear as either moulds or yeasts depending upon certain environmental factors (e.g., *Histoplasma capsulatum* is a yeast at body temperature [35° C to 37° C]) and

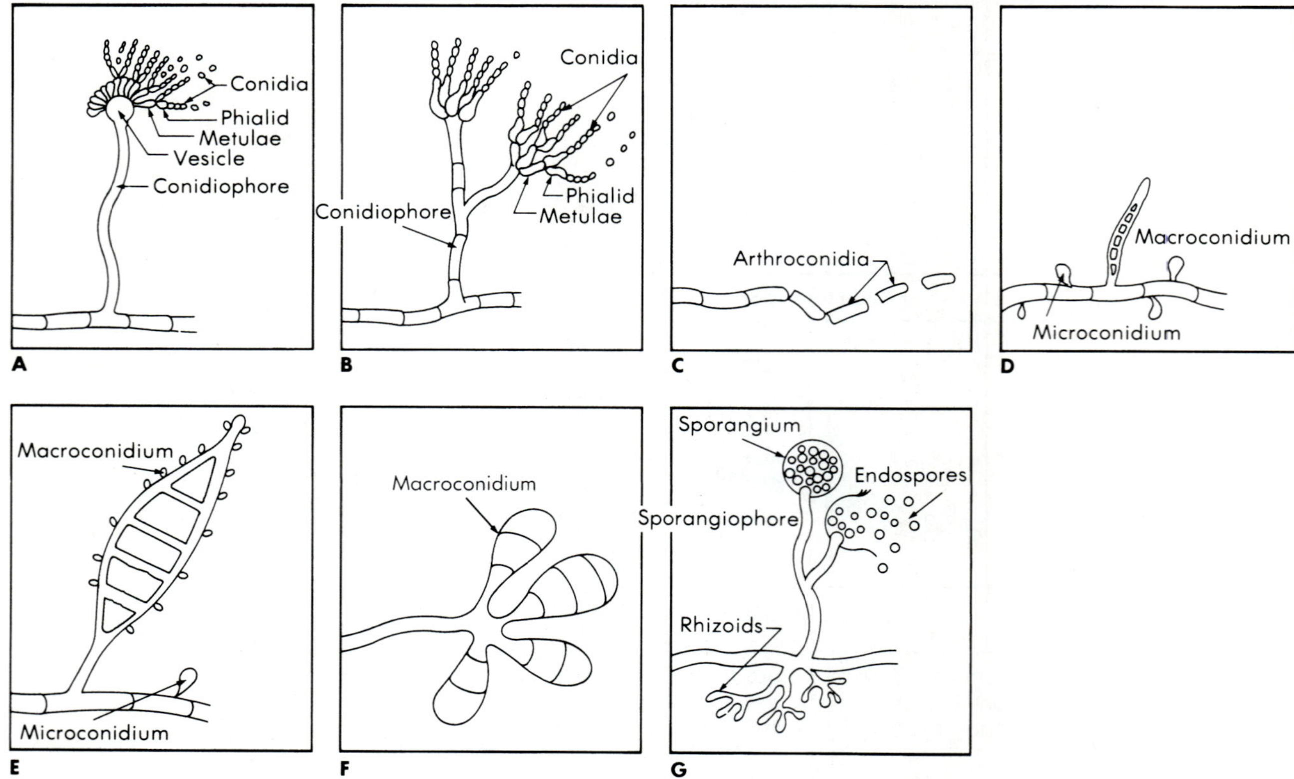

Fig. 4.2 Conidial development in **A,** *Aspergillus;* **B,** *Penicillium;* **C,** *Geotrichum;* **D,** *Trichophyton;* **E,** *Microsporum;* **F,** *Epidermophyton;* and **G,** *Rhizopus.*

mouldlike at room temperature (25° C). *Candida albicans* can appear dimorphic under certain conditions.

— ***Sexual reproduction*** The phase of sexual reproduction is called the teleomorph stage. It is a highly complex process, which is covered in necessary detail in Table 4.1.

Overview of Fungal Diseases

- **Mechanisms of disease** Fungi cause disease by three mechanisms.
  1. Colonization
  2. Development of hypersensitivity to the fungus
  3. Release of toxins

— ***Colonization and disease*** Almost all fungi are free living in nature. Humans get a disease after contact with and colonization of tissue by the fungus.

Classification of fungi according to site of diseases

- Superficial mycoses are infections of keratinized tissue, such as hair, skin, and nails (e.g., infections caused by dermatophytes).
- Cutaneous mycoses are infections of the epidermis and the deeper layers of the skin and the nails (e.g., some *Candida* infections).
- Subcutaneous mycoses are infections of the dermis, the subcutaneous tissues, the muscles, and the fascia (e.g., eumycotic mycetoma).

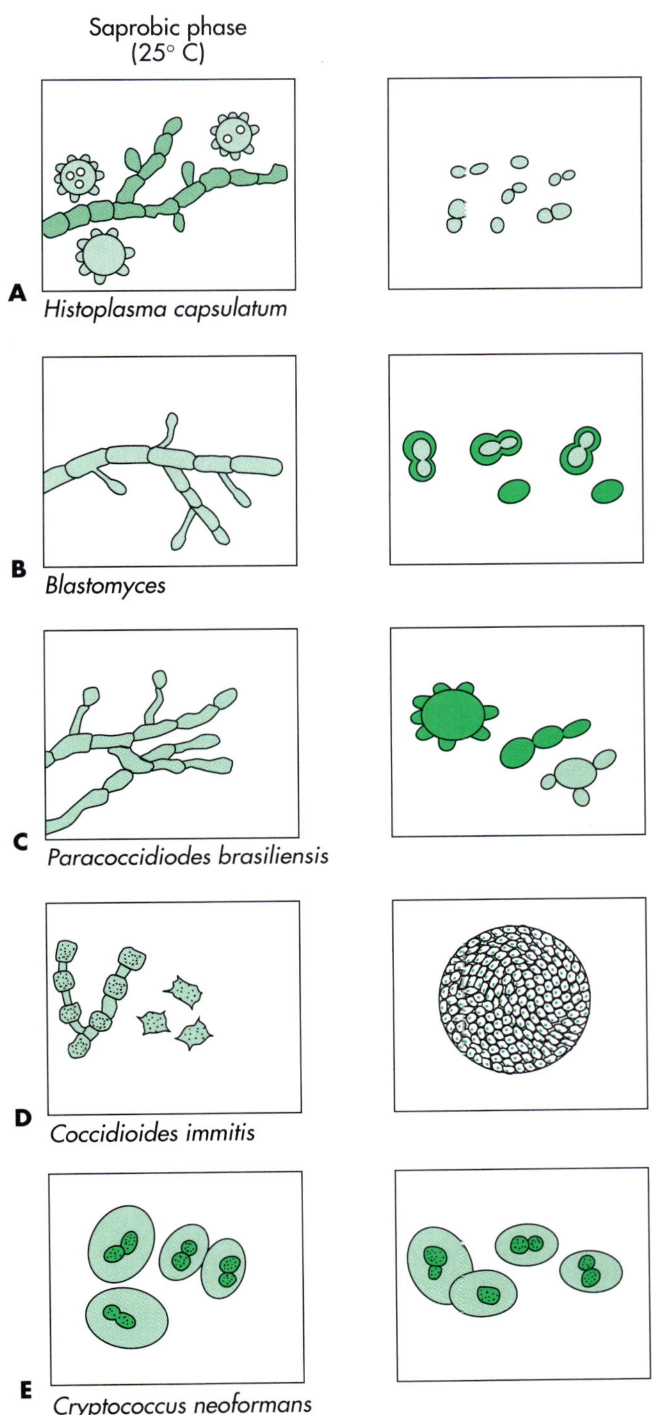

Fig. 4.3 Mould and yeast forms of systemic mycoses. Some fungi can grow as a yeast or as a mould depending upon the growth conditions and environment. All of the fungi shown are classified dimorphic except for *Cryptococcus neoformans.* **A,** *Histoplasma capsulatum,* **B,** *Blastomyces dermatitidis,* and **C,** *Paracoccidioides brasiliensis* exhibit mold-to-yeast transition when infecting susceptible species; **D,** *Coccidioides immitis* exhibits mold-to-spherule transition when it infects susceptible species; **E,** *Cryptococcus neoformans* is not dimorphic and is an encapsulated yeast at 25° C, 37° C, or in infected tissues.

• Systemic mycoses are infections of the deep organs of the body, often originating in the lungs (e.g., histoplasmosis).

• Opportunistic mycoses are infections that occur in immunosuppressed patients (e.g., fungal infections in cancer patients and patients with acquired immunodeficiency syndrome [AIDS]).

Host defenses

• Physical, chemical, and biologic barriers, such as intact skin, pH, fatty acids in the skin, the normal bacterial flora, and various humoral factors, normally prevent establishment of fungal infections.

• Only a few fungi can cause disease in healthy persons.

• **Most fungal infections are opportunistic:** *C. albicans* and even *Saccharomyces cerevisiae* (baker's yeast) are normal flora but can cause disease under certain conditions (e.g., after immunosuppression). Environmental organisms such as *Aspergillus* are also opportunistic.

• Use of antibacterial antibiotics can disrupt the normal bacterial flora and sometimes allow colonization by fungi.

• Immunity to fungal infections is conferred by delayed-type hypersensitivity (DTH). *Fungal infections are seen in individuals with T cell deficiencies, either genetic or induced (by chemotherapy or in AIDS).*

■ **Diagnostic Procedures** Diagnostic procedures are discussed more fully under the discussion of specific organisms.

A. Culture and microscopic diagnosis

• Specimens can be cultured up to 30 days at 25° C and 35° C on appropriate media often containing antibacterial antibiotics to inhibit bacterial over-growth.

• Slide cultures can be set up.

• Various histologic stains can be used for direct visualization of fungi in tissue specimens.

• Fungi in skin scrapings can be visualized after treatment of the specimen with 10% to 15% KOH.

• Yeasts can often be identified by sugar assimilation tests (somewhat similar to the fermentation tests for Enterobacteriaceae). Commercial tests kits are available.

B. Serologic tests

• Fungal antigen detection (ouchterlony, ELISA) in blood or CSF is an important tool for identifying and detecting fungal infections.

■ **Antimycotic Antibiotics** The most commonly used antifungal agents are the polyene antibiotics, including amphotericin B and nystatin, the azoles, including ketoconazole, fluconazole, itraconazole, and the older drug, miconazole. Also important is the nucleotide analog 5-fluorocytosine. Table 4.2 summarizes the modes of action of the most commonly used antimycotic agents.

● **Resistance** As with the antibacterial antibiotics, resistance is observed with all of the antimycotic agents. Certain specific instances are noted under the sections on the various agents of mycotic disease.

Section 4.2 Superficial Cutaneous and Subcutaneous Mycoses

■ **Superficial Mycoses** Superficial mycoses are infections of only the outermost layers of the skin and hair (Fig. 4.4).

Table 4.2 ***Antifungal Agents and Primary Sites of Activity***

Antifungal Agents	Target
Polyenes (e.g., amphotericin B, nystatin)	Membrane sterols (binds to ergosterol)
Azole derivatives (e.g., miconazole, ketoconazole, fluconazole, itraconazole)	Ergosterol biosynthesis (inhibits cytochrome-P450–dependent enzymes)
Nucleotide (e.g., 5-fluorocytosine)	Inhibits DNA and RNA synthesis
Grisans (e.g., griseofulvin)	Microtubules (inhibits microtubular function)
Allylamines (e.g., naftifine, terbinafine)	Squalene epoxidase
Thiocarbamates (e.g., tolnaftate, tolciclate)	Squalene epoxidase
Morpholines (e.g., amorolfine)	Ergosterol biosynthesis (inhibits Δ_{14}-reductase and Δ_7-Δ_8-isomerase)
Potassium iodide (e.g., SSKI)	Unknown (possibly activates lysomal enzymes and breaks down granulomas)

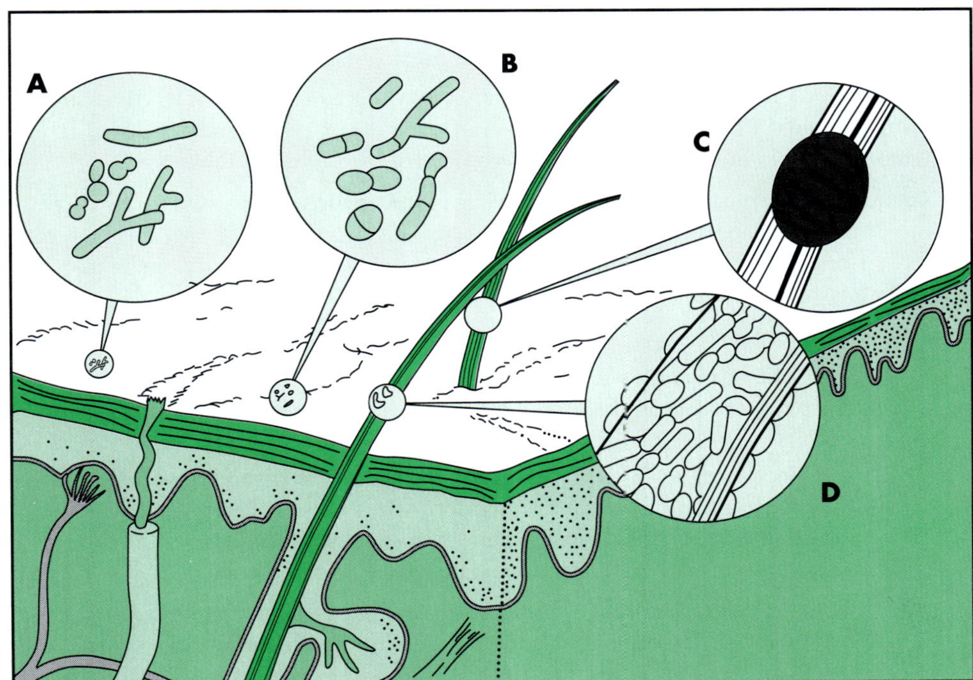

Fig. 4.4 Schematic illustration of superficial fungal infection and tissue involvement. **A,** Pityriasis versicolor. **B,** Tinea nigra. **C,** Black piedra. **D,** White piedra.

Table 4.3 *Dermatophytes*

Genus	Site of Infection
Microsporum	Hair and skin
Trichophyton	Hair, skin, and nails
Epidermophyton	Skin and nails

Table 4.4 *Cutaneous Mycoses*

Infection	Common Cause(s)
Tinea capitis (ringworm of the scalp)	*Trichophyton tonsurans, Microsporum audouinii*
Tinea favosa (favus of the scalp)	*T. schoenleinii*
Tinea corporis (ringworm of the body)	*T. tonsurans, M. audouinii, M. canis, T. rubrum, T. mentagrophytes*
Tinea cruris (jock itch)	*T. rubrum, Epidermophyton floccosum*
Tinea unguium (ringworm of the nail)	*T. rubrum, T. mentagrophytes*
Tinea manuum (ringworm of the hands)	*T. rubrum, T. mentagrophytes, E. floccosum*
Tinea pedis (athlete's foot)	*T. mentagrophytes, T. rubrum, E. floccosum*

- **Differential diagnosis** The differential diagnosis includes pediculosis and bacterial infections.
- **Treatment** For pityriasis versicolor and tinea nigra, treatment for cosmetic reasons consists of removal of the skin with agents that remove keratin. Topical miconazole can be used. For white or black piedra, the hair should be cut below the nodules. Personal hygiene should be discussed with the patient. (For a discussion of antifungal antibiotics see Section 4.1.)

Cutaneous Mycoses Cutaneous mycoses are infections of the hair, the skin, and the nails. They are restricted to keratinized layers of the body and will rarely cause systemic infections in immunosuppressed individuals (Table 4.3).

- **Clinical manifestations** Cutaneous mycoses include **ringworm** or **tinea** of various areas of the body. The type of infection is designated by the term tinea (wormlike) and the Latin term for the general body site of the infection (Table 4.4 and Fig. 4.5).

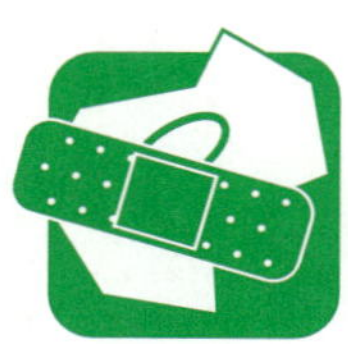

- **Pathogenesis**
  - The term *ringworm* describes the pattern of the infected skin. The organisms are viable on the periphery of the lesion, not in the center of the lesion.
  - In infections of the hair, *Microsporum* tends to invade the outside of the hair causing an *ectothrix* infection, while certain *Trichophyton* species tend to invade the inside of the hair shaft causing an *endothrix* infection. Infections with dermatophytes may be mixed with bacteria.

- **Laboratory diagnosis** For preliminary diagnosis, skin scrapings are placed on a slide with 10% potassium hydroxide, digested to remove skin tissue, and viewed under reduced light to observe *branching septate hyphae.* This procedure is useful, but less so for nails and hair. A potassium hydroxide preparation of hair will show spores and fragmented hyphae (arthrospores) (Table 4.5).

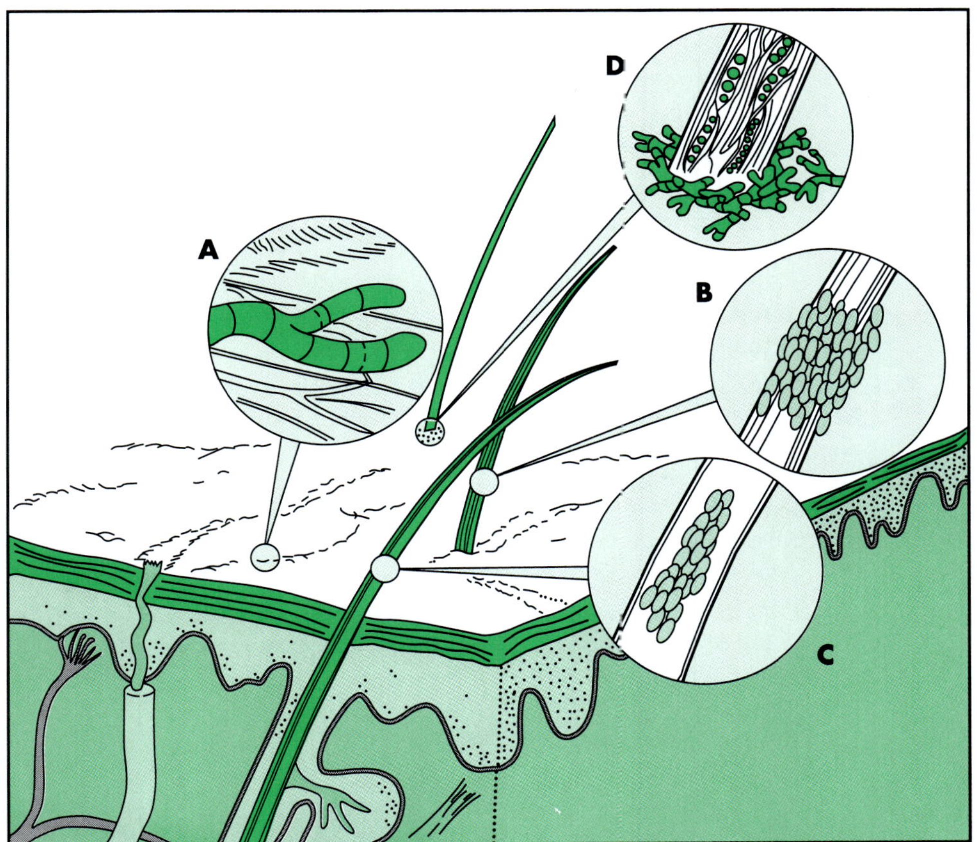

Fig. 4.5 Schematic of tissues colonized by dermatophytes. **A,** Stratum corneum. **B,** Ectothrix hair infection. **C,** Endothrix hair infection. **D,** Favic hair infection.

Table 4.5 ***General Characteristics of Macroconidia and Microconidia of Dermatophytes***

Genus	Macroconidia	Microconidia
Microsporum	Numerous, thick-walled, rough*	Rare
Epidermophyton	Numerous, smooth-walled	Absent
Trichophyton	Rare, thin-walled, smooth	Abundant†

**M. audouinii* is an exception.
†*T. schoenleinii* is an exception.

- **Differential diagnosis** Differential diagnosis includes infections with *Candida* species, bacterial infections, and sometimes viral (skin) infections. Other skin diseases must also be considered.
- **Treatment** For skin infections, a topical agent such as miconazole or clotrimazole may be used. Many over-the-counter agents are available. For hair

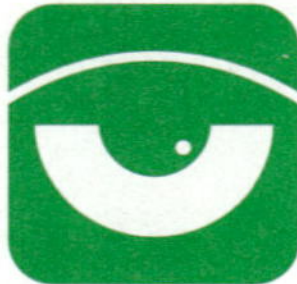
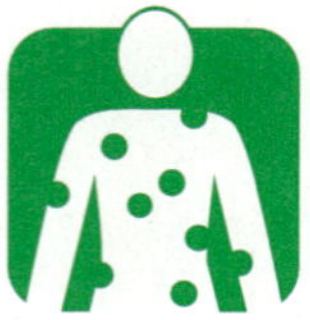

infections, azole antibiotic-containing shampoos and griseofulvin may be used. For infection involving the nails, the azole antibiotics (topical or systemic) are effective. Surgical or chemical removal of the infected nail may be necessary.

Subcutaneous Mycoses

- **General considerations** The subcutaneous mycoses are caused by a mixed group of agents that cause infections of the subcutaneous tissues. Infections usually occur through cuts, punctures, or stabs with soil-contaminated thorns or sharp tools or by other trauma. The organisms are often pigmented fungi that are loosely referred to as *dematiaceous (melanin-containing)* fungi.
- **Sporotrichosis** Lymphocutaneous sporotrichosis consists of chronic nodular and ulcerative lesions that develop and line up along the lymphatics that drain the primary site. Lesions often appear pink at first but later turn purple or black (Fig. 4.6).

  The causative organism is *Sporothrix schenckii* (a dimorphic fungus). It is inoculated by traumatic implantation. A frequent source is a rose thorn, thus the disease is sometimes referred to as "rose gardener's disease."

  — ***Laboratory diagnosis*** Tissue or pus is inoculated onto media at 25° C and 35° C. At 35° C, the organisms will grow as small yeastlike

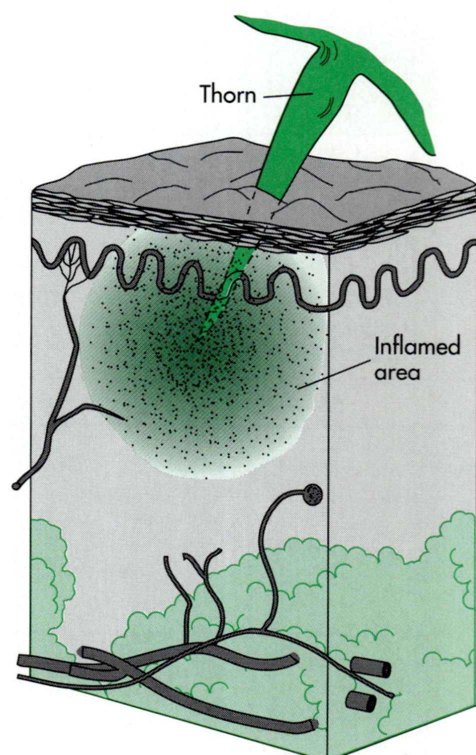

Fig. 4.6 *Sporothrix* and other soil fungi can be implanted by trauma (e.g., from a rose thorn) and establish infection. For sporotrichosis, lesions will erupt from the skin along the lymphatics that drain the site of the original lesion.

forms that look, microscopically, like tear-drop or banana-shaped cells. At 25° C (room temperature), the organism grows as a moist, white mould.

Histology: *Sporo (spores)* or numerous conidia form a flowerlike array on the end of a tiny hairlike conidiophore.

— ***Differential diagnosis*** A number of bacterial diseases can give rise to lesions somewhat similar to lymphocutaneous sporotrichosis. These include tularemia, plague, and gangrene. Other fungal infections also need to be considered.

— ***Treatment*** Subcutaneous infection responds to oral potassium iodide. Extracutaneous sporotrichosis requires amphotericin B or an azole, such as itraconazole.

- **Chromoblastomycosis** Chromoblastomycosis is a chronic infection caused by a variety of dematiaceous **soil fungi.**

The disease is characterized by *verrucoid (warty) nodules* at the site of inoculation that look like tumors of the skin or subcutaneous tissue. The lesion looks cauliflowerlike.

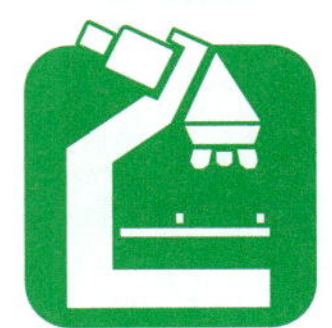

— ***Laboratory diagnosis***

Histology: Examination of tissue reveals abnormal multiplication of otherwise normal host cells, a condition called pseudoepitheliomatous hyperplasia. Tissue forms of the fungus contain copper-colored spherical cells often crisscrossed with division lines called sclerotic or Medular bodies.

Culture: Culture is not very useful for diagnosis.

— ***Differential diagnosis*** The differential diagnosis includes sporotrichosis and bacterial infections, such as tularemia, plague, and gangrene.

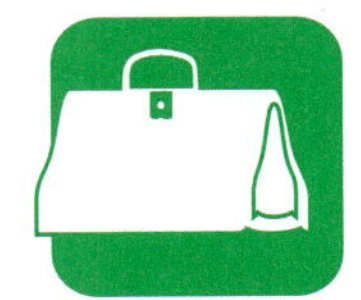

— ***Treatment*** Surgical removal is the treatment of choice for early disease. Advanced infections are treated with 5-fluorocytosine or the newer azoles, especially itraconazole and fluconazole.

- **Mycetoma**

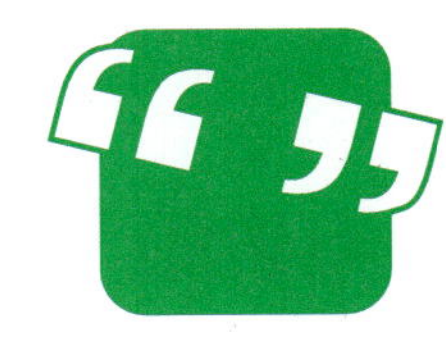

• Mycetoma is a chronic infection caused by dematiaceous (soil) fungi or bacteria and is characterized by (1) presence of swollen, deforming (tumorlike) lesions, (2) production of grains or granules, and (3) draining sinus tracts.

• The infection is seen most often in the hand or the foot because of contact with the soil.

• The most common fungal agents of mycetoma are *Pseudallescheria boydii* and *Madurella grisea.*

— ***Laboratory diagnosis***

• Approximately 50% of all mycetomas are caused by fungi and the other 50% by bacteria (e.g., Nocardia). It is, therefore, important to differentiate between fungal and bacterial causes of the disease by culture.

• The characteristic grains contain small, hyphal elements that can be picked off the lesions or removed from saline-soaked gauze pads which are removed from the lesions, crushed, and planted on media. The grains from *P. boydii* tend to be white or yellow, whereas those from *M. grisea* are gray to black.

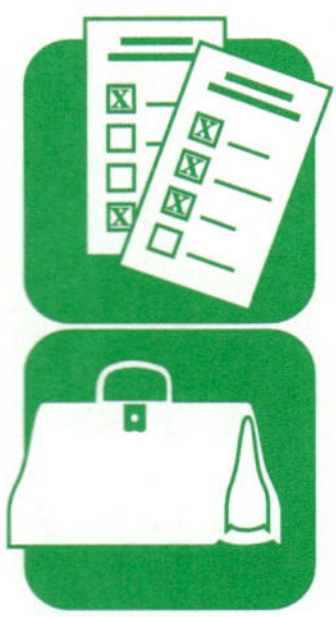

— ***Differential diagnosis*** The causative agent (whether bacterial or fungal) needs to be defined. Other bacterial infections and subcutaneous fungal infections need to be considered.

— ***Treatment***

- Antibacterial antibiotics are useful for mycetoma caused by bacteria. Fungal causes are difficult to treat. Physicians often resort to total excision or amputation of the limb.
- Amphotericin B, nystatin, and the azoles have limited activity.

Section 4.3 Opportunistic Fungal Infections

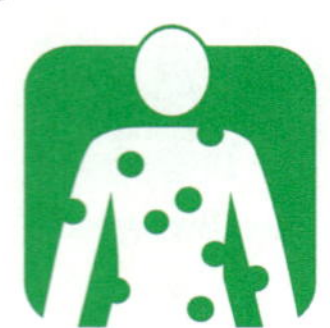

Immunocompromised patients, including patients with AIDS, patients undergoing chemotherapy, and transplant patients, are at increased risk for fungal infections (Table 4.6). The loss of neutrophil or T cell function (especially $CD4^{+}$ DTH cells) eliminates a major antifungal line of defense.

■ **Candidiasis (Moniliasis)** *Candida albicans* cause as many as 80% of *Candida* infections.

● **Spectrum of infections**

1. Normal flora: *C. albicans* is part of the normal flora in mucous membranes of the body in 10% to 20% of individuals.

2. Cutaneous candidiasis *(vaginal infections, oral thrush):* This is a self-limited infection of the skin, nails, or mucous membranes and is often the result of the local disruption of the immune system (such as after administration of local antiinflammatory agents), breaks in the integument, or disruption of the normal flora by use of antibacterial antibiotics (e.g., vaginal infections). Other correlations are less obvious, such as the correlation of obesity with infections of the folded skin areas of the body.

3. Chronic mucocutaneous candidiasis: This is an extensive cutaneous disease. Dissemination is rare, but the infection is resistant to treatment. It involves some T-cell deficiency or endocrine defects, such as hypoparathyroidism, hypothyroidism, or hypoadrenalism, or a thymoma. The physiologic defect needs to be corrected.

4. Disseminated disease: Disseminated candidiasis results from severe neutropenia or a T-cell deficiency. Most immunosuppressed patients, such as cancer patients and transplant patients, develop disseminated disease. AIDS patients tend to develop severe infections of the oropharynx and the upper

Table 4.6 ***Comparison of the Properties of Systemic and Opportunistic Fungal Agents***

Agents That Cause Systemic Infection	Agents That Cause Opportunistic Infection
Elicit disease in normal and compromised hosts	Elicit disease usually in compromised hosts
Cause disease that is often quickly resolved or asymptomatic disease	Often cause serious disease in compromised hosts
Elicit a strong immune response that resolves infection	Elicit a poor immune response
Cause diseases that are often geographically limited	Cause diseases worldwide
Are not normal flora	Are often normal flora, with a few exceptions
Are dimorphic (except for *Cryptococcus*)	Are not dimorphic

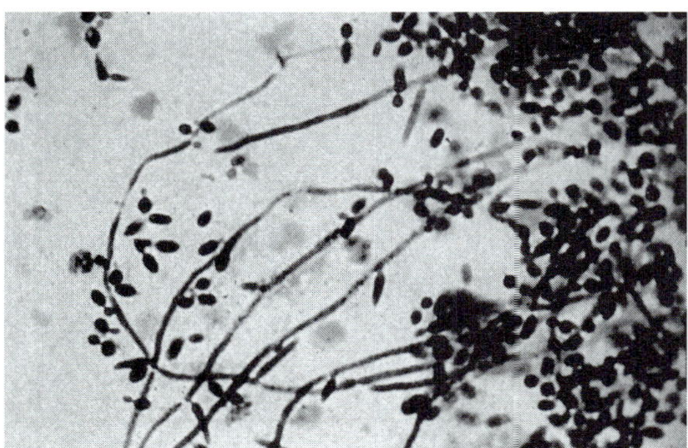

Fig. 4.7 Sputum specimen illustrating budding yeast cells and pseudohyphae of *Candida.*

gastrointestinal tract but, rarely, disseminated disease. Development of oral candidiasis is a common, early symptom of AIDS.

- **Laboratory diagnosis**

  Histology: *C. albicans* produces budding yeasts, pseudohyphae, and septate true hyphae (Fig. 4.7).

  Culture: The organisms grow on most laboratory media and produce opaque, cream-colored colonies.

  Serology: Serology is not useful because precipitins are found in normal individuals.

- **Differential diagnosis** Other bacterial and fungal infections must be ruled out.

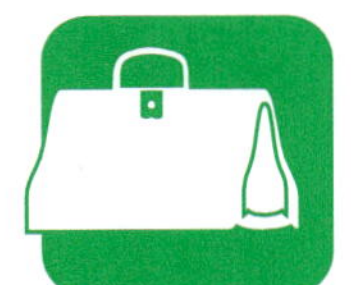

- **Treatment** Topical ketoconazole is used for cutaneous infections. For deep or systemic infections, oral ketoconazole or fluconazole are useful substitutes for amphotericin B treatment (except for *C. Krusei,* which is often resistant).

Aspergillosis

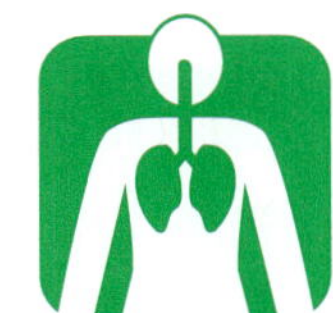

- **Laboratory diagnosis**

  Histology: A spherical mass of intertwined septate, branching hyphae called a *fungus ball* can be seen in lung tissue. Aspergillosis should be suspected if any septate branched hyphae are seen in any deep tissue. The organisms invade the tissue and blood vessels.

  Culture: Although *Aspergillus* grows easily, interpretation is difficult because the organisms are found in the environment. (A distinction of contamination versus colonization versus infection must be made.)

- **Differential diagnosis** Zygomycoses and infections by other moulds must be ruled out.

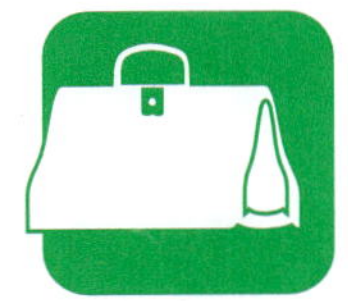

- **Treatment** If there is an underlying disease, it must be corrected. Infected tissue should be surgically removed when possible. Amphotericin B is commonly used to treat systemic infections.

Zygomycosis

The organisms that cause zygomycosis are zygomycetes and are commonly found in the environment. The most common genera involved in disease are *Rhizopus* and *Mucor.* All zygomycetes are coenocytic (aseptate).

- **Clinical disease**
  - The disease is similar to that caused by *Aspergillus.*

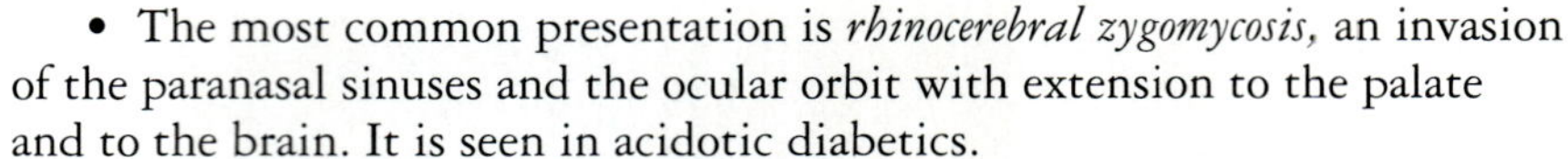

- The most common presentation is *rhinocerebral zygomycosis,* an invasion of the paranasal sinuses and the ocular orbit with extension to the palate and to the brain. It is seen in acidotic diabetics.
- A characteristic of this mycosis is the formation of hyphal emboli.

- **Laboratory diagnosis**

  Histology: This is the usual method of diagnosis. Coenocytic hyphae that tend to be broad can be seen penetrating tissues.

- **Differential diagnosis** Aspergillosis and other mould infections may mimic the disease.

- **Treatment**
  - Treatment consists of correction of the physiologic deficiency.
  - Antibiotics are often useless.
  - The infection is often a terminal event in a long-standing, debilitating disease.

SECTION 4.4 SYSTEMIC MYCOSES

The agents of systemic mycoses can cause disease in otherwise healthy individuals. These agents include the dimorphic fungi and *Cryptococcus* (a **nondimorphic fungus**) (Box 4.1).

Box 4.1

AGENTS CAUSING THE SYSTEMIC MYCOSES
Histoplasma capsulatum
Blastomyces dermatitidis
Paracoccidioides brasiliensis
Coccidioides immitis
Cryptococcus neoformans

Diseases Caused by Dimorphic Agents

- **Histoplasmosis (Darling's Disease; Reticuloendothelial Cytomycosis; Cave Disease; Spelunker's Disease)**
  - The organism is endemic in the Ohio and Mississippi river valleys and is found in **bird and bat droppings.**
  - The mould (saprophytic) form in the soil produces conidia or hyphal fragments that are inhaled, phagocytized by pulmonary macrophages, and converted to the yeast (parasitic or tissue) form (Fig. 4.8 and Table 4.7).

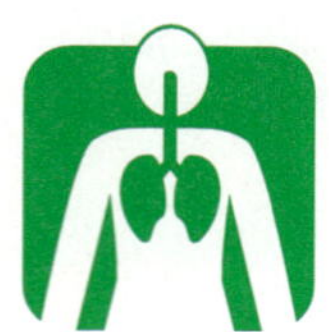

— *Diseases (Table 4.8)*

- Histoplasmosis is a self-limited respiratory infection.
- Approximately 1% of infected individuals develop progressive disseminated disease.
- Immunocompromised persons are at risk for disseminated reactivation disease or **central nervous system disease.**

— *Laboratory diagnosis*

Specimens: Histoplasma can be isolated from sputum, bone marrow, and blood.

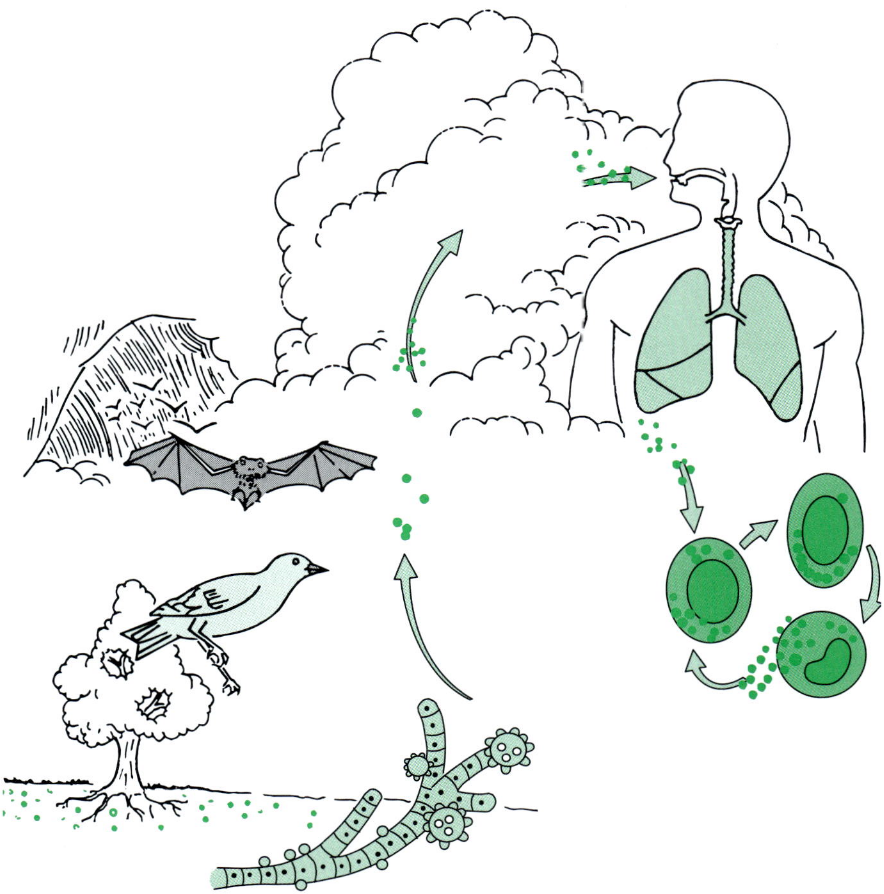

Fig. 4.8 Schematic illustration of the natural history of the saprobic and parasitic cycles of *Histoplasma capsulatum.*

Table 4.7 ***Summary of Histoplasmosis***

Etiologic Agent	Mycology	Epidemiology and Ecology	Clinical Disease
Asexual phase: *Histoplasma capsulatum* Sexual phase: *Ajellomyces capsulatus*	Dimorphic; mycelia at 25° C; tuberculate macroconidia; microconidia. At 37° C and in tissue this organism is a budding yeast. Found predominantly in histiocytes.	Occurs throughout temperate, subtropical, and tropical areas of the world. Endemic areas include the **Ohio and Mississippi River Valleys** and parts of Central and South America. The organism has been isolated from numerous soil samples, particularly those contaminated by **bat, chicken, and starling droppings.** Bats are naturally infected, but birds are not.	The clinical symptoms vary depending on the degree of individual exposure and immunological state of the patient. Less than 1% of infections become progressive and require therapy. An underlying condition of debilitation or immunosuppression makes these individuals prone to life-threatening disease.

Table 4.8 *Classification of Histoplasmosis*

TYPE OF INFECTION	SPECIFIC DISORDER	COMMENTS
Histoplasmosis in normal hosts	Asymptomatic or mild flu-like illness	Occurs with normal exposure
	Acute pulmonary histoplasmosis	Occurs with heavy exposure
	Rare complications	Pericarditis, mediastinal fibrosis
Opportunistic infection	Disseminated histoplasmosis	Occurs in individuals who have an immune defect
	Chronic pulmonary histoplasmosis	Occurs in individuals who have an anatomical defect

Histology: Small intracellular yeasts can be seen in macrophages (see Table 4.7). Culture may take several weeks. DNA probes are available for diagnosis.

Serology: Skin testing is of little value for histoplasmosis. The histoplasma exoantigen test is an immunodiffusion test for fungal antigens (Fig. 4.9).

— ***Differential diagnosis*** Other agents of systemic fungal diseases and bacterial and viral agents of pneumonia must be considered. Intracellular *Histoplasma* organisms (especially within histiocytes) may be mistaken for *Leishmania* or *Toxoplasma* organisms.

— ***Treatment*** Most patients recover without treatment and are never diagnosed with active disease. Patients requiring treatment will usually receive amphotericin B, although ketoconazole is effective in non-immunocompromized patients without CNS lesions. AIDS patients, who often undergo a relapse, may receive long-term suppressive therapy with itraconazole.

- **Blastomycosis (Chicago Disease; Gilchrist's Disease; North American Blastomycosis)** The **yeast** cells are very **large.**

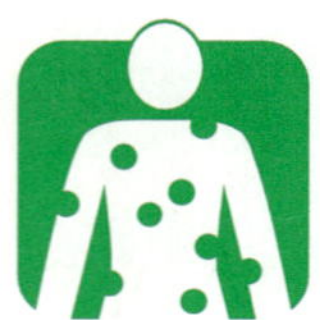

— ***Disease*** The primary lung infection is usually a benign, self-limited infection. More rarely, blastomycosis develops into a chronic infection that disseminates to other areas of the body, especially the skin and bones (Fig. 4.10).

— ***Laboratory diagnosis*** Diagnosis is by identification of the organisms either in infected tissue or in culture.

Specimens: Organisms can be isolated from skin lesions, sputum, and biopsy material from skin or bone.

Histology: In tissue, the yeast cells are large with broad-based buds.

Serology: An exoantigen test is available.

— ***Differential diagnosis*** Other agents of systemic, cutaneous, and subcutaneous fungal diseases, bacterial and viral agents of pneumonia, and agents of skin infections must be ruled out. The skin lesions could be misdiagnosed as chancres from syphilis; drainage tracks may cause the disease to be mistaken for sporotrichosis.

— ***Treatment*** Uncomplicated disease may respond to ketoconazole. Amphotericin B is used in more extensive disease. Itraconazole and fluconazole are also useful.

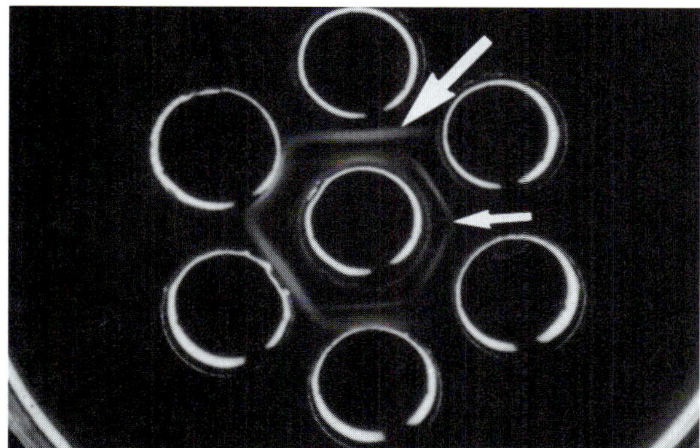

Fig. 4.9 Immunodiffusion illustrating H *(short arrow)* and M *(long arrow)* precipitin bands that form when histoplasmin is tested against sera containing reactive antibodies.

- **Paracoccidioidomycosis (South American Blastomycosis; Lutz-Splendore-Almeida Disease)**

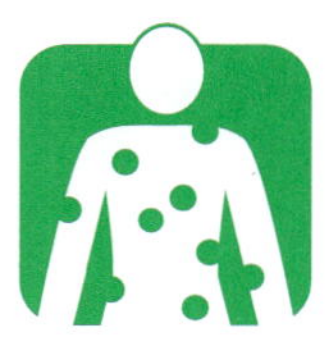

  — ***Disease*** Paracoccidioidomycosis is a primary pulmonary infection that is often asymptomatic. Common forms of the disease include ulcerative lesions of the oral and nasal mucosa.

  — ***Differential diagnosis*** Other agents of systemic, cutaneous, and subcutaneous fungal diseases, bacterial and viral agents of pneumonia, and agents of skin infections cause similar disease.

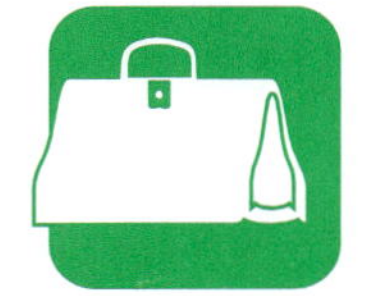

  — ***Treatment*** Long-term therapy with antifungal agents is necessary. Sulfa drugs have been used, but treatment failures are common. Azoles appear to be effective. Amphotericin B is too toxic to be used long term.

Coccidioidomycosis (Posadas-Wernicke Disease; San Joaquin Fever; Valley Fever; Desert Fever; Desert Rheumatism)

- **Disease**

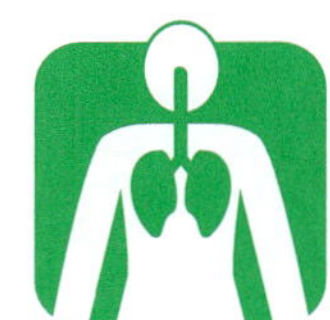

  • In 40% of the cases, coccidioidomycosis manifests as an acute, self-limited respiratory infection (cough, fever, and chest pain). Night sweats and joint pain may also occur.

  • The fungus is endemic to the **desert** areas of the **southwestern United States.** In desertlike areas, where the organism is endemic, the hyphae fragments form arthroconidia that are inhaled. In the lungs, spherules form, giving rise to the tissue phase of the organism. **The organism is highly infectious and culture of the mould phase can be hazardous.**

- **Laboratory diagnosis**

Histology: Analysis can be difficult. Spherules may be seen on hematoxylin and eosin-stained tissue. There is a useful exoantigen test available.

Serology: Serologic diagnosis is probably the easiest means of diagnosis. Skin testing may be prognostic of the eventualoutcome of the disease (Fig. 4.11).

Culture: This may be the only means of diagnosis of coccidioidomycosis in immunosuppressed patients. Culture of this organism poses a hazard.

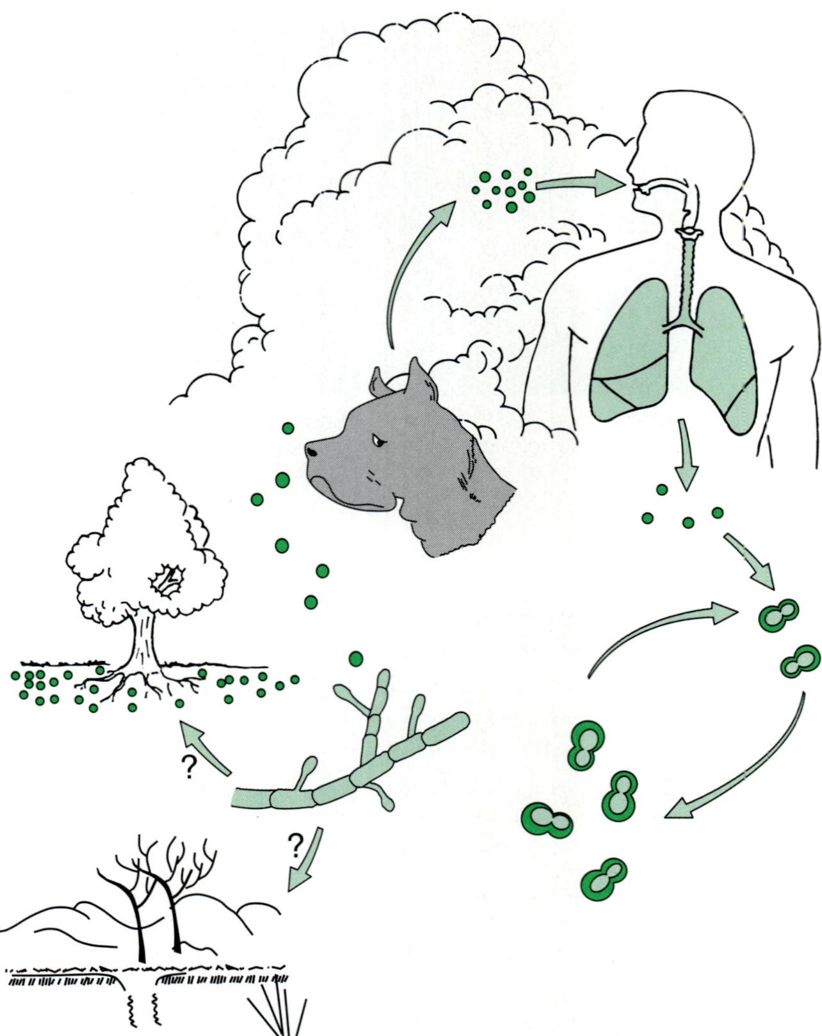

Fig. 4.10 Schematic illustration of the natural history of the saprobic and parasitic cycle of *Blastomyces dermatitidis.*

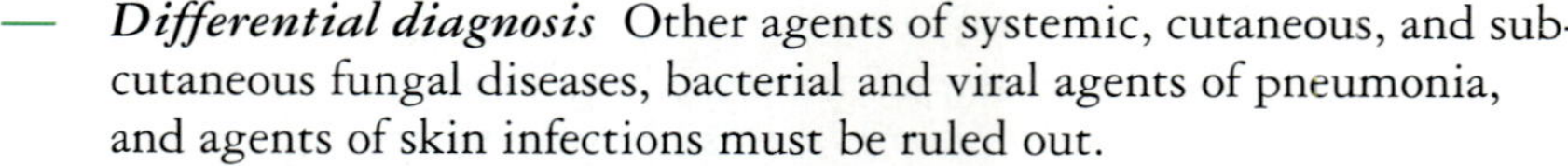

— ***Differential diagnosis*** Other agents of systemic, cutaneous, and subcutaneous fungal diseases, bacterial and viral agents of pneumonia, and agents of skin infections must be ruled out.

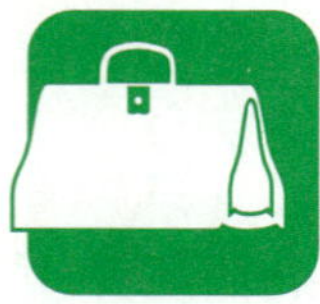

— ***Treatment*** Amphotericin B is the treatment for severe disease, but it penetrates poorly into cerebrospinal fluid. Ketoconazole is useful for long-term therapy. Fluconazole appears to be useful as an alternative.

Diseases Caused by Nondimorphic Systemic Agents

Cryptococcosis (Busse-Buschke Disease; Torulosis; European Blastomycosis) The organism *Cryptococcus neoformans* produces a large **capsule** that inhibits phagocytosis and, antigenically, is useful in diagnosis.

— ***Disease***

- Cryptococcosis is a chronic infection that originates in the lungs but has a strong predilection for the central nervous system.

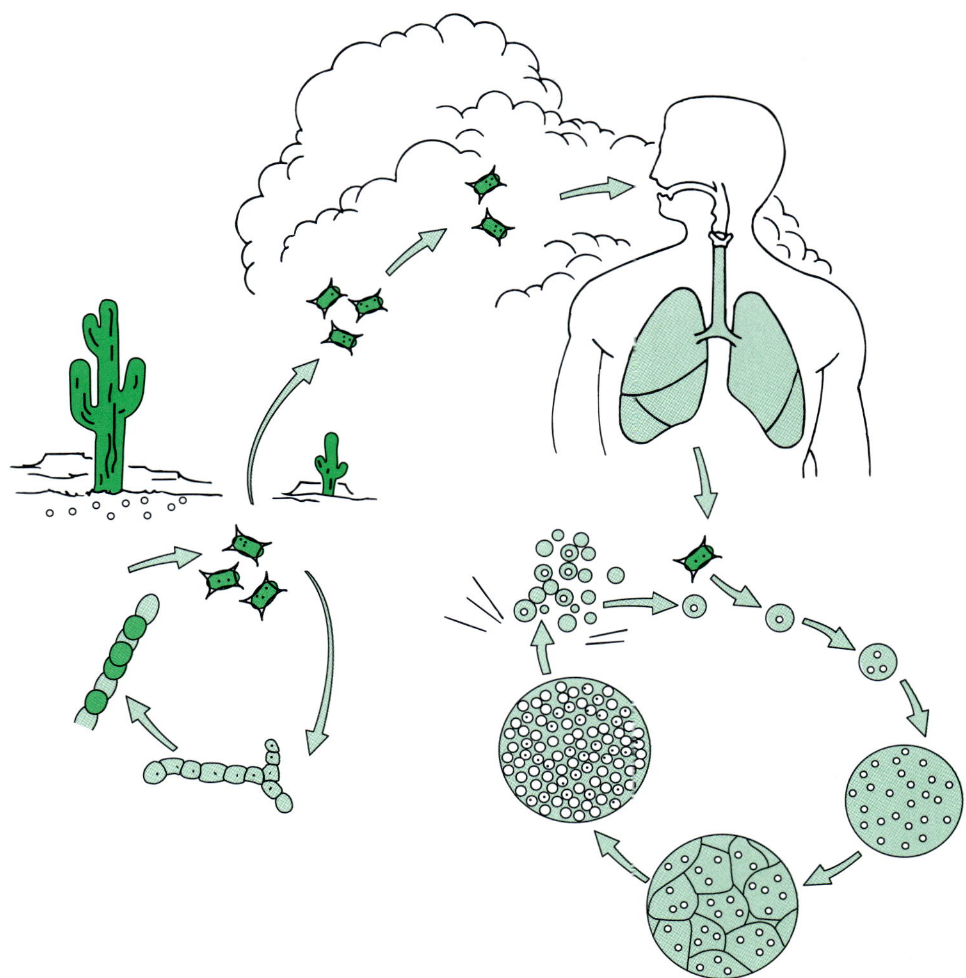

Fig. 4.11 Schematic illustration of the natural history of the saprobic and parasitic cycles of *Coccidioides immitis.*

- Asymptomatic primary pulmonary infections are the most common form of the disease. The infection is often discovered coincidentally as a solitary pulmonary nodule that may mimic carcinoma.
- *The most frequently diagnosed form of the disease is meningitis.*
- Skin and bone lesions may also occur.
- Cryptococci cause systemic disease in normal individuals, but AIDS patients and other immunosuppressed individuals are at increased risk (see Fig. 4.9).

— ***Laboratory diagnosis*** Laboratory diagnosis is based on the detection of antigen in body fluids. The latex agglutination test is performed for capsular antigen in CSF and serum. *India Ink preparations of spinal fluid can be viewed for the presence of capsules.*

Culture: The organisms may be cultured on routine laboratory media. Identification is based on carbohydrate assimilation tests, urease activity, and capsule production.

- *Cryptococcus* does not fit morphologically with the other systemic fungi because it is not dimorphic.
- An old, but useful, medium for differential isolation is "bird-seed" agar. The medium contains phenolic compounds that will cause colonies of *C. neoformans* to turn dark brown or black as they produce melanin (because of phenoloxidase production).

— ***Differential diagnosis*** Other systemic fungal agents (especially *Histoplasma*) and other agents of meningitis must be eliminated. Lung cancer must also be considered.

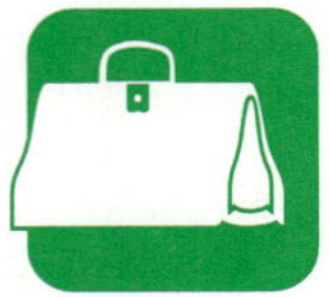

— ***Treatment*** Historically, amphotericin B and 5-fluorocytosine (5-FC) have been used together in the treatment of cryptococcosis. Currently, the use of fluconazole in place of 5-FC in primary treatment is being investigated. Use of fluconazole after initial treatment for long-term control, especially in AIDS patients, is becoming routine.

Section 4.5 Summary and Correlations of the Mycoses

Organism	Site of Infection	Symptoms/Disease	Other Features
Agents Causing Superficial Mycoses			
	Skin, hair	Pityriasis versicolor	
	Skin, hair	Tinea nigra	
Agents Causing Cutaneous Mycoses (Dermatophytes)			
Trichophyton spp.	Beard, face	Tinea barbae	
Microsporum spp.	Scalp	Tinea capitis	
	Skin	Tinea corporis	
	Groin	Tinea cruris	
	Feet	Tinea pedis	
	Body	Tinea veriscolor	
Agents Causing Subcutaneous Mycoses			Many of these fungi are found in the soil
Sporothrix schenckii	Hands, feet	Nodular lesions along lymphatics	Acquired from rosethorns, by trauma, or by gardening
Dematiaceous fungi or bacteria	Hands, feet	Mycetoma; tumorlike lesions	Grains containing hyphal elements present in lesions
Dematiaceous soil fungi	Hands, feet	Chromoblastomycosis: cauliflowerlike warty nodules	
Agents Causing Opportunistic Mycoses			
Candida albicans	Common: mucous membranes of the mouth and vagina Also: systemic	Thrush; vaginal yeast infections in normal and compromised patients	Normal flora; occurs in normal, diabetic, and AIDS patients
Aspergillus	Lungs	Fungus ball; allergies	Produces aflatoxins
Rhizopus spp.	Paranasal sinuses, eyes, brain	Zygomycosis	Aseptate hyphal emboli
Mucor spp.	Paranasal sinuses, eyes, brain		
Pneumocystis carinii	Lungs	Pneumonia	Diagnostic characteristic for AIDS
Agents Causing Systemic Mycoses			Normal individuals can be infected; immunosuppressed individuals are at higher risk of infection by these fungi
Cryptococcus neoformans	Lungs, CNS	Meningitis	*Nondimorphic; encapsulated;* spread by pigeon droppings
Histoplasma capsulatum	Lungs, CNS, reticuloendothelial system	Addison's disease; flulike symptoms	Present in soil and bird droppings; endemic in Ohio/Mississippi River valleys
Coccidiodes immitis	Lungs and disseminated infection	Coccidiodomycosis; San Joaquin fever; valley fever; cough, fever, and joint pains	Southwestern United States; desert areas; very infectious
Blastomyces dermatitides	Lungs, CNS, skin, bone	Tuberculouslike pneumonia	

Multiple Choice Review Questions

1.-5. Match the correct organism, disease, or group of organisms with each of the following statements. An organism may be used more than once or not at all.

a. Dermatophytes
b. *Sporothrix*
c. *Histoplasma*
d. *Coccidioides*
e. Mycetoma
f. *Cryptococcus*
g. *Candida* spp.

1. This organism can be confused with *Toxoplasma.* It is associated with disease in the Ohio and the Mississippi River valleys and with areas contaminated with bird-droppings, e.g., from pigeons.

2. These organisms are keratinophilic and infection is generally limited to superficial areas of the body.

3. A gardener was seen in the emergency room with nodular eruptions on her arm along the route of the draining lymphatics but not in the lymph node. A dimorphic fungus was isolated from the lesion.

4. A traveling salesman returns from a trip to Arizona with respiratory disease followed by the development of red tender nodules over the shin. A highly infectious organism which produces large spherules in tissue and arthrospores when grown at 25° C is isolated but great precautions were taken.

5. A yeast that produces a large capsule and is urease positive was isolated from an AIDS patient diagnosed with meningitis.

Chapter 5

Parasitology

Overview

Overview Although parasites are not stressed on the Boards, there will be several questions on the important parasites. This information is highlighted in Tables 5.1 and 5.2.

Special Notes

1. Creeping eruption or serpigenous (serpentlike) lesions are caused by migrating larva in the skin and are observed with the following parasites:

- Dog hookworms *(Ancylostoma braziliense, A. caninum)*
- *Strongyloides*

2. Infection of subcutaneous tissue is expressed as a subcutaneous swelling or nodule (not commonly seen in the United States) and is observed in infections with the following parasites:

- *Onchocerca volvulus*
- *Loa loa*
- *Gnathostoma spinigerum*
- *Dracunculus medinensis*
- *Spirometra* spp.
- Parasites that cause myasis

3. Pulmonary infiltrates with eosinophilia are caused by passage of migrating larva through the lungs. These infiltrates are cbserved in infections with the following parasites:

- Hookworm *(Ancylostoma duodenale, Necatcr americanus)*
- *Strongyloides*
- *Ascaris*
- Less common (depending on geographic location): *Toxocara, Echinococcus, Paragonimus*

4. Central nervous system involvement is observed in the following infections:

- *Cystircercus* (*Taenia solium* larva) infection
- *Toxoplasma* infection (especially in AIDS patients)
- *Trichinella spiralis* infection
- *Schistosoma mansoni* and *S. japonicum* infecrion (ova deposition)
- *Echinococcus* infection
- *Paragonimus* infection
- Toxocariasis (visceral larval migrans)

Text continued on p. 283

Table 5.1 *Description of Selected Parasites Intestinal Nematodes*

Scientific and Common Name	Epidemiology	Disease-Producing Form and Its Location in Host	How Infection Occurs	Major Disease Manifestations, Diagnostic Stage, and Specimen of Choice	Diagnostic or Characteristic Morphology
Enterobius vermicularis (pinworm)	Worldwide	Adult worms in colon; eggs on perianal region	Infective eggs are discharged by the gravid female on perianal skin; eggs are transferred from hand to mouth	Perianal itching caused by local irritation from scratching Diagnosis: eggs found by cellophane test	
Ascaris lumbricoides (large intestinal roundworm)	Worldwide, especially in moist, warm climate	Larval migration through lungs Adult worms in small intestine	Ingestion of eggs containing mature larvae from infected soil or food	Light infection—asymptomatic Heavy infection—pneumonia from larval migration Diarrhea and bowel or appendix obstruction Diagnosis: eggs (or adults) in feces	Unfertilized egg Fertilized egg
Strongyloides stercoralis (threadworm)	Cosmopolitan warm areas	Larval migration; pulmonary signs Adults in small intestine	Immature (rhabditiform) larvae are shed in feces, and become mature in soil or intestine Infective (filariform) larvae penetrate host skin, especially feet Autoinfection by maturing larvae in intestine	Repeated infection results in larval dermatitis with later pulmonary symptoms Heavy infections—abdominal pain, vomiting, and diarrhea Moderate eosinophilia Immunosuppressed host may suffer severe symptoms or death from heavy worm burdens as autoinfection may occur Diagnosis: rhabditiform larvae in feces	(See fig.)

Trichinella spiralis (trichinella worm)	Cosmopolitan	Adults in small intestine Larval migration; larvae encyst in striated muscle	Ingestion of encysted larva in undercooked meat (pork or bear)	Gastric distress, fever, eye edema, acute muscle pain, eosinophilia Diagnosis: encysted larvae in muscle biopsy; serology	Larva in muscle
Necator americanus (New World hookworm)	U.S., West Africa, Asia, and South Pacific	Larval migration; ground itch Adults in small intestine	Eggs shed in feces, mature into larvae in soil Infective (filariform) larvae penetrate host skin, especially feet	Repeated infection results in larval dermatitis with later pulmonary symptoms Microcytic hypochromic anemia from chronic blood loss if heavy infection and poor diet Diagnosis: eggs in feces	
Ancylostoma duodenale (Old World hookworm)	Europe, Brazil, Mediterranean area, and Asia	Larval migration; ground itch Adults in small intestine	Eggs shed in feces, mature into larvae in soil Infective (filariform) larvae penetrate host skin, especially feet	Repeated infection results in larval dermatitis with later pulmonary symptoms Microcytic hypochromic anemia from chronic blood loss if heavy infection and poor diet Diagnosis: eggs in feces	(See fig.)

Larva

Continued.

Table 5.1 *Description of Selected Parasites—cont'd* *Blood and Tissue Nematodes*

Scientific and Common Name	Epidemiology, Periodicity, and Intermediate Host	Disease-Producing Form and Its Location in Host	How Infection Occurs	Major Disease Manifestations, Diagnostic Stage, and Specimen of Choice	Diagnostic or Characteristic Morphology
Wuchereria bancrofti (Bancroft's filaria)	Tropics Nocturnal periodicity *Culex, Aedes,* and *Anopheles;* mosquitoes	Adults live in the lymphatics (microfilariae in blood)	Filariform larvae are injected into the blood when the mosquito bites a human to take a blood meal	Invades lymphatics and causes granulomatous lesions, chills, fever, eosinophilia, and elephantiasis Diagnosis: microfilariae in blood; serology	(See fig.)

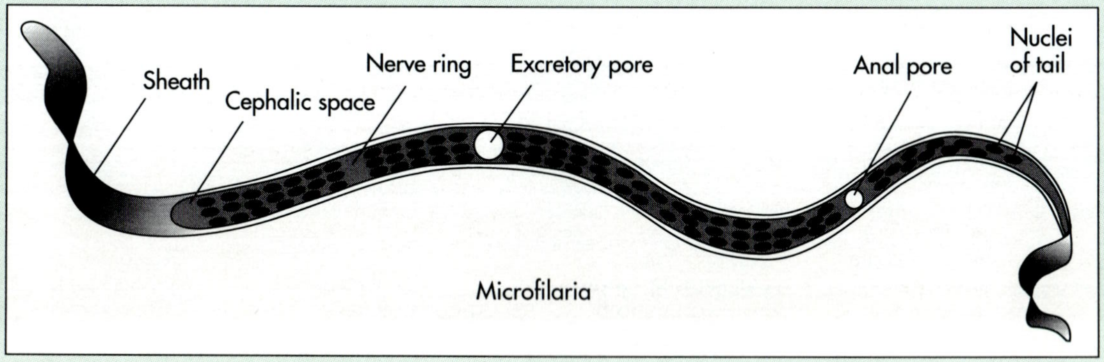

Microfilaria

Table 5.1 *Description of Selected Parasites—cont'd* *Important Zoonotic Nematodes*

Scientific and Common Name	Geographic Location	Normal Animal Host	Disease	Symptoms in Humans	Method of Infection of Humans
Ancylostoma braziliense *A. caninum* (dog hookworms)	Southern U.S., Central and South America, Africa, Asia, Northern Hemisphere	Dog	Cutaneous larval migrans (CLM) Creeping eruption	Allergic response to the migration of larvae under the skin Red, itchy tracts, usually on legs	Penetration of the skin by filariform larvae
Toxocara canis *T. cati* (large intestinal roundworms of dogs or cats)	Worldwide	Dog, cat	Visceral larval migrans (VLM)	Eosinophilia, hepatomegaly, pulmonary inflammation with cough and fever, possible encystment of the larvae in the eye, which mimics a malignant tumor All symptoms due to migration of larvae in the tissues of humans	Ingestion of infective stage larvae in developed eggs from soil
Dirofilaria spp. (filariae of canines)	Various species worldwide	Dog, racoon, fox	Tropical eosinophilia, eosinophilic lung	High eosinophilia, chronic cough, pulmonary infiltrates, high levels of IgE Microfilariae are rarely present in peripheral blood	Bite of insect vector carrying infective filaria larvae

Continued.

Table 5.1 *Description of Selected Parasites—cont'd* *Cestoidea: Tapeworms*

Scientific and Common Name	Epidemiology	Disease-Producing Form and Its Location in Host	How Infection Occurs	Major Disease Manifestations, Diagnostic Stage, and Specimen of Choice	Diagnostic or Characteristic Morphology
Taenia saginata (beef tapeworm)	Cosmopolitan in beef-eating countries	Adult lives in small intestine	*Cysticercus bovis* larva eaten by human in undercooked beef	Most people are asymptomatic Can experience abdominal pain, diarrhea, weight loss Diagnosis: eggs or proglottid in feces	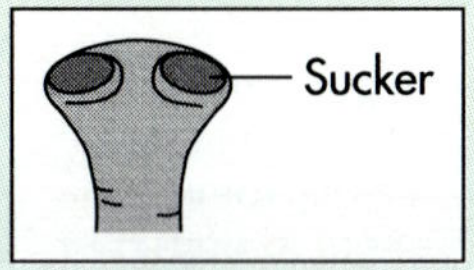 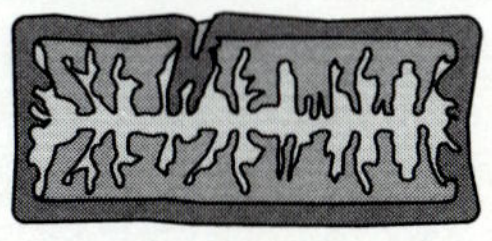 Sucker Gravid proglottid
Taenia solium (pork tapeworm)	Worldwide (rare in U.S.)	Adult lives in small intestine	*Cysticercus cellulosa* larva eaten by human in undercooked pork	Same as *Taenia saginata*	
(cysticercosis)		Racemose, cysticercus in brain	Accidental ingestion of egg	Death can occur	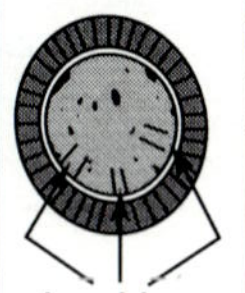 hooklets Egg

Diphyllobothrium latum (broad fish tapeworm)	Temperate areas where freshwater fish is eaten	Adult lives in small intestine	Larva ingested by human in undercooked freshwater fish	Can cause intestinal obstruction and macrolytic anemia due to B_{12} deficiency; abdominal pain and weight loss Diagnosis: eggs in feces	
Echinococcus granulosus (dog tapeworm)	Worldwide in sheep-raising areas	Adults live in the intestine of dogs or other wild canines	Human accidentally ingests eggs by close contact with an infected dog	Cyst can be found in the liver (most commonly) or lung of human Lung symptoms include coughing and pain Leakage of hydatid fluid causes allergy and eosinophilia Diagnosis: radiography, serology	(See fig.)

Continued.

Table 5.1 *Description of Selected Parasites—cont'd Trematoda: Flukes*

Scientific and Common Name	Epidemiology	Disease-Producing Form and Its Location in Host	How Infection Occurs	Major Disease Manifestations, Diagnostic Stage, and Specimen of Choice	Diagnostic or Characteristic Morphology
Clonorchis sinensis (Oriental or Chinese liver fluke)	Far East	Adults live in bile ducts	Ingestion of encysted metacercariae in uncooked fish	Jaundice and eosinophilia in acute phase; long-term heavy infections lead to functional impairment of liver Diagnosis: eggs in feces	
Schistosoma mansoni (Manson's blood fluke) (Bilharzia; swamp fever)	Africa, Middle East, and South America; snail is intermediate host	Adults in venules of the colon Eggs trapped in liver and other tissues	Free-swimming cercariae in snail-infested water burrow into skin and spread in blood	Granuloma formation around eggs (i.e., in liver, intestine and bladder) Toxic and allergic reactions Diagnosis: eggs in feces	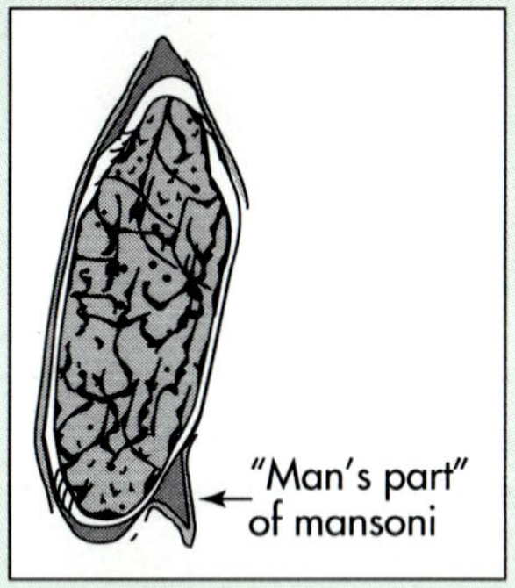 "Man's part" of mansoni
Schistosoma japonicum (Oriental blood fluke)	Far East	As above	As above	As above, but symptoms are more severe due to greater egg production Diagnosis: eggs in feces	
Schistosoma haematobium (bladder fluke)	Africa, Middle East, and Portugal	Adults in venules of bladder and rectum Eggs caught in tissues	As above	Bladder colic with blood and pus Systemic symptoms are mild Diagnosis: eggs in urine	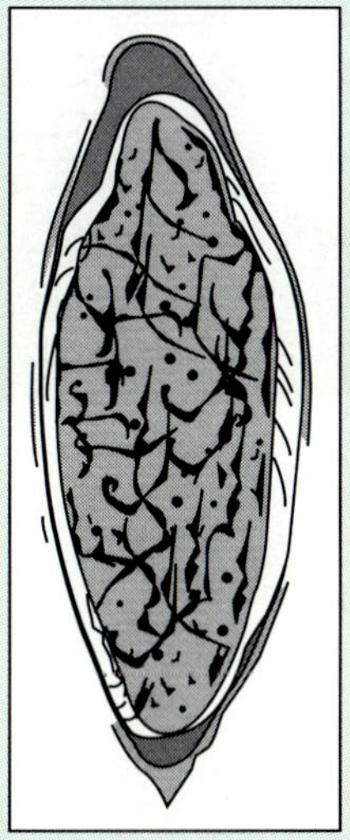

Table 5.1 *Description of Selected Parasites—cont'd* *Protozoa*

Scientific and Common Name	Epidemiology	Disease-Producing Form and Its Location in Host	How Infection Occurs	Major Disease Manifestations, Diagnostic Stage, and Specimen of Choice	Diagnostic or Characteristic Morphology
Entamoeba histolytica (amebic dysentery)	Worldwide	Trophozoites in large intestinal mucosa, liver, or other tissues	Ingestion of cyst in fecally contaminated food or water	Enteritis with abdominal pain and bloody dysentery Diagnosis: cysts and trophozoites in feces	Cyst
Giardia lamblia (traveler's diarrhea)	Worldwide Campers and hikers at risk	Trophozoites in large intestinal mucosa	Ingestion of cysts in fecally contaminated food or water, streams cyst	Mild to severe dysentery; malabsorption syndrome Diagnosis: cysts and trophozoites in feces	Axoneme Troph
Trichomonas vaginalis (trich)	Worldwide	Trophozoites in urethra or vagina	Sexual contact	Irritating, frothy vaginal discharge; men usually asymptomatic Diagnosis: trophozoites in urine or vaginal smear (no cysts formed)	
Leishmania braziliensis (New World leishmaniasis espundia)	Central and South America	Leishmania in macrophages in skin lesion and mucocutaneous tissue	Bite of *Phlebotomus* spp.	Self-healing skin lesion, later ulceration of cephalic mucocutaneous tissue Diagnosis: recovery of leishmania forms from lesion	

Continued.

Table 5.1 *Description of Selected Parasites—cont'd* *Protozoa*

Scientific and Common Name	Epidemiology	Disease-Producing Form and Its Location in Host	How Infection Occurs	Major Disease Manifestations, Diagnostic Stage, and Specimen of Choice	Diagnostic or Characteristic Morphology
Trypanosoma cruzi (Chagas' disease)	South America	Early trypanosomal and crithidial forms in blood; later LD bodies in heart and other tissues	Infected feces of *Triatoma* spp. (kissing bug) rubbed into bite site	Fever, enlarged spleen and liver, Romaña's sign (edema around eyes), chronic damage to heart and alimentary tract Acute death, especially in children Diagnosis: trypanosomes in blood xenodiagnosis	
Plasmodium ovale (none)	West Africa	Initial hypnozoites in liver; schizogony and gametocytes in red blood cells (RBCs)	*Anopheles* spp. mosquito transmits sporozoites	Cyclic fever, chills, enlarged spleen, parasites in RBCs Diagnosis: malarial forms in blood smear	
Plasmodium vivax (benign tertian malaria)	Tropics, subtropics, some temperate regions	Initial hypnozoites in liver; schizogony and gametocytes in RBCs	*Anopheles* spp. mosquito transmits sporozoites	Cyclic fever, chills, enlarged spleen, parasites in **only young** (larger) RBCs Diagnosis: malarial forms in blood smear	

Plasmodium malariae (quartian malaria)	Tropics	Initial hypnozoites in liver; schizogony and gametocytes in RBCs	*Anopheles* spp. mosquito transmits sporozoites	Cyclic fever, chills, enlarged spleen, parasites in **only old** (small) RBCs; relapses Diagnosis: malarial forms in blood smear
Plamodium falciparum (malignant malaria)	Tropics	Initial hypnozoites in liver; trophozoites and gametocytes in peripheral RBCs	*Anopheles* spp. mosquito transmits sporozoites	(See fig.) Cyclic fever, chills, enlarged spleen, parasites in **old and young** (large and small) RBCs Blackwater fever from hemoglobin in urine, blockage of capillaries, death Diagnosis: malarial forms in blood smear

Ring Troph Schizont Macro gametocyte

Continued.

Table 5.1 *Description of Selected Parasites—cont'd Protozoa*

Scientific and Common Name	Epidemiology	Disease-Producing Form and Its Location in Host	How Infection Occurs	Major Disease Manifestations, Diagnostic Stage, and Specimen of Choice	Diagnostic or Characteristic Morphology
Toxoplasma gondii (toxoplasmosis)	Worldwide; cats are hosts; neonates and AIDS patients at risk	Trophozoites intracellularly in all organs; pseudocysts in brain and other tissue	Ingestion of oocysts; ingestion of trophozoites or pseudocysts in undercooked meat; congenital passage of trophozoites	Fever, enlarged lymph nodes In fetus or neonate; damage (TORCH) Can cause acute infection in immunosuppressed patient Diagnosis: serology	
Cryptosporidium (none)	Worldwide	Invades GI tract mucosa	Ingestion of fecally contaminated food or water	Diarrhea Diagnosis: trophozoites and schizonts in biopsy of jejunum and/or oocysts in stool	oocyst
Babesia spp. (none) (zoonosis)	Worldwide	*Babesia* trophozoites in RBC	Tick bite	Fever; symptoms can resemble malaria Diagnosis: trophozoites in blood smear	(See fig.)

Sporozoites mature on the surface of the intestinal epithelium.

Trophozoite

Diagnostic stage

Table 5.2 ***Parasites and Keywords***

Parasite	Keywords
Protozoa	
Entamoeba histolytica	Dysentery, liver abscess
Giardia lamblia	Traveler's diarrhea
Cryptosporidium parvum	Diarrhea, waterborne outbreak, AIDS, acid-fast
Isospora belli	Diarrhea, AIDS
Microsporidium	Diarrhea, AIDS
Trichomonas vaginalis	Vaginitis, sexually transmitted
Babesia spp.	Erythrocyte infection, asplenia, tick-borne
Plasmodium spp.	Malaria; ring form; hemolysis; mosquito-borne; sporozoite is acquired, merozoites infect erythrocytes, gametocytes are given back to the mosquito (Fig. 5.1)
Naegleria, Acanthamoeba	Meningoencephalitis, swimming pools, fresh water lakes
Toxoplasma gondii	Mononucleosis syndrome, CNS and AIDS, cat litter, undercooked hamburger
Leishmania spp.	Sandfly, phlebotomus, chronic ulcer, visceral
Trypanosome, African	Sleeping sickness, tsetse fly
Trypanosome, American	Reduviid bug, Chagas disease, orbital edema, megasyndromes
Pneumocystis carinii (fungus not a protozoon)	Pneumonia, AIDS
Nematodes (Round Worms)	
Ascaris lumbricoides	Pneumonia with eosinophilia, intestinal obstruction
Trichuris trichura	Whipworm, rectal prolapse
Enterobius vermicularis	Pinworm, anal itching, scotch tape
Strongyloides stercoralis	Autoinfection, hyperinfection, pneumonia with eosinophilia, larvae in the stool
Necator and *Ancylostoma* spp. (hookworm)	Iron deficiency anemia, pneumonia with eosinophilia
Wuchereria and *Brugi* spp. (filaria)	Mosquito, elephantiasis
Onchocerca spp.	Black flies, eyes, subcutaneous nodules
Loa loa	Tabanid flies, eyeworm
Dirofilaria spp.	Dog, heartworm, lungs
Dracunculus	Guinea worm, waterborne
Trichinella spiralis	Pork, muscle
Trematodes (Flukes)	
Opisthorchis (Clonorchis) sinensis	Liver, bile duct, cholangiocarcinoma, cholangitis, pancreatitis
Paragonimus spp.	Hemoptysis, pulmonary lesion, wheezing, ova in the sputum
Schistosoma spp.	Blood fluke, hematuria *(S. haematobium)*, spiny appendage (ova of *S. haematobium* and *S. mansoni)*, snails, ascites
Cestodes (Flatworms)	
Taenia saginata	Beef
Taenia solium	Pork, cysticercosis, brain, eye
Diphyllobothrium latum	Megaloblastic anemia, fish
Echinococcus spp.	Liver, lung, hydatid cyst

- *Strongyloides* infection (hyperinfection)
- *Angiostrongylus cantonensis* infection (eosinophilic meningitis)
- *Entamoeba histolytica* infection (amebic brain abscess)
- Ameboflagellates (*Acanthamoeba* and *Naegleria*) amebic meningoencephalitis
- Malaria
- African sleeping sickness

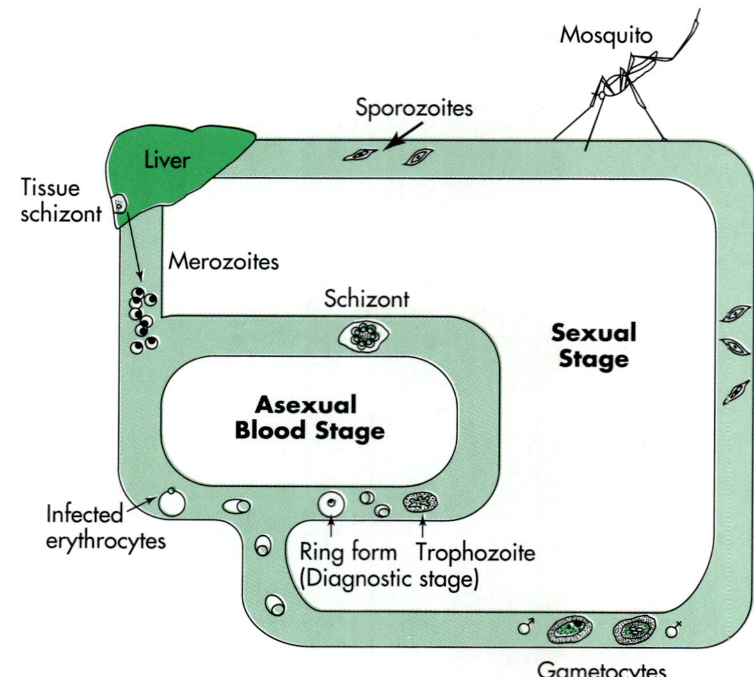

Fig. 5.1 Life cycle of plasmodia in humans. The female *Anopheles* mosquito injects the *sporozoite* into the blood. It infects the liver and produces *merozoites* which infect erythrocytes. Reproduction by both asexual (*ringform, trophozoite, schizont, merozoite*) and sexual (*gametocyte*) mechanisms occur in the blood at the same time. Mosquitos which acquire male and female gametocytes during a blood meal can produce sporozoites for human infection. ***P. falciparum*** **infect young and old erythrocytes; *P. vivax,* only young RBC; *P. malariae,* only old RBC.**

5. Lesions in the liver and the lungs are found in infections by the following organisms:

- *Echinococcus*
- *Schistosoma*
- *Entamoeba histolytica*

6. Hematuria is seen in infections with *Schistosoma haematobium.*
7. Eye lesions are found in the following parasitic infections:

- *Loa loa* infections
- Onchocerciasis
- Cysticercosis
- Toxoplasmosis
- Toxocariasis
- Gnathostomiasis
- Angiostrongyliasis

8. Autoinfections occur when the infective larval stage develop and spread within the host:

- Taenia solium
- *Strongyloides stercoralis*

Multiple Choice Review Questions

1. Which of the following statements is false?
   a. The presence of red cells in the ameba is diagnostic for *Entamoeba histolytica.*
   b. The presence of double crescent-ring forms in a red cell is diagnostic for *Plasmodium falciparum.*
   c. The gametocyte stage of *P. falciparum* is infective for humans.
   d. The infectious form of *Giardia lamblia* is the cyst.
   e. The presence of rhabditiform larvae in the stool is diagnostic for *Strongyloides* infestation.

2. Which of the following statements is characteristic of *Enterobius vermicularis?*
   a. A 5-year-old boy with perianal itching
   b. A 28-year-old woman with a serpigenous skin lesion on the bottom of her foot (history of walking barefoot on the beach)
   c. A 19-year-old man from the Caribbean with a chronic nonhealing skin ulcer
   d. A 45-year-old man with periorbital swelling and muscle ache
   e. A 24-year-old Laotian woman with jaundice but no fever

3-6. Match the clinical information with the parasite:
   a. Magnetic resonance imaging shows a space-occupying lesion in the brain
   b. Lesions in the liver and lungs
   c. Megaloblastic anemia
   d. Chronic diarrhea
   e. Hemolysis

   3. Toxoplasmosis in an AIDS patient
   4. Cysticercosis *(Taenia solium)*
   5. *Diphylobothrium latum*
   6. *Giardia lamblia*

Chapter 6

Infectious Disease Correlations

Overview This chapter integrates much of the information presented in earlier chapters. The tables in this chapter present the pathogens (bacteria, viruses, fungi, and parasites) associated with specific diseases and syndromes.

Section 6.1 Common Infection Syndromes

Common syndromes of infections are listed in Table 6.1

Section 6.2 Infections of the Immunocompromised Host

Immunosuppression increases risk to specific infectious agents (Table 6.2). AIDS patients are at increased risk to viruses, fungi, and intracellular infections (see below).

PRINCIPAL OPPORTUNISTIC PATHOGENS IN AIDS PATIENTS

Bacteria

Listeria monocytogenes
Nocardia asteroides
Mycobacterium tuberculosis
Mycobacterium avium-intracellulare
Salmonella spp.
Legionella pneumophila

Fungi

Candida spp.
Cryptococcus neoformans
Histoplasma capsulatum
Coccidioides immitis
Pneumocystis carinii

Parasites

Toxoplasma gondii
Strongyloides stercoralis

Table 6.1 *Common Syndromes of Infection*

Common Syndromes of Infection	Common and Less Common Pathogens	Laboratory Diagnosis
Endocarditis		
Native valve	Viridans group streptococci, *Enterococcus* spp., *Streptococcus pneumoniae, Staphylococcus aureus,* HACEK* organisms	Blood culture
Prosthetic valve: <60 days	Coagulase-negative staphylococci, *S. aureus, Enterococcus* spp., *Corynebacterium* spp.	
Prosthetic valve: >60 days	Viridans group streptococci, coagulase-negative staphylococci, *Enterococcus* spp.	
Central Nervous System Infections		
Acute bacterial meningitis	*S. pneumoniae, Neisseria meningitidis, Haemophilus influenzae,* and less commonly, *Listeria monocytogenes* In neonates: *Streptococcus agalactiae* and *Escherichia coli*	Blood and (CSF) cultures; antigen detection in spinal fluid, blood, and urine
Aseptic meningitis	Viral agents: Enterovirus, herpes simplex virus (HSV), adenovirus, mumps virus, lymphocytic choriomeningitis virus, Epstein-Barr virus (EBV), arbo-encephalitis virus	Viral culture; viral serology
	Mycoplasma pneumoniae	Mycoplasma antibody
	Treponema pallidum	Syphilis serology
	Leptospira spp.	Leptospiral antibody
	Borrelia burgdorferi	
Chronic meningitis	*Mycobacterium tuberculosis, Cryptococcus neoformans, Coccidiodes immitis, T. pallidum, B. burgdorferi*	CSF smear and culture for mycobacteria or fungi
Encephalitis	HSV, bunyaviruses, togaviruses, picornaviruses, measles virus, rabies virus, *Toxoplasma*	Viral culture, brain biopsy
Brain abscess	Mixed infection: streptococci, anaerobes, *S. aureus,* Cysticerosis *(Taenia)*	Direct needle aspiration
Progressive multifocal leukoencephalopathy	Papovaviruses	
Diarrheas (Tables 6.3 and 6.4)		
Bacterial		
Watery	*Vibrio cholerae, E. coli*	
Bloody	*Shigella* spp., *Salmonella* spp., *Campylobacter* spp., *E. coli, Clostridium difficile, Vibrio parahemolyticus*	
Nonbloody	*E. coli*	
Toxin-mediated	*V. cholerae, Clostridium perfringens, E. coli, S. aureus, Bacillus cereus*	
Viral	Norwalk agent, reovirus, rotavirus, adenovirus	
Parasitic	*Giardia, Cryptosporidium, Entamoeba histolytica, Stronglyloides stercoralis*	
Intraabdominal Infections		
Spontaneous peritonitis	*E. coli, Klebsiella pneumoniae, S. pneumoniae, Enterococcus* spp., *M. tuberculosis*	Peritoneal fluid culture
Secondary peritonitis or intraabdominal abscess	*E. coli, Bacteroides fragilis* and other anaerobes, *Enterococcus* spp., *Pseudomonas aeruginosa*	
Peritoneal dialysis-associated peritonitis	Coagulase-negative staphylococci, *S. aureus, Streptococcus* spp., less often aerobic gram-negative rods	

**HACEK:* Haemophilus aphrophilus, Actinobacillus actinomycetemcomitans, Cardiobacterium hominis, Eikenella corrodens, Kingella kingii.

Continued.

Table 6.1 *Common Syndromes of Infection—cont'd*

Common Syndromes of Infection	Common and Less Common Pathogens	Laboratory Diagnosis
Upper Respiratory Tract Infections		
Common cold	Rhinoviruses and other picornaviruses, coronaviruses, influenza viruses, paramyxoviruses, adenoviruses	Symptoms, isolation from nasal washings or sputum
Pharyngitis	*S. pyogenes,* adenoviruses, EBV, HSV	Throat culture, streptococcal serology
	Less common: *M. pneumoniae, Chlamydia pneumoniae, Corynebacterium diphtheriae, Corynebacterium ulcerans, Arcanobacterium haemolyticum, Yersinia enterocolitica, Neisseria gonorrhoeae,* mixed anaerobes	
Croup	*Parainfluenza* virus	
Otitis externa	*P. aeruginosa* (swimmer's ear)	Culture of the ear exudate
Malignant external otitis	*P. aeruginosa* (found in diabetic patients)	
Otitis media and sinusitis	*S. pneumoniae, H. influenzae, Moraxella catarrhalis,* anaerobes	Culture of exudate (culture is generally not necessary)
Lower Respiratory Tract Infections		
Bronchitis	*S. pneumoniae, H. influenzae, M. catarrhalis, M. pneumoniae, C. pneumoniae, Bordetella pertussis,* parainfluenza viruses, respiratory syncytial virus (RSV), adenoviruses	Sputum culture; nasopharyngeal culture for *B. pertussis*
Pneumonia, community acquired	*S. pneumoniae, H. influenzae, M. catarrhalis, M. pneumoniae, C. pneumoniae, Legionella* spp., influenza viruses, parainfluenza viruses, adenoviruses, RSV, varicella-zoster virus (VZV), hantavirus	Sputum culture; viral culture serology; *Legionella* antigen in urine for serotype I
Pneumonia, nosocomial	*S. aureus,* gram-negative bacilli, mixed aerobic/anaerobic infection	Same as above
Pneumonia, chronic	*M. tuberculosis,* mixed aerobic/anaerobic infection, *Nocardia* spp., *Histoplasma capsulatum, Coccidiodes imitis, Blastomyces dermatitidis*	Culture of respiratory secretion
Eye Infections		
Conjunctivitis	*S. pneumoniae, S. aureus,* Coagulase-negative staphylococci, *H. influenzae, N. gonorrhoeae, C. trachomatis,* measles virus, adenovirus, enterovirus	Culture from the site of infection
Keratitis	*S. aureus, S. pneumoniae, P. aeruginosa, Moraxella* spp., HSV, mycobacteria	Culture from site of infection
Endophthalmitis	*S. aureus, P. aeruginosa, Bacillus* spp.	Culture of vitreous humor
Joint Infections		
Arthritis (pyarthrosis)	*S. aureus, N. gonorrhoeae, Streptococcus* spp.	Joint aspirate for culture; blood culture
	In children: *H. influenzae* Less common: mycobacteria, *Brucella* spp., *Nocardia* spp., fungi	
Prosthetic joint	*S. aureus,* Coagulase-negative staphylococci, *Streptococcus* spp., diphtheroids, anaerobes	Direct aspiration or operative culture; blood culture has a low yield
Arthritis (immunologic or reactive)	*S. pyogenes* (rheumatic fever)	Clinical and laboratory criteria
	B. burgdorferi (Lyme disease)	Clinical criteria; serology; PCR
	Yersinia, Salmonella, Shigella, Mycoplasma, Ureaplasma, C. trachomatis	High antibody titer
Viral arthritis	Parvovirus, hepatitis B virus (immune complexes), rubella virus, mumps virus	Viral isolation; antibody titer

Table 6.1 ***Common Syndromes of Infection—cont'd***

Common Syndromes of Infection	Common and Less Common Pathogens	Laboratory Diagnosis
Bone Infections		
Osteomyelitis	*S. aureus,* Enterobacteriaceae, *P. aeruginosa, M. tuberculosis,* other mycobacteria anaerobes	Direct bone culture; blood culture
Urinary Tract Infections	*E. coli, Proteus mirabilis, Klebsiella* spp., *P. aeruginosa, Enterococcus* spp., *Staphylococcus saprophyticus*	Urine culture
Genital Tract and Sexually Transmitted Infections		
Urethritis	*N. gonorrhoeae, Chlamydia trachomatis, Ureaplasma, Mycoplasma*	Urethral smear and culture
Cervicitis	*N. gonorrhoeae, C. trachomatis,* HSV, actinomycetes (intrauterine devices)	Culture
Genital ulcers	HSV, *T. pallidum, H. ducreyi, C. trachomatis* (lymphogranuloma venereum [LGV])	Culture and serology
Warts (condyloma acuminatum)	Papilloma virus	Cytology; immunofluorescent and immunoperoxidase staining
Skin and Soft Tissue Infections		
Impetigo	*S. pyogenes, S. aureus*	Smear and culture
Furuncle, carbuncle	*S. aureus*	
Paronychia	*S. pyogenes, S. aureus, P. aeruginosa*	
Erysipelas	*S. pyogenes*	
Cellulitis	*S. pyogenes, S. aureus, H. influenzae*	
Necrotizing fasciitis	*S. pyogenes, C. perfringens,* mixed anaerobic/aerobic organisms	
Molluscum contagiosum	Poxvirus	Histology
Rashes		
Bacterial: Scarlet fever, meningococcemia	*S. pyogenes, N. meningitidis*	
Rickettsial: typhus, Rocky Mountain spotted fever	*Rickettsia prowazeki, Rickettsia rickettsiae*	
Vesicular	HSV, VZV, Coxsackie viruses, echo viruses and other picornaviruses	
Maculopapular	Measles virus, rubella virus, human herpes virus 6 (roseola), parvovirus B19 (erythema infectiosum)	

CSF, Cerebrospinal fluid; *PCR,* polymerase chain reaction.

Viruses
Herpes simplex virus
Cytomegalovirus
Varicella-zoster virus
Measles virusJC virus
Adenovirus
Epstein-Barr virus

Section 6.3 Arthropod-Borne Diseases

Tick-borne Diseases

- Rocky Mountain spotted fever *(Rickettsia rickettsii)*

Table 6.2 ***Infections Associated with Defects in Immune Responses***

Defect	Pathogen
Induced by physical means (e.g., burns, trauma)	*Pseudomonas aeruginosa* *Staphylococcus aureus* *Staphylococcus epidermidis* *Streptococcus pyogenes* *Aspergillus* spp. *Candida* spp.
Granulocytes/monocytes defects in movement, phagocytosis, killing or decreased number (neutropenia)	*Staphylococcus aureus* *Streptococcus pyogenes* *Haemophilus influenzae* Gram-negative bacilli *Escherichia coli* *Klebsiella* spp. *Pseudomonas aeruginosa* *Nocardia* spp. Aspergillus spp. *Candida* spp.
Complement system individual components	*Staphylococcus aureus* *Streptococcus pneumoniae* *Pseudomonas* spp. *Proteus* spp. *Neisseria meningitidis* *Neisseria gonorrhoeae*
T cells	Cytomegalovirus Herpes simplex virus Herpes zoster virus *Listeria monocytogenes* *Mycobacterium* spp. *Nocardia* spp. *Aspergillus* spp. *Candida* spp. *Cryptococcus neoformans* *Histoplasma capsulatum* *Pneumocystis carinii* *Strongyloides stercoralis*
B cells	Enteroviruses *Staphylococcus aureus* *Streptococcus* spp. *Haemophilus influenzae* *Neisseria meningitidis* *Escherichia coli* *Giardia lamblia* *Pneumocystis carinii*
Combined immunodeficiency	As for T and B cells

- Lyme disease *(Borrelia burgdorferi)*
- Babesiosis (*Babesia* spp.)
- Ehrlichiosis (*Ehrlichia* spp.)
- Endemic relapsing fever (*Borrelia* spp.)
- Colorado tick fever (Colorado tick fever virus [orbivirus])
- Hemorrhagic fever
    - Crimean-Congo hemorrhagic fever (Crimean-Congo hemorrhagic fever virus [bunyavirus])
    - Omsk hemorrhagic fever (Omsk hemorrhagic fever virus [flavivirus])

Table 6.3 *Infectious Diarrheas**

Characteristics	Non-Inflammatory	Inflammatory	Inflammatory and Invasive
Site of Lesion	Small intestine	Colon	Peyer's patches
Fever	Not common	Common	Prolonged
Bacteremia	No	Uncommon	Common
Fecal Leukocytes	Absent	Usually present	Usually present
Etiologic Agents	**Toxin Related** *S. aureus* (preformed toxin) *Bacillus cereus* *Clostridium perfringens* *Vibrio cholerae* *E. coli* (toxogenic) **Non-Toxin Related** *Giardia lamblia* *Cryptosporidium* *Cyclospora*	*Shigella* *Salmonella* *Campylobacter jejuni* *Clostridium difficile* *Aeromonas* *Plesiomonas* *Vibrio parahaemolyticus* *Entamoeba histolytica* (fecal leukocytes usually absent)	*Salmonella typhi* *Yersinia*

*Clinical questions will often list the characteristics provided in this table and Table 6.4.

Table 6.4 *Key Words for Diarrheas*

Diarrhea Agent	Key Words
Clostridium difficile	Antibiotics Pseudomembranous colitis
E. coli 0157:H7	Hemorrhagic colitis, hamburger Shigalike toxin, verotoxin Hemolytic uremic syndrome Thrombotic thrombocytopenic purpura
Vibrio parahemolyticus	Marine product
Vibrio vulnificus	Shellfish
Aeromonas hydrophila	Fresh water, leech
Salmonella	Poultry
Cholera	Rice water stool
Yersinia	Cabbage
Listeria	Unpasteurized dairy products
Toxogenic *E. coli*	Traveler's diarrhea
Bacillus cereus	Fried rice
Staphylococcus aureus *Clostridium perfringens*	Custard, picnics, sandwich meats, potato salad
Giardia lamblia	Contaminated stream water, camping, trophozoite with a face
Cryptosporidium	Water supply, immunocompromised patient
Entamoeba histolytica	Amoebic dysentery

Mite-transmitted Diseases

- Tsutsugamushi disease *(R. tsutsugamushi)*
- Rickettsialpox *(R. akari)*

Flea-transmitted Diseases

- Plague *(Yersinia pestis)*
- Murine typhus *(R. typhi)*
- Tapeworm disease *(Dipylidium caninum)*
- Tapeworm disease *(Hymenolepis diminuta)*

Louse-borne Diseases

- Epidemic typhus *(R. prowazekii)*
- Epidemic relapsing fever *(Borrelia recurrentis)*

Reduviid Bug-transmitted Diseases

- Chagas disease *(Trypanosoma cruzi)*

Sandfly-transmitted Diseases

- Leishmaniasis (*Leishmania* spp.)
- Sandfly fever (phleboviruses)
- Bartonellosis (Oroya fever and veruga peruana *[Bartonella bacilliformis]*)

Mosquito-borne Diseases

- Malaria (*Plasmodium* spp.)
- Filariasis (*Filaria* spp.)
- Dengue (dengue virus [flavivirus])
- Yellow fever (yellow fever virus [flavivirus])
- Chikungunya (chikungunya virus [alphavirus])
- Japanese B encephalitis (Japanese encephalitis virus [flavivirus])
- St. Louis encephalitis (St. Louis encephalitis virus [flavivirus])
- Epidemic polyarthritis (Ross River virus [alphavirus])
- California encephalitis (La Crosse virus [bunyavirus])

Deer Fly-transmitted Disease

- Eye infection *(Loa loa)*

Tsetse Fly-borne Disease

- Trypanosomiasis (*Trypanosoma* spp.)

Multiple Choice Review Questions

1. A 76-year-old man who has been a smoker since his teenage years was admitted with a right lower lung lobe infiltrate. A diagnosis of pneumonia was strongly considered and the patient was admitted to the hospital. Which of the following agents is not associated with adult community-acquired pneumonia?
   a. *Streptococcus pneumoniae*
   b. *Mycoplasma pneumoniae*
   c. *Chlamydia trachomatis*
   d. *Hemophilus influenzae*
   e. *Legionella pneumophila*

2. Which of the following tests is least useful in making the etiologic diagnosis in Question 1?
   a. Blood culture
   b. Gram stain of the sputum
   c. Culture for routine bacteria using blood agar or chocolate agar
   d. Culture for *Mycoplasma pneumoniae*
   e. Urinary antigen detection for *Legionella*

3. A Gram stain of a sputum sample showed many epithelial cells, no polymorphonuclear cells, many gram-positive cocci, and some gram-negative rods. What is your interpretation?
   a. The sample is invalid
   b. *S. pneumoniae* mixed with *H. influenzae* infection
   c. *S. pneumoniae* infection
   d. *Staphylococcus* infection
   e. *Escherichia coli* infection

4. A 5-year-old boy was admitted for fever and a stiff neck. Meningitis was suspected. A Gram stain of the cerebrospinal fluid was performed. Which of the following results is most likely?
   a. Many leukocytes and gram-positive cocci in clusters
   b. Many leukocytes and gram-positive diplococci
   c. Many leukocytes and small gram-negative rods
   d. Many leukocytes and gram-positive branching rods
   e. Many leukocytes and gram-positive bacilli

5. A 46-year-old woman was seen in the doctor's office because of vomiting and diarrhea. She had attended a picnic 4 hours earlier. Which of the following is most likely?
   a. Staphylococcal food poisoning
   b. *Bacillus cereus* food poisoning
   c. *Clostridium perfringens* food poisoning
   d. *Salmonella* food poisoning
   e. Acute chemical poisoning

6. Which of the following statements about meningitis is *false?*
   a. Mycobacteria and *Cryptococcus* can cause chronic meningitis.
   b. Syphilis may be associated with aseptic (bacterial culture negative) meningitis.
   c. Herpes meningitis is invariably fatal.
   d. Aseptic meningitis is one of the manifestations of Lyme disease.
   e. All cases of bacterial meningitis should be considered acute emergencies.

7. Which of the following vaccines is recommended for patients with AIDS?
   a. Oral polio
   b. Oral typhoid
   c. Pneumococcal
   d. Yellow fever
   e. Varicella-zoster

8. Which of the following statements is *false?*
   a. Opportunistic infections occur when $CD4^+$ T cell levels fall below 200 cells per cubic millimeter.
   b. The key indicators of AIDS are *Pneumocystis carinii* and mycobacterial infections and Kaposi's sarcoma.
   c. The blood supply in the United States is screened by ELISA for HIV virions.
   d. HIV is transmitted in blood, semen, saliva, sweat, and tissue.
   e. HIV dementia is caused by HIV infection of the central nervous system.

Answers and Explanations to Multiple Choice Review Questions

Chapter 1: Immunology and Basic Concepts in Pathogenesis

Matching questions 1-5

1. e: The $CD4^+$ helper T cell recognizes antigenic peptides presented by antigen-presenting cells that have phagocytized antigen (by the exogenous pathway) in the context of MHC class II antigens.

2. b: Natural killer cells and activated macrophages kill virus-infected and tumor cells in a non-MHC restricted manner.

3. c: Neutrophils are phagocytic cells and a major line of defense against bacteria but are not antigen-presenting cells.

4. d: The mast cell has Fc receptors for IgE. Crosslinking of the cell surface, by the binding of allergen to IgE, activates the release of histamine from granules.

5. h: The plasma cell is a terminally differentiated B cell with a small nucleus and a large cytoplasm, a factory dedicated to antibody production.

Matching questions 6-10

6. b: Chronic granulomatous disease (CGD) of children is characterized by the inability of neutrophils to kill certain bacteria, especially those that make catalase, e.g., *Staphylococcus aureus.*

7. g: AIDS results in a decrease in $CD4^+$ T helper cells, DTH reactions, and subsequent immune responses, thereby increasing the risk for opportunistic infections, especially those that are brought under control by DTH (e.g., herpesvirus and Candida infections).

8. f: Systemic lupus erythematosus is an autoimmune disease, and the presence of anti-DNA antibodies is a key diagnostic feature.

9. e: C3 deficiency is associated with serious recurrent infection with *Streptococcus pneumoniae* and *Neisseria meningitidis.* Deficiency in the terminal components of the complement cascade are associated with life-threatening neisserial infections.

10. a: Antibody deficiency syndromes are more predisposed to respiratory infections, such as otitis, sinusitis, and pneumonia and also to chronic diarrhea caused by viruses, bacteria, or parasites.

11. Answer c:
    Addition of the J chain makes IgA a dimer, and addition of the secretory component promotes IgA secretion.

    a: Surface IgM and IgD are present on early B cells and are the only isotypes that can be expressed in the same cell.
    b: Differentiation of the B cell promotes recombination of the Ig gene that juxtaposes V, D, and J units and deletes the heavy chain genes preceding the ϵ chain gene.
    d: The Fab fragment of IgG lacks the Fc portion of antibody. The Fc portion is responsible for binding to complement and Fc receptors on macrophages, B cells, and killer cells.
    e: The IgM heavy chain gene segments and IgD segments are adjacent and are transcribed as one RNA. The IgM sequences are deleted from the RNA by splicing to produce the IgD mRNA and protein.

12. **Answer d:**
The neutrophils are attracted by chemotaxis to the site of infection by C3a and C5a not by C8 or C9. C8 and C9 are components of the membrane attack complex.

a: Neutrophils are the first cells to arrive at the infected site. Neutrophils are a characteristic response to bacterial infections. The neutrophils attach to the invading bacteria and phagocytize them.
b: Neutrophils have a very short life span. Activation of the neutrophil by ingestion of bacteria leads to the death of the cell.
c, e: The phagosome containing the ingested bacteria fuses with a lysosome that contains antibacterial enzymes and toxic substances, such as myeloperoxidase and hydrogen peroxide.

13. **Answer c:**
The proper complement cascade along the classical pathway is as follows: C1 binds to antibody; C1-antibody complex cleaves C4 and then C2; C4bC2a complex cleaves C3; C4bC2aC3b complex cleaves C5.

a: The alternative (properdin) pathway is activated by surface structures of bacteria.
b: The classical pathway is activated by antigen-antibody complexes.
d: C5a is chemotactic for macrophages and neutrophils, induces smooth muscle contraction, mast cell degranulation, and increases capillary permeability.
e: C9 is the terminal component of the complement cascade, similar to perforin; activation of this protein results in a hole in the membrane.

14. **Answer c:**
$CD4^+$ T cells also become activated and produce lymphokines (e.g., IL-2) that activate the $CD8^+$ T cells.

a: T lymphocytes transferred in the graft recognize the new host as foreign and become activated.
b, d: Rejection of the graft implies tissue incompatibility, which promotes allotypic T cell activation.
e: The strongest rejection reactions are directed against HLA-A, HLA-B, and HLA-DR antigens and, therefore, matching at these loci is important. A mismatch could be responsible for the rejection.

15. **Answer a:**
Binding of the T cell receptor to the antigen-presenting cell is **not** sufficient for activation. Interleukin-1 or another co-activator is also required.

b, c: Several cascades are activated to promote activation of the T cell, including cleavage of phosphatidyl inositol and activation of calcium-dependent protein kinases, protein kinase C, and tyrosine kinases.
d: The CD3 portion of the T cell receptor contains subunits responsible for activation of phospholipase C and cleavage of phosphatidyl inositol.
e: Adhesion proteins on the target cell and on the T cell tighten the interaction between the two cells and contribute to the crosslinking and activation reactions.

Matching questions 16-20

16. c: IgM is a pentamer of dimers, consisting of 10 heavy and 10 light chains.

17. e: IgD is found on the cell surface of early B cells and is not readily secreted.

18. a: Secretory IgA antibody is important in protecting epithelial surfaces from infection.

19. b: IgG (subclasses 1, 3, and 4) is the only form of antibody that can cross the placenta.

20. d: IgE promotes allergic reactions, which are defined as Type 1 hypersensitivity reactions.

Chapter 2: Bacteriology

1. **Answer d:**
Plasmids are extrachromosomal segments of DNA, and do not encode essential genes and are dispensable.

a: Antibiotic resistance or lack of sensitivity can be caused by a mutation in the gene for the antibiotic target structure or the porin proteins important for permeability of the drug.
b: Some toxin genes are encoded on plasmids; others are encoded by the chromosome.

c: Transposons can integrate themselves either into a plasmid or into the chromosome. Transposons in a plasmid may promote integration of the plasmid.
e: Plasmids and chromosomal DNA are both replicons because they contain the appropriate sequences to support replication.

2. **Answer d:**
Erythromycin binds to the 50S subunit of the bacterial ribosome and inhibits elongation of the peptide chain.

a: Ampicillin is a beta-lactam antibiotic and inhibits the D-ala-D-ala transpeptidase enzyme involved in cross-linking the peptidoglycan.
b: Ciprofloxacin is a quinolone and inhibits topoisomerase action.
c: Rifampin prevents RNA polymerase action.
e: Chloramphenicol binds to the 50S subunit of the bacterial ribosome and inhibits peptidyl transfer and elongation.

3. **Answer a:**
Manifestations of infective endocarditis are not caused by the toxin but by vegetations.

b, e: Scalded skin syndrome and bullous impetigo are caused by exfoliatin.
c: Toxic shock syndrome toxin (TSST-1), a superantigen, has been found to cause toxic shock syndrome.
d: Gastroenteritis is caused by an enterotoxin and is related to the other enterotoxins that cause gastroenteritis in staphylococcal food poisoning.

Matching questions 4-6

4. c: Acute poststreptococcal glomerulonephritis and acute rheumatic fever are nonsuppurative complications of streptococcal infections. Glomerulonephritis may occur after either skin or pharyngeal infections.

5. a: Rheumatic fever occurs only after pharyngitis.

6. d: Reiter's syndrome is a postinfection reaction involving the joints (reactive arthritis) and mucous membranes.

Matching questions 7-10

7. c: *Streptococcus pneumoniae* can be identified by serotyping, optochin sensitivity (P disk), and bile solubility.

8. a: Group A streptococcus is bacitracin sensitive (A disk).

9. b: Group B streptococcus hydrolyzes hippurate.

10. c: See answer to question 7.

11. c:
a: *Neisseria* and *Moraxella* are both oxidase positive organisms. *Neisseria* is differentiated from *Moraxella* by the ability of *Neisseria* to ferment glucose.
b: "M" is for maltose and *Neisseria meningitidis.* "G" is for glucose and for *N. gonorrhoeae.*
c: See a.
d: Asymptomatic gonococcal infection is common and provides the greatest reservoir of infection.
e: Three major factors allow *N. meningitidis* to cause disease: (1) ability to colonize the nasopharynx (mediated by pili), (2) ability to spread systemically and escape antibody-mediated phagocytosis (protection provided by polysaccharide capsule), and (3) ability to exert toxic effects (mediated by endotoxin).

Matching questions 12-16

12. a: Unlike *Salmonella* and *Shigella* organisms, *Escherichia coli* is a lactose fermenter.

13. a: *E. coli* O157:H7 can be isolated by using sorbitol medium and is thus distinguished from other *E. coli.*

14. b: *Shigella, Salmonella, Campylobacter,* and *Clostridium difficile* are known to be associated with fecal leukocytes; *E. coli* is not.

15. d: Bacteremia is uncommon in *Shigella* and *E. coli* O157:H7 infections.

16. c: Both agents can cause bloody diarrhea.

17. b: *Bacteroides fragilis*
All the organisms are facultative, anaerobic gram-negative rods, except for *B. fragilis,* which is a strict anaerobe and requires prereduced media and anaerobic conditions for growth.

18. Answer a:

a, b: Cholera is characterized by severe watery diarrhea with rice-water stools (containing mucous flecks). The disease is caused by cholera toxin that binds to the GM1-ganglioside receptor on the intestinal cell membrane via subunit B. Subunit A1, which is the active portion of the toxin, activates adenylate cyclase, which results in accumulation of cyclic AMP along the cell membrane. Cyclic AMP is responsible for the active secretion of water and electrolytes out of the cell into the intestinal lumen. *Intestinal fluid absorption is not impaired.* Therefore, the oral administration of fluids containing glucose and electrolytes is used to replace the increased secretory loss.

c, e: Without aggressive resuscitation measures using fluid replacement and tetracycline therapy (of secondary importance), the mortality has been extremely high.

d: Although cholera epidemics continue to be reported in many other parts of the world, such as India, Southeast Asia, and parts of South America, cholera is also found on the gulf coast of the United States.

19. Answer d:

Pseudomonas aeruginosa is a long, thin gram-negative rod that grows aerobically. These organisms grow on MacConkey medium as non–lactose fermenters and react in the oxidase test. Mucoid strains of *P. aeruginosa* are frequently isolated from cystic fibrosis patients. Key words here are *cystic fibrosis, non-lactose fermenter, and oxidase positive.*

a: Staphylococci are gram-positive cocci.

b: *Klebsiella pneumoniae* may appear mucoid, but generally not as much as the true mucoid strains isolated from cystic fibrosis patients. *K. pneumoniae* is a non–lactose fermenting aerobe but is oxidase negative.

c: *Haemophilus influenzae* is an oxidase negative, gram-negative cocco-bacillus.

e: *Bacteroides fragilis* is an anaerobe.

20. Answer d:

Bacteroides fragilis is also bile resistant, while the other anaerobic bacteria are bile sensitive.

a, c, and e: *Prevotella, Veillonella, Capnocytophaga,* and *Bacteroides* grow better anaerobically.

b: *Escherichia coli* is a gram-negative rod that grows aerobically.

21. Answer d:

Penicillin is effective against *Actinomyces.*

a, b: *Actinomyces* organisms are anaerobic gram-positive bacilli that appear as branching filaments.

c: Sulfur granules recovered from the drainage are composed of colonies of the bacteria.

e: *Actinomyces* organisms normally colonize the upper respiratory tract, the gastrointestinal tract, and the female genital tract. Hence, infections can involve the cervicofacial region, the thoracic region, the abdominal region, and also include pelvic infections. Central nervous system involvement has been reported. In women using an intrauterine device, actinomycosis of the pelvic organs is more common.

Matching questions 22-24

22. b: *Pasteurella multocida* has been associated with infections from animal bites. Such infections are seldom due to a single organism. Most common Pasteurellaceae are associated with human disease.

Table A.1

Organism	Primary Diseases
Haemophilus influenzae	Meningitis, epiglotitis, cellulitis, otitis, sinusitis, pneumonia, conjunctivitis, arthritis, bacteremia
Haemophilus parainfluenzae	Bacteremia, endocarditis, opportunistic infections
Haemophilus ducreyi	Chancroid
Haemophilus aphrophilus	Endocarditis, opportunistic infections
Actinobacillus actinomycetemcomitans	Endocarditis, juvenile periodontitis

23. d: *H. influenzae* B causes epiglottitis and meningitis but is preventable by vaccination.

24. c: Chancroid is a sexually transmitted disease characterized by an ulcer, symptomatic for males.

25. a: Legionellae are intracellular organisms, and therefore, medications that concentrate intracellularly are preferred. Beta-lactam agents, such as ampicillin are not effective. Macrolides, such as erythromycin, azithromycin, and clarithromycin are effective. Quinolones, such as ciprofloxacin and ofloxacin are also effective. Doxycycline has been shown to have clinical efficacy. Rifampin is effective and is recommended to be used in combination with another agent in seriously ill patients.

26. **Answer a:**

Mycobacteria can be isolated using broth culture and egg-based or agar-based media. Chlamydiae require tissue culture for isolation.

b: Tuberculosis is transmitted most commonly by infectious aerosols. For example, a patient with laryngeal tuberculosis is most contagious.

c: Humans are the natural host and reservoir for tuberculosis. The organism can remain dormant and is reactivated when host conditions are optimal.

d: Patients with tuberculous leprosy have an immune response to the infection. Therefore, the number of organisms are fewer than in lepromatous leprosy.

e: Reactivation may be seen in the elderly and in patients who are treated with immunosuppressive agents.

27. e: Syphilis in the primary stage is not very contagious. Dark-field microscopy of exudate from the chancre will show the presence of treponemal organisms in the chancre, which is contagious. Disease may be acquired through sexual contact or through any mucous membrane contact. The secondary stage, disseminated disease, is characterized by bacteremia, mucocutaneous rash, and lymphadenopathy. The skin rash contains treponemal organisms and is very contagious. Transfusion of blood infected with treponemes is another method of transmission. Inanimate objects, such as toilet seats do not transmit disease.

28. **Answer b:**

Treponema pallidum is a strict anaerobe and does not grow in culture.

a: The Venereal Disease Research Laboratory (VDRL) test and the rapid plasma reagin (RPR) test are diagnostic but do not directly assay treponemal antigens and, therefore, may be associated with biologic false-positive results.

c, d, e: Two direct microscopic techniques are used on exudates from skin lesions, namely, darkfield microscopy and direct fluorescent antibody staining. Specimens from oral lesions should not be examined using these techniques because oral spirochetes can contaminate the specimen.

29. **Answer d:**

See Table A.2.

Table A.2

Disease	Organism	Vector	Reservoir
Rocky Mountain spotted fever	*R. rickettsii*	Ticks	Ticks, wild rodents
Ehrlichiosis	*E. chaffeensis*	Ticks	Ticks
Rickettsialpox	*R. akari*	Mites	Mites, wild rodents
Scrub typhus	*R. tsutsugamushi*	Mites	Mites, wild rodents
Epidemic typhus	*R. prowazekii*	Lice	Humans, squirrels, fleas, flying squirrels
Trench fever	*R. quintana*	Lice	Humans
Lyme disease	*Borrelia burgdorferi*	Tick	Deer, rodents, pets
Babesiosis	*Babesia microti* (protozoon)	Ticks	Rodents, humans
Murine typhus	*R. typhi*	Fleas	Rodents, cats, raccoons, skunks

Chapter 3: Virology

1. c: Detergent sensitivity indicates the presence of an envelope and only DNA or (+) sense RNA viral genomes are infectious.

Table A.3

Virus	Family	Structure
A. Adenovirus	Adenoviridae	Naked capsid, DNA
B. Influenza virus	Orthomyxoviridae	Enveloped, (–) sense RNA
C. Yellow fever virus	Flaviviridae	Enveloped, (+) sense RNA
D. Mumps virus	Paramyxoviridae	Enveloped, (–) sense RNA
E. Papilloma virus	Papovaviridae	Naked capsid, DNA

2. **Answer c:**

During a latent infection, the genome remains in the cell but without production of viral proteins.

a: Production of SV40 would cause lysis of the cell rather than immortalization.
b: Unlike DNA viruses, retroviruses transform cells and continue to produce virus.
d: The HBsAg is an indicator of infection with HBV.
e: The immune system cannot eliminate human immunodeficiency virus and the virus continues to replicate and kill the $CD4^+$ target cells.

Matching questions 3-7

3. **a, b:** DNA and (+) RNA viral genomes resemble host components, and therefore, the cellular enzymes can recognize the genome and transcribe and replicate the structure. Only DNA replicates in the nucleus.

4. **c, d:** Interestingly, hepadnaviruses would also be included. Even though they are DNA viruses, a full length (+) RNA is used as a template for a viral reverse transcriptase to make DNA.

5. e: Retroviruses must integrate into the host chromosome to replicate.

6. a: The simpler DNA viruses (parvoviruses and papovaviruses) are too small to encode their own polymerase and therefore depend on the host. There are no host enzymes that can replicate RNA.

7. **c, d:** A polymerase must be brought into the cell to convert the (–) RNA viral genome into mRNA because the (–) RNA cannot bind to the ribosome. It does not encode proteins either (the code is backwards). The (–) RNA genome is a template for mRNA. The double-stranded RNA genome acts like a (–) RNA genome and is transcribed within the subviral capsid.

8. **Answer a:**

$CD4^+$ T cells recognize antigen in the context of MHC class II but not MHC I antigens. In general, the $CD4^+$ T cells are helper and DTH T cells, rather than direct cytolytic cells ($CD8^+$ T cells).

b: Measles is not very cytolytic. The rash associated with measles virus is primarily due to host immunopathogenesis.
c: Interferon action is accompanied by the fever, myalgia, and fatigue that are associated with interferon activation of the immune system. Influenza virus is a good inducer of interferon.
d: The presence of large amounts of HBsAg in the blood stream promotes antigen-antibody complex formation. These complexes can get trapped in the kidneys, causing glomerulonephritis.
e: Cell-mediated immunity is required to control most enveloped viruses. Cell-mediated immunity causes tissue damage. Also, all (–) RNA viruses are enveloped and are also good inducers of interferon.

9. c: Foscarnet (phosphonoformate) looks like pyrophosphate, not like a nucleotide analogue.

10. **Answer a:**

Amantadine inhibits the uncoating of influenza A virus, not influenza B virus. The target for amantadine is the M2 matrix protein.

b: Amantadine prevents establishment of infection and therefore is prescribed for prophylactic treatment. It can also limit the spread of the virus within the first 3 days, after which the symptoms and tissue damage will be due largely to host immunopathogenesis.

c, d: Ganciclovir and acyclovir are nucleotide analogues with truncated sugars. Acyclovir requires a viral thymidine kinase (encoded by herpes simplex virus, [HSV] and varicella-zostar virus [VZV]) for activation. Ganciclovir is also activated by a cytomegalovirus (CMV) enzyme.

e: Zidovudine (AZT), dideoxyinosine (DDI), and dideoxycytidine (DDC) inhibit the reverse transcriptase of HIV.

11. c: Epstein-Barr virus (EBV) latency is established in B lymphocytes. EBV cannot infect neurons because they do not express a viral receptor.

12. b: VZV causes a vesicular rash similar to HSV.

13. c: The papilloma virus is not readily produced and tissue culture systems are not available for its growth.

Matching questions 14-18

14. b-e: All of these picornaviruses can cause coldlike symptoms.

15. c: For coxsackie virus, B is for body.

16. b: Hand-foot-and mouth disease and herpangina.

17. d: Echovirus usually causes benign diseases except in neonates.

18. a: Use of the killed (Salk) and the live (Sabin) polio vaccines have led to the elimination of this disease in the Western hemishphere.

19. **Answer d:**

Influenza virus undergoes antigenic shift by *reassortment* of the genome segments, not by recombination. Upon infection of a cell by two strains of influenza virus, the genome segments can be shuffled and then packaged into hybrid viruses. Antigenic drift occurs by mutation of the segments.

a: Influenza has eight segments of (–) RNA in its nucleocapsid, surrounded by an envelope containing the hemagglutinin (HA) and neuraminidase (NA) and lined by the matrix proteins.

b: Influenza utilizes host mRNA as a primer for transcription, thus stealing a 5′cap for its mRNA. Replication also occurs in the nucleus.

c: Amantadine and the related agent rimantadine inhibit uncoating of influenza virus.

e: The HA binds to sialic acid on target cells. Antibodies to HA block infection.

Matching questions 20-23

20. b: Croup is a subglottal swelling characterized by a "seal bark" cough.

21. a: Koplik's spots (appearance of grains of salt surrounded by a red halo) are usually observed on the buccal mucosa and precede the classic symptoms of measles.

22. c: Mumps causes glandular swelling. Use of the MMR vaccine has virtually eliminated this disease in the United States.

23. a, b, d: Parainfluenza, respiratory syncytial, and measles viruses cause pneumonia in children, with immunocompromised individuals being at highest risk. With the use of the MMR vaccine, measles pneumonia has become rare in the United States but remains a serious complication of measles.

Matching questions 24-27

24. b, d: Both the yellow fever virus and the St. Louis encephalitis virus can establish a viremia in humans that allows human-mosquito-human transmission.

25. a: Rubella is a normally benign disease but is teratogenic.

26. c, d: Both of these flaviviruses damage the endothelial cells of the vasculature.

27. e: All of these viruses are enveloped, (+) RNA viruses and good interferon inducers. They all also induce viremia, which exposes the viruses to interferon-producing leukocytes.

28. **Answer a:**

There are two types of oncogenic retroviruses: acute viruses, which encode oncogenes and chronic viruses, such as HTLV-1, which do not. HTLV-1 activates cell growth, and subsequent mutation promotes leukemogenesis.

b: By turning on IL-2 and IL-2 receptor production, the virus makes the cell more receptive to stimulation. This facilitates virus growth.

c: Once integrated into the host chromosome, retroviruses are transcribed similarly to host genes.

d: The major mRNAs produced are the gag, pol, and env mRNAs. These are subsequently cleaved into individual proteins.

e: The cleavage of the gag-pol polyprotein occurs after assembly and results in maturation of the virion. The protease is a target for antiviral drugs.

29. **Answer e:**

Src is the name of a protein kinase viral oncogene. HIV does not encode Src.

a: HIV predominantly infects CD4-expressing cells and is capable of all three types of infection.

b: Syncytia (multinucleated giant cells) result from cell-cell fusion. The formation of syncytia is lethal to the infected cells.

c: HIV mutates readily enough that differences can be observed during the course of disease in a single individual. Mutations promote antiviral drug resistance, enhance the infection of macrophages, and help the virus escape immune control.

d: HIV p24 is the earliest marker of HIV infection and is present in serum before antibodies can be detected.

30. **b:** This profile resembles that of a vaccinated individual. A person who was infected with virus at some time would have antibodies to other viral antigens.

Chapter 4: Mycology

Matching questions 1-5

1. **c:** *Histoplasma* is a dimorphic fungus that is inhaled and can cause pneumonia in normal and immunocompromised individuals.

2. **a:** Dermatophytes live on the skin and can digest keratin. They cause infections, such as tinea (ringworm) and include the genera *Microsporum* and *Trichophyton.*

3. **b:** *Sporothrix schenkii* is a soil fungus that is injected under the skin. Gardeners are at risk for infection upon being scratched by thorns.

4. **d:** *Coccidiodes immitis* is endemic to the dry regions of the southwestern United States. The mycelia are very fragile, break off the colony, and spread easily to cause a disease that ranges from a mild febrile illness (unlike *Histoplama*) to severe lung disease. (It is also known as San Joaquin valley fever, Posadas disease, or desert rheumatism.)

5. **f:** *Cryptococcus neoformans* infects the lungs but can spread and cause infections of the brain and meninges in normal and immunocompromised patients. The capsule is required for virulence and is of diagnostic importance.

Chapter 5: Parasitology

1. **c:** The sporozoite form is injected into the blood by the bite of the *Anopheles* mosquito. The gametocytes are the male or the female forms that are transmitted back to the mosquito.

2. **Answer a:**

Enterobius vermicularis (pinworm)

b: Dog hookworm infection
c: Leishmaniasis
d: Trichinosis
e: Clonorchiasis

Matching questions 3-6

3. **a:** *Toxoplasma gondii* is an opportunistic pathogen for AIDS patients and neonates. In AIDS patients, it causes cerebral masses leading to neurologic symptoms.

4. **a:** *Taenia solium* is the pork tapeworm and can establish infection in and cause damage to the brain.

5. **c:** *Diphylobothrium latum* is a freshwater fish tapeworm acquired by eating raw fish, e.g., sushi or uncooked gefilte fish.

6. **d:** *Giardia lamblia,* a flagellate, has a charac-

teristic appearance, resembling an old man. *Giardia* is acquired from water contaminated by beaver or muskrat feces.

Chapter 6: Infectious Disease Correlations

1. **Answer c:**

   Chlamydia pneumoniae, not *C. trachomatis,* is associated with adult pneumonia. *C. trachomatis* can cause pneumonia in infants following acquisition during the passage through an infected birth canal.

   a, b: *Streptococcus pneumoniae* and *Mycoplasma pneumoniae* are by far the most common causes of community acquired pneumonia.
   d: *Haemophilus influenzae* is commonly associated with chronic lung disease.
   e: *Legionella pneumophila* is common in certain geographic areas and has also been associated with outbreaks.

2. **Answer d:**

   Culture of *Mycoplasma* organisms is difficult, requires a long growth period, has a very low yield, and is not recommended for use in a non–research laboratory environment.

   a: Pneumococcus may not be isolated from the sputum but would be present in the blood.
   b: Sputum examination is important in helping to establish the etiology of infection. A Gram stain and an acid-fast stain are good screening tools for *Streptococcus pneumoniae, Haemophilus influenzae, Moraxella catarrhalis* (and less common causes of pneumonia including gram-negative rods and *Staphylococcus aureus*) and mycobacteria.
   c: Sputum cultures for routine bacteria using blood and chocolate agar are commonly used to detect *S. pneumoniae, H. influenzae,* and *Moraxella.* spp.
   e: The urinary antigen test for *Legionella* subgroup 1 is useful.

3. a: The specimen was probably a saliva sample. A good sputum sample should contain leukocytes and minimal numbers of epithelial cells. A culture of this sample will yield information that is misleading and not useful.

4. **Answer b:**

   Streptococcus pneumoniae is a gram-positive diplococcus. This organism is the most frequent cause of bacterial meningitis in adults. *S. pneumoniae* can also cause meningitis in children.

   a: When gram-positive cocci occur in clusters, the bacteria are most likely to be staphylococci. Meningitis from these organisms is not common.
   c: Before the introduction of the *Haemophilus* type b vaccine, *Haemophilus influenzae* was the most common organism causing meningitis in children. *H. influenzae* appears as a gram-negative coccobacillus. Meningococcal meningitis may occur sporadically or with outbreaks. It may be accompanied by meningococcemia (purpuric skin lesions may be observed). Meningococci appear as gram-negative cocci.
   d: Meningitis resulting from large gram-negative rods, branching rods, or gram-positive bacilli is not common.
   e: *Listeria monocytogenes* can cause meningitis but is less common among normal hosts.

5. **Answer a:**

   Staphylococcal food poisoning is the most likely cause because it is characterized by an incubation period that is between 1 to 6 hours and is associated with picnics.

   b: *Bacillus cereus* food poisoning may mimic the incubation period of *C. perfringens* and *Staphylococcus* but is associated with rice dishes.
   c: *Clostridium perfringens* food poisoning has an incubation period of greater than 6 hours.
   d: *Salmonella* food poisoning has an incubation period of about 2 days.
   e: Acute chemical poisoning usually manifests within 30 minutes of ingestion.

6. **Answer c:**

   Herpes meningitis may be found in newborns as well as in adults. In adults, herpes meningitis may occur in association with herpes genitalis. The prognosis is good. In contrast, herpes encephalitis is known to result in neurologic complications and has a high mortality.

a: Mycobacteria and *Cryptococcus* spp. are common causes of chronic meningitis. Fungal diseases, such as coccidiodomycosis and histoplasmosis may also cause chronic meningitis.
b: Syphilis may present as aseptic meningitis during the secondary stage.
d: Lyme disease has neurologic manifestations that include neuropathy and aseptic meningitis.
e: When bacterial meningitis is suspected, it should be considered an emergency. Antimicrobial therapy should be started as soon as possible.

7. c: As a rule, live vaccines are not recommended for patients who are immunocompromised, including AIDS patients and pregnant women. These vaccines include oral polio, oral typhoid, yellow fever, and varicella-zoster vaccines. The measles and mumps vaccines, both live, attenuated vaccines, may be given to AIDS patients (there are exceptions). Measles vaccination is not recommended during pregnancy. Inactivated pneumococcal vaccine, meningococcal vaccines, diphtheria-tetanus vaccine, influenza vaccine, Salk polio vaccine, hepatitis B vaccine, and rabies vaccine are not live vaccines and are considered safe.

8. **Answer d:**

HIV is transmitted in blood, semen, and tissue (e.g., transplants), not in saliva or sweat.

a: The reduction of $CD4^+$ T cell levels to below 200 per cubic millimeter reduces DTH responses below effective levels, increasing the risk for fungal and mycobacterial infections.
b: *Pneumocystis carinii* and mycobacterial infections are classic opportunistic infections. AIDS patients are at unusually high risk for Kaposi's sarcoma.
c: ELISA detection of HIV antibody is the primary screening method, with western blot used to confirm HIV infection.
e: HIV infects astroglial cells (cells of the macrophage lineage) and neurons causing dementia.

INDEX

Pages in italics indicate figures; pages with *t* indicate tables.

D

Q

R

T